Tissue Viability

The prevention, treatment and management of wounds

SYLVIE HAMPTON, MA, BSc(HONS), DPSN, RGN
and
FIONA COLLINS, MSc, DIPCOT, SROT

with contributions from

Katherine Martyn, BSc, BED, DipNS, SRN, RNT
Kate Springett, BSc, BED, DipNS, SRN, RNT
Mathew Philip, BSc(Hons), PhD, CEng, CPhys,
M Inst, MIM
and
Leyton Stevens, MBA

D1065571

W
WHURR PUBLISHERS
LONDON AND PHILADELPHIA

British Library Cataloguing in Publication Data

A catalogue record for this book
is available from the British Library.

ISBN 1 86156 237 3

Printed and bound in the UK by Athenaeum Press Ltd,
Gateshead, Tyne & Wear.

Tissue Viability

The prevention, treatment and management of wounds

Acknowledgement

The editors and publisher are grateful for the support of the following companies.

Sareo Health Care

and

Smith and Nephew

Contents

Preface

There are many excellent books written on wound management, mainly for nurses with basic knowledge of tissue viability, or, on a higher level, for tissue viability specialists and doctors. This book provides a comprehensive and extensive view of wound prevention, management and treatment and will be useful to all tissue viability enthusiasts, whether requiring basic or advanced information. The nursing student will be able to obtain the information they require at a level that suits them, whilst nurses with previous knowledge of wound management, specialist nurses, physiotherapists, occupational therapists and doctors will find useful and advanced information and tips. There are 14 chapters with each chapter devoted to a different aspect within tissue viability. It will be up to the individual reader to select where their level is at present and use the chapters accordingly. The book is a mixture of evidence-based nursing and the reality of wound care, and is based on the authors' and contributors' years of experience and knowledge gained acting as Tissue Viability Nurse and Tissue Viability Consultant, a Senior Lecturer in Occupational Therapy and Tissue Viability Consultant, a Senior Lecturer in Nursing, a Senior Lecturer in Podiatry and a Senior Lecturer at the University of Brighton.

Whilst this book concentrates on the technical and scientific aspects of wound healing, it also investigates the philosophy of holistic patient assessment, providing the practitioner with guidance in treatment or prevention of individual patient wounds. The information is derived from researched evidence and also draws on the experiences of the authors, with examples provided in the form of case studies and anecdotes. The contents cover every aspect of wound management, such as prevention and treatment of pressure ulcers, wound treatment, undertaking clinical audit, the role of the specialist nurse, ethics and treatment of leg ulcers.

Discussion of audit and how audit of wound and pressure injury prevention can be used to develop research and good practice in tissue viability is included. An audit tool is provided, which has been developed to offer a method of prevalence audit and will be useful to tissue viability nurses or hospital trusts, nursing homes and community nurses wishing to undertake audit in pressure ulcers.

Advances in wound management are covered along with the authors' own experiences in using leeches, maggot therapy and vacuum-assisted closure. Bacterial resistance to antiseptics and antibiotics, use of antiseptics in wound care, infection and the future for treatment of methicillin-resistant *Staphylococcus aureus* is included. The microbiology of wounds, how wounds heal and the part that wound dressings play in the provision of the optimum wound healing environment in colonized or infected wounds are reviewed.

The broad scope of this book is designed to enable practitioners, whether nurse, doctor, physiotherapist or occupational therapist, to develop knowledge of wound management, how pressure ulcers may be prevented and to develop understanding, practice and research appreciation. The purpose of the book is to probe deeper than just practical issues in wound management and to enable practitioners to provide high quality service in tissue viability. Dedication and knowledge *can* made a difference to healing in a wound.

Introduction

Tradition, lack of education and convenience has dictated wound management, possibly for centuries, and certainly since Florence Nightingale's time on the wards. Florence laid down rules for nursing, but wound management still relied on a mishmash of old wives' tales and doctors' experiences and was not a recognized science in its own right. Cow dung, spiders' webs, herbs, maggots and leeches were among the many dressings used for healing wounds. It was even a belief that wounds should produce pus to heal; if pus was not found in the wound, the doctor would introduce it by taking it from another patient's wound. It was then known as 'laudable pus'.

Over 40 years ago, wound management began to be developed as a science when Winter (1962) discovered that a wound heals faster if provided with a moist environment. This led to other studies such as Lock's study (1979) which demonstrated that any drop in wound bed temperature would delay healing for up to four hours. Nurses and doctors appeared to be slow in taking up the research evidence and there are still indications today that dry and often inappropriate dressings are used indiscriminately by a small number of nurses and doctors who are reluctant to change their practice and ideas. Nevertheless, wound management is becoming a powerful science; it will soon be difficult to continue with old methods when efficacy of new methods are being proven beyond question and clinical governance demands that a rationale is provided for all care. Wound healing is an art as well as a science and the immensely complex processes of wound healing are only just being identified and understood. However, this art (the enormous experience of some practitioners) has the potential to be lost within the search for the 'holy grail' that is research.

Dressings do not contain miracle substances that 'heal' wounds and dressing companies that claim their dressings can 'heal' are bending the truth. Dressing selection relies on the practitioner's knowledge of the optimum wound healing environment and how that can be achieved through use of appropriate dressings or equipment. Assessment of nutritional and medical status and use of modern interactive dressings, which control the microenvironment of the wound, will lead to rational selection. 'Blanket' treatment of wounds, such as potassium permanganate soaks or the use of hypochlorites for every leg ulcer (as was once the case), whilst successful in certain instances, is no longer acceptable. Each individual wound has different requirements for provision of an optimum healing environment; skilled assessment of the wound will lead to informed decisions in wound care. Wound management must be based on individual, holistic patient assessment with the chosen wound product providing such an environment. Provision of the optimum wound healing environment can only be made by a practitioner or clinician with a working knowledge of the stages of wound healing and the ability to assess the state of the wound. Therefore, it is essential to have knowledge of dressings and the environment those dressings can provide for different types of wounds.

Decisions about equipment for the prevention of pressure ulcers is another vital area and the practitioner requires knowledge of skin and the pathology that occurs following sustained pressure. This book will provide that knowledge.

CHAPTER 1

The skin and wound healing

The skin

The primary function of the skin is to serve as a protective barrier against the external environment. Therefore, preserving skin integrity is one of the primary jobs of the nurse with involvement, co-operation and advice of the medical team and other professions allied to medicine (PAMs). Therefore, education in the structure and function of skin is vital if excellence in wound prevention and treatment is to be achieved.

The skin is the largest organ in the body, weighing 2.7 kg in the average adult. It is vital to the maintenance and balance of the body and is an indispensable structure for human life. The skin has a stratified, impermeable and avascular layer of dead keratinized skin scales (epidermis), which is waterproof, prevents water loss and acts as a barrier against bacterial invasion of dermis. Healthy skin has a top layer of stratum corneum (horny layer), which comprises dead cells that have been propelled away from the base of the epidermis by layers of cells growing below in the dermis. The flattened dead cells are grouped around lipids and proteins and this mixture makes up the skin's main barrier to water loss. Any break in this layer can pose a threat to the system.

The epidermis system is complete and invaginates at the surface, forming hair follicles and exocrine glands. It is this continuous line of epidermis that allows islands of epithelium to appear in healing leg ulcers. The migration of epidermal cell from hair follicles begins at 24 hours (Winter 1962).

Underlying the epidermis (see Figure 1.1) are the viable dermis and subcutaneous layers consisting of nerves, glands, fatty (adipose) tissue and muscular tissue. These structures are maintained and

1

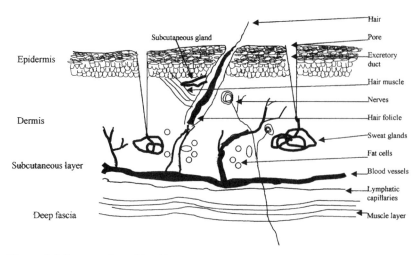

Figure 1.1 Cross-section of the skin.

supported by fibrous and elastic connective tissue with each structure
having a special role to play in maintaining homeostasis. The principle functions will be maintenance of body temperature, perception
of stimuli, protection and excretion. The dermis has a fibrous
component of collagen and elastin. Collagen gives the dermis its
structural stability and strength to healing wounds (which is
discussed in detail later in this chapter), whilst elastin provides
elasticity and resilience.

   Within the dermis are sensory nerve endings that respond to the
sensation of touch, temperature, pressure and pain. Motor nerve
fibres control the rate of blood flow by controlling the constriction or
dilation of blood vessels. Body temperature is carefully balanced by a
combination of the skin thermoreceptors and the hypothalamus in
the brain. Increases in body temperature will lead to dilation of the
blood vessels and to sweating, whilst decreases will lead to blood
vessel constriction and shivering. Both mechanisms are designed to
bring the body to homeostasis.

   Beneath the dermis is a subcutaneous layer of adipose tissue
containing a plexus of blood vessels. This layer connects the dermis
to lower structures, provides protection between bony prominences
and the skin surface, provides energy when required and maintains
warmth of the lower structures. The plexus of blood vessels consist
of arterioles and venules, both of which are innervated by the

sympathetic nervous system and are capable of contraction although the venules have a much weaker muscle coat. It is this ability to contract and dilate that provides the body with warmth, blood pressure control and blood volume control (Bliss 1998). There are 10 billion capillaries in the body, providing 500 square metres of surface area for fluid and nutrient exchange (Bliss 1998).

The skin is covered with a microorganism environment with the most common inhabitants being bacteria. These bacteria are generally part of the natural balance and are, on the whole, harmless. However, within a wound, the organisms can multiply and can become pathogenic when they enter the host (resulting in clinical infection) (see Chapter 4). As a general rule, however, the organisms will live within the wound exudate (colonization) and cause little disturbance to wound healing – particularly in the later stages of healing.

Keeping the skin clean

The skin has been described as a vast empire in which contrasts of terrain and climate are as varied as those of the earth itself (Hallett 1994). Skin flora is generally harmless to human beings, although it can become pathogenic if allowed to enter a wound. Therefore, it is important to keep skin reasonably clean around peri-wound areas.

The use of soap can destroy the natural oils produced in the sebaceous glands of the skin and it is advisable not to use soap for skin cleansing. An alternative to soap can be emollients, which can soothe and hydrate the skin, keeping the natural oils intact. However, the action of the emollient is often short lived and a barrier cream or ointment may be required to maintain hydration of the skin. The author usually soaks leg ulcers in a bucket (lined with polythene) of tap water containing emollients. The skin is then left undried but a lanolin free cream or ointment is applied over the skin (paying particular attention to between the toes) to 'lock' the oil and moisture into the skin.

Use of antiseptic wipes for cleansing

There has been debate for some time on the efficacy of alcohol wipes in cleansing the skin prior to injection. Lawrence revisited the problem in 1994 and found that iosopropanol-impregnated paper wipes could reduce normal skin flora by at least 97 per cent. However, to achieve this higher kill, the alcohol wipe needed to be in contact with the skin for five seconds. Lawrence found that some instances, the wiping lasted less than one second. There is also a strong potential for the alcohol in the wipes to enter the skin with the needle, thereby increasing pain from the injection. This research would lead us to question the use of antiseptics in cleansing the skin, particularly as the lotion would not be on the skin long enough to reduce bacterial count.

Physiology of wounds

Partial thickness wounds

The most painful wounds are those that are shallow with exposed nerve endings. These wounds are generally caused by trauma, are surface damage only and are likely to be bright red with serous fluid immediately apparent or deeper loss with a lighter pink base.

Partial thickness wounds extend to the dermis and, providing hair follicles remain undamaged, epithelial tissue can grow outward from the follicles like 'islands' of tissue. If the wound is left untouched, it will form a scab. The scab will dehydrate and will draw fluid from the wound beneath so continuing the dehydration process. This dries the wound beneath the scab, delaying healing (Winter 1962). However, in minor injuries such as a finger cut, this drying is of little consequence as the wound will continue to heal in spite of the desiccation. It is the larger, acute injuries that will suffer from the dehydration process.

Full thickness wounds

This is loss of the epidermal and dermal layers and, possibly, extending to subcutaneous layers involving the fascia and muscle layer and even bone. Bryant (1992), Torrance (1983) and Reid and Morrison (1994) gave definitions of pressure ulcer grading that can be used to determine the size of the wound (see Chapter 9). Full thickness wounds involving infective necrosis and bone can be life threatening and sinus tract formation can occur because of infection and can prove very difficult to heal. Full thickness wounds will pass through several phases of healing.

Moist wound healing

Torrance described the ideal wound healing environment and included 'moist wound healing' as a prerequisite condition. The concept was originally formed in 1962 when Winter described the post-surgical behaviour of wounds measuring 2.5 cm^2 by 0.01–0.03 cm deep in young pigs. Three days post-operatively, wounds that had been exposed to air were showing half the epithelialization of those covered with polythene film. Wounds that were kept moist, allowed the epithelial tissue to migrate, unimpeded, across the moist wound surface. Wounds that were allowed to dry formed a scab, moisture evaporates from the scab and the scab then draws moisture from the wound bed, drying it further. Winter found that epithelial tissue had to burrow below the scab to find enough moisture to allow it to migrate across the wound surface, thereby delaying healing.

Work completed by Svensio et al. (1998) demonstrated that wounds kept 'wet' healed faster than moist or dry wounds. A saline container was used for wet wounds, hydrocolloid for moist and gauze for the dry wounds. They found that 12 days post-operatively the dry wounds were zero per cent healed, moist wounds 20 per cent healed and wet wounds 86 per cent healed.

Dyson et al. (1988) studied cellular changes in 42 dry wounds and 42 moist wounds created on seven domestic pigs. After three days the moist wounds contained almost twice as many macrophages as the dry wounds and by seven days the wounds had mainly epithelialized whereas the dry wounds remained largely unhealed.

Healing by primary intention

A wound that has the edges brought together in approximation will heal through primary intention (Figure 1.2). Within 24–48 hours the surface of the surgical wound will be sealed and the dressing can be removed (Cruse and Ford 1980). The phases of healing will progress hidden beneath the sealed surface. Once the wound margin is 'sealed' the wound requires little care.

Clinical infection in a sealed wound is likely to be primary with the bacteria having entered the tissues when the wound bed was exposed in theatre possibly entering the wound from the skin flora with the cut of the scalpel.

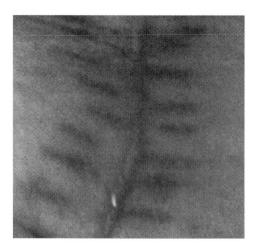

Figure 1.2 Wound healing through primary intention (see Plate 1).

Healing can be undermined and dehiscence an outcome in the presence of:

- clinical infection;
- obesity;
- haematoma formation;
- malnourishment;
- repeated surgery.

The wound is likely to be left to heal through secondary intention unless there is an abdominal burst suture with the body organs exposed. This is an emergency situation and the patient will be returned to theatre for deep tension sutures (see Chapter 7).

Healing by secondary intention

A wound that is open (wound bed exposed), will heal by secondary intention (Figure 1.3). This presents a high risk of wound contamination and possible clinical infection. Therefore, wound dressings should protect the wound from the surrounding environment.

Skin changes and wounds can occur for many reasons and can be intrinsic or extrinsic in origin.

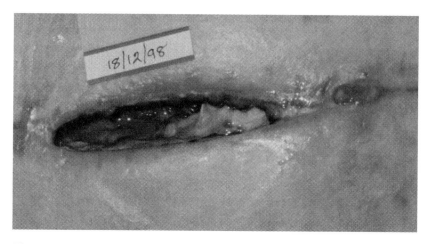

Figure 1.3 This wound will heal through secondary intention (see Plate 2).

Wound healing

Wound healing is a cellular and biochemical process, which relies essentially on an inflammatory reaction. Iocono et al. (1998) described wound healing as overlapping phases of inflammation, proliferation and remodelling. The components of blood that are responsible for the inflammation and proliferation contain chemical mediators that encourage wound repair.

There are many phases of wound healing, with differing descriptions of the process suggesting between three and eight phases. This chapter restricts the process to four phases to enable the reader to understand the process: inflammation, destruction, proliferation and maturation.

Inflammation phase

Inflammation is a response to the injury of vascularized tissues. Its purpose is to deliver defensive materials (blood cells and fluid) to the site of injury. It is a process rather than a state (Majno and Joris 1996). The purpose of the inflammation is to defend the tissues against bacterial invasion and at the same time, deliver mediators to stimulate the wound healing process.

The moment an injury occurs to the skin a clotting cascade is established. Vasoconstriction takes place within the vessels surrounding the injured site. Stickiness, initiated through the clotting cascade, occurs within the platelets. The platelets cling to each other and to the subendothelial components of the vessels, forming a 'plug' and preventing blood loss (Figure 1.4). This process will be prevented or delayed in patients who are receiving heparin, which prevents coagulation, or warfarin, which prevents absorption of vitamin K, or aspirin, which reduces platelet adhesion. The vascular response immediately post injury, with the initiation of the clotting cascade, involves 13 different coagulation factors (Flanagan 1997). This is accompanied by release of chemical mediators such as adenosine triphosphate and platelet derived growth factors (PDGF) (van de Kerhof 1996), which promote cell migration and repair at the injured site. (The use of such growth factors in the healing of wounds is under investigation.)

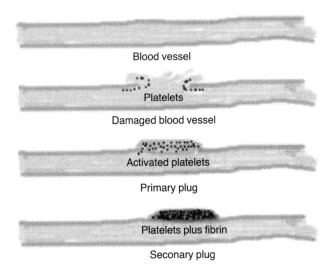

Blood vessel

Platelets

Damaged blood vessel

Activated platelets

Primary plug

Platelets plus fibrin

Seconary plug

Figure 1.4 Formation of an endothelial plug by platelets.

The clotting cascade stimulates the release of histamine from mast cells, which results in vasodilation and increased capillary permeability. Bradykinins, derived from plasma, contribute to prolonged vascular permeability. Prostaglandins are released with any breach of cell membrane and are important to wound healing, with the main role being the control of an adequate blood supply. Medications (aspirin, non-steroidal anti-inflammatory drugs, steroids, etc.) that effect or lower the production of prostaglandins can lead to a delay in the wound healing process. The chemical response allows fluid to leak into the injured tissues and, within an hour post injury, neutrophils can be found at the wound site (Dealey 1994a).

The inflammatory process will cause redness, swelling, pain and heat to be apparent in the area of the injury and this can last for three days (see Figure 1.5). The signs of inflammation can be mistaken for clinical infection, although if the redness and swelling is present for less than three days, it is unlikely to be due to an infection. However, should the redness, pain and swelling continue after the three to five days, there is a possibility that a clinical infection is present and a swab may be required (see Chapter 4).

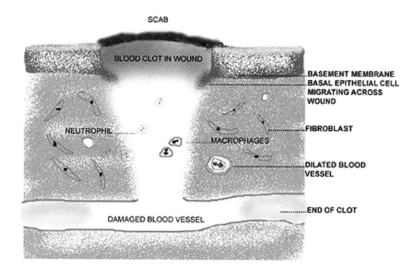

Figure 1.5 The inflammatory process.

Thompson (1998) writes: 'The inflammatory response to tissue injury plays an important role in combating infection by promoting clearance of bacteria.' The early cascade of effector molecules (chemokines; discussed later in this chapter) from injured skin cells is associated with endothelial damage, vascular leakage and oedema. These events may increase tissue injury and increase potential of bacterial infection. Leucocytes are known to rush toward necrotic tissue and to crawl into it as far as possible (Majno and Joris 1996). Majno and Joris report that when a single leucocyte dies, other leucocytes converge on it 'like sharks upon one of their number which has blood escaping from a wound'. Therefore, the presence of alien or dead tissue will result in swift and deadly action. Whilst cells are dying (as in the case of injury) they release chemotaxins. However, once this initial outburst is complete, no more messages are sent and the necrotic 'lump' ceases to attract the 'sharks'. It is therefore a fact that dying tissue elicits an intense but transient inflammatory reaction (Majno and Joris 1996).

The presence of microbial antigens perpetuates the inflammatory process so that the mechanism, which should promote wound repair, becomes detrimental and leads to further tissue damage. This process will increase exudate production (due to vascular leakage and oedema) leading to possible stress for the patient.

Macrophages and polymorphonuclear leucocytes are the 'workhorses' at this point as they are attracted, during the first 24 hours, to the injured site. They lyse clots and debris, destroy and remove bacteria through phagocytosis and allow fluid-filled cavities to form, into which fibroblasts and endothelial cells can grow. As macrophages scavenge, they become activated and secrete a number of polypeptide factors (cytokines or growth factors) and, in this manner, direct the activities of all other cells (Majno and Joris 1996). Macrophages continue to play a vital role in wound healing but require a moist wound environment to enable interaction with, and migration across, the wound surface. Therefore, provision of a moist wound bed is vital for this important player to accomplish the task.

Within hours there is the beginning of migration of squamous epithelial cells toward the area of cell deficit (Westaby 1981) and contraction and the route to final healing has begun. Mitotic activity is activated by the presence of released peptide growth factors (Garrett 1998). Winter (1962) found that wound surface moisture must be maintained. Epithelial tissue can only migrate over viable tissue and dry, dessicated tissue will necessitate the epithelial tissue to move into the layer below, thereby delaying healing. This 'burrowing' of epithelial tissue will occur in areas such as pin sites, around sutures and under dry dressings, which cause a dry wound bed, and, therefore, extended closure time.

Inflammation is an important, normal and necessary prerequisite to wound healing. It is this phase of healing that will successfully initiate healing and will prepare the wound for the next phase of healing through removal of debris such as necrotic tissue and bacteria. A prolonged inflammatory phase, however, can delay the healing process, resulting in a chronic wound. Macrophages and mast cells, both with a high responsibility in wound healing, will stop migration to the injured site when inflammation becomes chronic and the wound will become 'stuck' (or may even, eventually, produce overgranulation). Therefore, the inflammatory stage is not only important at the beginning but may also be important in 'kick-starting' a wound to heal (see Chapter 3).

Within 24 hours, the inflammatory phase will have produced fibrinogen and, with the assistance of thrombin, fibrinogen will convert to a fibrin monomer, which then assembles into fibrin filaments. Fibrin forms a network with filaments that are coated with the plasma protein fibronectin (Majno and Joris 1996) and it is this network that provides a 'climbing frame' for the use of epidermal cells and migrating fibroblasts – the collagen matrix (Figure 1.6).

Once the initial vasoconstriction is not longer required, vasodilation occurs and results in loss of fluids. Within this fluid are growth factors and white cells and the fluid loss can also include serum albumin, thus emphasizing the importance of a high calorie and high protein diet to replace this loss (see Chapter 6).

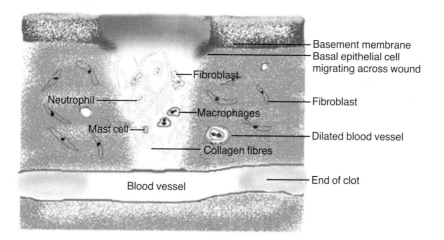

Figure 1.6 Collagen matrix.

Destruction phase

The destructive phase can last from one to seven days, when poly-morphs and macrophages ingest and destroy bacteria and dead cells (phagocytosis) (Figure 1.7). At the same time, macrophages stimulate the release of fibroblasts and a factor that stimulates angiogenesis within the wound. It is this process that makes the macrophage so vital in wound healing; without macrophage involvement the wound is unlikely to heal.

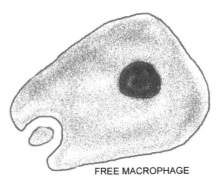

FREE MACROPHAGE

Figure 1.7 Phagocytosis.

Any drop in temperature affects macrophage activity and this will delay wound healing. Therefore, wound dressings should be selected to promote maintenance of wound temperature and dressings should be removed infrequently if possible. Macrophages also require oxygen to enable the burst of energy required for phagocyto-sis. Patients with anaemia, or chronic obstructive airways disease, may find wound healing delayed. There may also be an advantage in warming a wound and/or patients, using mechanical or natural processes, as this will encourage vasodilation which in turn will bring nutrients and oxygen to the area and promote removal of bacteria, thereby reducing the potential of infection. Scientists culture human cells at 36–37°C. Raising or lowering the temperature by just two degrees can delay healing, with mitotic activity delayed for four hours (Lock 1979), fibroblast activity delayed for up to eight hours (Sato et al. 1999) and leucocyte activity delayed for up to 12 hours. There is a dressing (see Chapter 3) that can warm the localized area; there may also be an argument for warming intravenous fluids and warming patients on theatre tables in order to prevent infection and promote healing (Scott et al. 1999a).

The presence of necrotic tissue will prevent healing and will encourage bacterial proliferation, thereby prolonging inflammation. This may also prohibit epithelialization and lead to overgranulation. It is important, therefore, to remove necrotic tissue to enable the natural healing process to occur within the microenvironment of the wound.

Proliferation phase

At this stage, lasting between three and 24 days, there is an intense proliferation of fibroblasts and endothelial cells. Proliferating fibroblasts respond to growth factors and begin to synthesize collagen fibrils and a collagen matrix is laid down. Endothelial buds grow into the space cleared by macrophages (Torrance 1986) and the fibroblasts carry on the process of repair by laying down fibrous tissue. However, fibroblasts must be stimulated to synthesize collagen and the primary stimulants are ascorbate (ascorbic acid) and lactate. Therefore, there is evidence that administration of vitamin C is beneficial to wound healing. There is a balance at this stage of the newly forming capillaries and the nutrients required for tissue repair and reformation.

A wound that is in this stage of healing will have a pink wound bed with dark red raised bumps in the surface to the wound. The dark red bumps have the appearance of granules and the tissue is, therefore, named granulation tissue. It is at this point that the wound can be seen to be in a healing state as angiogenesis (growth of new blood vessels) is apparent in the form of the granules (the newly formed capillary loops) in the base of the wound. The capillary buds will grow towards low oxygen tension within the wound (Dealey 1994a) and Partridge (1998) confirms this by stating that an initial low oxygen tension at the wound site causes macrophages to stimulate angiogenesis. Therefore, anoxia is a major factor in stimulating vascular ingrowth (Majno and Janis 1996). The wound adaptation to anoxia may explain why occlusive dressings, vacuum-assisted closure (VAC) and dispersion therapy dressings appear to increase angiogenesis within a wound (see Chapter 3). Macrophages will also suffer anoxia and this causes them to secrete a factor that stimulates capillary outgrowth (Majno and Joris 1996).

As the wound bed advances level with the good tissues, the epithelial cells will begin to migrate over the wound surface in a 'leapfrog' manner and require a mixture of fibrin and fibronectin in order to freely glide at a rate of 0.5 mm/day (Majno and Joris 1996). As myofibroblasts shorten, the wound begins to contract and can be seen to be drawing closer together the edges of the wound. Among the substances most active in inducing contraction are (Tejero-Trujeque 2001):

- serotonin;
- angiotensin;
- vasopressin;
- bradykinin;
- epinephrin;
- prostaglandin.

Although the exact mechanism of wound contraction is still not fully understood (Tejero-Trujeque 2001) the above explanation assists toward comprehension.

Maturation phase

The final stage of healing involves wound contraction, full epithelialization and reorganization. Epithelial tissue will continue to migrate over the surface of raw and viable (moist) tissue within the wound; a reason for keeping the wound in a constant healing state with granulation rather than allowing bacterial contamination to promote slough and necrotic tissue. Even at this stage, macrophages are important to collagen lysis and synthesis and there will be a mass of fibrous tissue. Contractile fibroblasts will pull the wound edges together and the wound will change its appearance to become pale or white. Tensile strength is increased, although it will always remain below normal, and the wound will continue to form and change over the next 24 months.

   The healing phases apply to both acute and chronic wounds. However, in chronic wounds the process is visible with changes, or non-changes, in the wound bed being obvious. In surgical wounds, which are healed by primary intention with the wound edges approximated, the healing is not obvious. This leads to the question, when does an acute wound become a chronic (unhealing) wound? Many experts have attempted to answer this question and have not yet fully reached a conclusion. However, it is generally accepted that a wound of greater than six weeks duration can be described as a chronic wound (Dale et al. 1983). It is possible that a wound reaches a stage of delayed healing when various factors interrupt the healing process. The body then may accept the presence of the wound and perceive it as 'normal'. Macrophage/leucocyte activity would cease, bacteria can proliferate and proteolytic enzymes delay healing further.

In reality, the four phases of wound healing overlap and a wound can pass from one phase to another and then return to the previous phase. In wound healing, it is important to provide an environment to encourage a natural transition from one phase to the next preventing a return to the previous phase through the art and science of wound management.

Complexities of wound healing

Growth factors are a subclass of cytokines, discovered in the late 1970s. They are an assortment of small, naturally occurring proteins (peptides), which are thought to direct a variety of biological processes including embryological development, tumour growth and wound repair (Hart 1999). Chronic wounds may be deficient in one or more growth factors, which may be partly responsible for the delay in healing.

Cytokines are complex and bind to specific receptors to act as hormones. The effect of a given cytokine relies on the presence of other cytokines and one cytokine may produce another (Majno and Joris 1996). They are produced by many cells such as macrophages, leucocytes, mast cells, keratinocytes and platelets and are mediators that direct the processes involved in wound healing, the control of inflammation, communication between cells and the subsequent repair of the tissues. Cytokines, particularly TGF-beta, are believed to be instrumental in sustaining the fibrotic process that leads to scarring (Parekh et al. 1999) and they could be considered the conductors in the orchestration of wound healing. They appear to play a central role among the messengers of the complex process of wound repair and more than 20 types have been identified (Ganong 1995). Growth factors are being reviewed by scientists for their effect on the wound healing process with the hypothesis that growth factors introduced to a wound will increase healing. Being polypeptides, they may be degraded by proteases, although little is known about the reality of growth factor activity in chronic wounds.

Proteases are enzymes that have the ability to cleave proteins and, in certain conditions, can lead to widespread destruction of proteins within the wound. A pathological feature associated with some leg ulcers is the abnormally high level of proteolytic activity in the wound fluid compared with the activity in wound fluid of normally healing wounds (Hoffman and Eagle 1999). Fluid from chronic wounds contains abnormally high concentrations of proteases, which may cause excessive degradation of extracellular matrix components, growth factors and growth factor receptors and thus contributes to the refractory nature of chronic wounds.

Vascular permeability factor, also known as vascular endothelial growth factor, is a multifunctional cytokine that is over-expressed in many human cancers, healing wounds, psoriasis and rheumatoid arthritis (Dvorak et al. 1995). These growth factors play an important role in angiogenesis.

There are different growth factors for each required wound healing action. Fibroblast growth factor released following injury and is responsible for promotion of angiogenesis. Platelet derived growth factor is responsible for cellular proliferation, is involved in the chemotaxis of monocytes, neutrophils and fibroblasts (Hart 1999) and is one of the first growth factors released at the site of injury. Transforming growth factor has a role in fibrosis, immunosupression, the promotion of extracellular matrix synthesis and regulates growth factors synthesis by a variety of cells (Hart 1999).

Epidermal growth factor stimulates the production of epithelial cells, accelerating epidermal regeneration (Hart 1999).

Interleukin is thought to be associated with inflammation and tissue repair. Nerve-growth factor (NGF) has several biological activities both *in vitro* and *in vivo* (Bernabei et al. 1999). Fibroblasts and epithelial cells not only produce NGF but are also receptive to the action of NGF and accelerate healing on mouse skin (Bernabei et al. 1999).

Some growth factors are thought to signal wound healing to cease. The effect of growth factors on healing has led scientists to add recombinant human growth factors to chronic wounds in an attempt to replace factors that are lacking within the chronic wound. This science is still in its infancy but there is some evidence that platelet derived growth factor may stimulate healing. Growth factors are most highly researched at the time of writing and the topical use of growth factors in wound healing is a new and exciting field.

Hyaluronan

Rheinwald and Green (1975) discovered a method of culturing human epidermal keratinocytes. Today, these keratinocytes are cultured and seeded on hyaluronic acid impregnated membranes. Hyaluronan is a major carbohydrate component of the extracellular matrix. It is found in most parts of the body and is generally accepted as being associated with wound repair (Chen and Abatangelo 1999). Generally, wound tissues show an increase in hyaluronic acid in the early stages of wound repair (Bentley 1967). Hyaluronic acid is a negatively charged glycosaminoglycan that is composed of repeating disaccharide units of D-glucuronic acid and N-acetylglucosamine; it is the major glycosaminoglycan of the foetal dermis (Iocono et al. 1998).

The reports of the benefits of the application of hyaluronan in wound care has led to the production of hyaluroran based dressings. Chen and Abatangelo (1999) write:

> Hyaluronan solutions are highly osmotic and control tissue hydration during periods of change such as the inflammatory process. When hyaluronan synthesis contributes to tissue hydration, the result is a weakening of cell anchorage, allowing temporary detachment from the matrix and facilitation of cell migration and division. The highly viscous nature of hyaluronan contributes to the retardation of bacterial passage through the pericellular zone.

Hyaluronan is also thought to be associated with the scarless quality of foetal wound healing (West et al. 1997).

Prostaglandins

All mammalian cells produce prostaglandins if stimulated and these have a role in pain and vasodilation. Prostaglandins are released from phospholipids in the cell membrane through hormonal stimulation. The action of prostaglandins varies for the area in which it is expected to work.

Prostaglandins have the following roles:

1 Promoters of the inflammatory process (drugs that interfere with the production of prostaglandins will reduce inflammation).
2 Some are vasoconstrictors and this reduces blood loss until the clotting cascade has formed a plug.

3 Others are vasodilators and this increases blood flow to the injured site.
4 All are initiators of the clotting cascade by causing platelet aggravation.
5 All influence cell activity by acting as messengers between cells and/or modulating intracellular activity.
6 They are initiators of sensitivity to painful stimuli.

Therefore, prostaglandins are important factors that influence wound healing and administration of drugs (NSAIDs, steroids, aspirin) that inhibit their production will reduce the healing status of the wound. At the same time, administration of these drugs will dampen down the inflammation and reduce pain and swelling initiated in part by prostaglandins.

Collagen

Collagen is the most abundant protein in the animal world and is responsible for holding the body together, skeleton included (Majno and Joris 1996). The term collagen is frequently used to mean collagen fibres, but actually relates to a family of glycoproteins found in a range of histological entities including collagen fibres, reticulin fibres and basement membranes (Fletcher 2000). Collagen may be detected in a wound within the first 10 hours post injury.

Connective tissue proper is a loose connective tissue forming the dermis of the skin. This tissue consists of scattered collagen, a fibrous protein with the tensile strength of steel wire. The fibres lie together in the dermis and offer wound repair strength, protection and binds with water (Hinchcliffe and Montague 1988).

A second type of connective tissue is a compact irregular tissue with a densely packed meshwork of collagen. This tissue forms tough sheaths around organs and becomes tendons connecting bones together. There are 14 genetically distinct collagens, encoded by 30 different genes, and they account for 70–80 per cent of the dry weight of the dermis (Hopkinson 1992) and contain 18–40 per cent of the body's water. Approximately six of the 14 types are thought to be important in wound healing and are dispersed throughout the dermal matrix. Collagen is formed within the ribosomes of fibroblasts and a collagen molecule is a triple helical structure consisting of three polypeptide α chains (Hopkinson 1992). Ascorbic acid is essential for the formation of collagen and a patient with a wound is advised to ensure vitamin C is in the diet or supplemented.

Collagen acts as a chemoattractant for fibroblasts to the wound area and may be responsible for providing the signal to remodel the matrix (Fletcher 2000). The water binding properties of collagen decreases with age and the wrinkling appearance of old age is now thought to be due to loss of the water carrying properties rather than loss of elastin as was once thought (Hinchcliffe and Montague 1988).

Elastin

Elastin tissues are protein fibres found in the dermis of the skin, which have an important function in provision of elasticity and resilience for the skin and arteries. Elastin fibres are produced by fibroblasts and, when matured, form the elastic fibre network, which is stabilized by enzymatically-generated covalent cross-links (Hopkinson 1992). The role of elastin in wound healing is not clear although it is known to have an undefined function (Hopkinson 1992). The elastin deteriorates with age and the tissues become less elastic. Elastin's resistance to chemical agents is astounding and it tends to survive in necrotic tissue long after all other structures have disappeared (Majno and Joris 1996).

With age, elastin becomes stiffer due to cross-linking and the amount of calcium bound to the elastin fibres increases. In some atherosclerotic arteries the internal elastic lamina is specifically and strikingly calcified (Majno and Joris 1996).

Plasminogen

Plasminogen activators are produced within the blood, tissues or body fluids. Activation of clotting factor 2 leads to the generation of plasminogen activator and red and white blood cells produce plasminogen activators that act locally (Hinchcliffe and Montague 1988). Plasminogen is the pro-enzyme of plasmin and promotes fibrinolysis and cell migration during normal wound healing. Hoffman and Starkey (1998) found that plasminogen is degraded by wound fluid, specifically due to neutrophil elastase activity. They claim that keratinocyte migration is impaired in leg ulcers because of reduced availability of plasminogen for plasmin generation.

Granulation tissue

Chemical mediators, serotonin, prostaglandins, bradykinins and histamine are important in the synthesis of granulation tissue. Small (1994) writes:

> It is likely that urogastrone, a growth factor, stimulates synthesis of granulation tissue. Urogastrone initiates DNA synthesis and (therefore) cell reproduction and RNS protein synthesis. A connective tissue activating peptide released from leucocytes may be responsible for activating wound fibroblasts and factors released by platelets are involved in the repair process.

Overgranulation

Overgranulation or proud-flesh, can occur in the later stages of healing, when the wound bed has filled with granulation tissue and normal epithelialization does not occur. The granulation tissue continues to fill the area until it is proud of the wound, preventing epithelial tissue from migrating over the surface. Overgranulation may occur for two reasons.

The first cause could be modern dressings which are possibly too clever in healing wounds. Hydrocolloids are sometimes blamed for this as the dressing provides the optimum wound healing environment encouraging angiogenesis and, perhaps over-accelerating cell growth (Table 1.1).

Chronic infection is a second cause. Over stimulation of the inflammatory reaction may cause the wound to progress beyond the edges of the epithelium by forgetting to 'switch off'. For treatment of overgranulation see Chapter 3.

Chronic wounds

Chronic wounds present the greatest challenge to clinicians. Acute wounds, if all healing factors are in place, will heal without interference from the clinician. A chronic wound requires all the art and science of wound healing to bring the wound back to inflammation and healing. Wounds that are chronic can progress to healing by the careful selection of dressings that provide an ideal environment. However, it is the body that heals itself and not the dressing (see Chapter 3).

Once healing commences, a chronic wound that is debrided of slough or necrotic tissue will appear to 'open' like a flower as the wound is cleaned. This may lead the clinician to believe that the

Table 1.1 Dressing requirements for providing an optimum wound healing environment

Moisture	Winter (1962) found that epithelial cells only migrate over viable tissue and wounds heal three times faster in a moist environment.
Thermal insulation	Any drop in temperature below 37° delays mitotic activity for up to four hours (Torrance 1986). Leucocytes will not function in a low temperature wound – increasing the potential for clinical infection.
Highly absorptive	Exudate can be harmful to good skin. Chronic wound exudate can delay healing (Phillips et al. 1998).
Bacterial impermeability	For protection of the wound against bacterial contamination. 'Strike through' of exudate allows passage for bacteria into, and out of, the wound.
Free of contaminants	Gravel, cotton wool, remains of dressings, necrotic tissue are foreign bodies and are foci for infection.
Non-adherent	Adherent dressings may tear dried exudate off the wound bed, causing trauma to newly forming tissues. Newly forming capillaries can grow through gauze loops and will be torn when the gauze is removed.
Non-toxic/harmful	Many antiseptics have been found to damage healthy tissue and hypochlorites may still be in use in some areas (Flanagan, 1997; Leaper 1988; Ferguson 1993). Hydrogen peroxide has been shown to cause air emboli when used to irrigate cavity wounds (Sleigh and Linter 1985; Morgan 1992).

wound is enlarging. However, as a collagen matrix is formed in the wound bed, the edges of the wound are 'pushed' outward. Myofibroblasts then initiate the contraction process and the wound edges begin to shrink inward making the wound obviously smaller.

A chronic wound that has granulation in the base is a healing wound and requires only minor support from the clinician. Once the healing commences, the outcome will generally be excellent providing clinical infection is prevented and trauma from inappropriate dressings is strictly avoided.

Summary of the wound healing process

When a wound occurs, the inflammatory reaction is initiated by the non-specific mechanisms of phagocytosis. Blood vessels immediately constrict for eight to ten minutes and then dilate causing redness over the injured site. Chemical mediators, such as histamine, serotonin and bradykinin, increase capillary permeability, allow fluid to leak into the injured site and form oedema. Prostaglandins and kinins are released from the granules of basophils and mast cells and are stimulated to enter the wound site. β-lymphocytes produce antibodies against bacterial antigens, thereby promoting phagocytosis and protecting against further bacterial invasion. Vasoconstriction of an injured arteriole or small artery (due to the release of serotonin, and other chemicals, released from damaged and adhered platelets) may be so marked, following injury, that its lumen is obliterated (Ganong 1995).

Macrophages, having entered the tissues 72 hours previously as monocytes, migrate in response to chemotactic stimuli from injured tissues, engulfing and killing bacteria, dead cells and foreign matter. They play a key role in immunity and wound healing and secrete up to 100 different substances including clot-promoting factors and factors that affect the production of prostaglandins (Ganong 1995).

Mast cells produce histamine and serotonin, and, therefore, are also important to wound healing. Neutrophils, lymphocytes and monocytes move out of the blood in large numbers as part of the inflammatory reaction, keeping wounds free from bacteria. When a wound becomes chronic, the inflammation becomes chronic and ceases to function as part of the healing mechanism. If the inflammatory action ceases to function, these transient cells cease to enter the wound. Bacteria can proliferate, the chemical chain reaction ceases and the wound becomes static.

When injury occurs, the clotting cascade forms a 'plug' to prevent blood loss and the inflammatory process begins to clear the site of potential infective agents and initiates the healing process (see Figure 1.4). A matrix is built within the wound bed and angiogenesis weaves through the fibres of the matrix. Healing occurs and maturation of the wound site can continue for up to two years.

This process occurs in the acute wound. However, a chronic wound has often passed through one or two of these phases and has become 'stuck' in that phase. The inflammatory phase, so vital to wound healing, is no longer active and this halts the production of growth factors.

Exudate

Exudate is a product of the inflammation process. It consists of dead and living leucocytes, tissue fragments and bacterial cells, all suspended in serum. Leucocytes pouring into the wound bed by billions, destroy bacteria and concentrate the exudate into pus. This is facilitated by plasma proteins coating foreign materials to make phagocytosis easily accomplished and antibodies are produced by β-lymphocyctes binding to the surface of bacteria.

Due to vasodilation, many of these components are leaked into the tissues at the site of trauma (which leads to localized swelling).

When newly forming in a wound, exudate is healthily essential with many growth factors to stimulate the wound to heal. However, once the wound becomes chronic the situation changes: macrophage activity decreases or ceases, bacterial colonization increases and proteolytic enzymes and the wound fluid become destructive leading to delayed healing.

Wysocki (1996a) found that fibronectin can be degraded in fluid from chronic wounds but remains intact in blood derived serum, plasma derived serum and mastectomy wound fluid, whereas matrix metalloproteinases are overexpressed in chronic wound fluid. The conclusion from Wysocki's study was that the two factors may contribute to delayed healing of chronic wounds.

Other factors involved in exudate production are:

- hydrostatic pressures in venous leg ulcers (see Chapter 5);
- vascular permeability caused by bacterial invasion (see Chapter 4);
- leg dependency in venous ulceration.

Eschar

Eschar is an undesirable component of a wound and must be removed (see Chapter 3) to promote healing. However, little is known about the composition of eschar and a study completed by Thomas, Harding and Moore (1999) recognized the importance of discovering eschar composition to enable common (empirically derived) methods of removal to be assessed for efficacy. The study found that chronic wounds are not amorphous masses but consist of structural elements in the form of collagen, chondroitin sulphate, fibronectin, fibrinogen and elastin, although it was noted that this varied between patients.

Factors that affect wound healing

The skin provides excellent protection for the body and serves very many complex functions. The numerous factors that affect these functions can be jeopardized if the skin's integrity is not maintained. Therefore, assessment and a comprehensive knowledge base of the skin and functions is an important part of patient care.

Intrinsic factors

Drugs

Drugs such as inotropes, steroids and non-steroidal anti-inflammatory drugs can all affect wound healing. Steroid therapy can produce paper-thin skin, causing the skin to be easily damaged with degloving injuries common, and tissues which are difficult to heal. Chemotherapy can lower immunological resistance leading to higher rates of infection and will kill new cells forming within the body, thereby, destroying new cells within the wound bed and delaying healing.

Diabetes

Diabetes can delay healing as viscous blood, functional impairment of polymorphonuclear neutrophils, low delivery of nutrients and oxygen to the wound will all increase the risk of clinical infection and slow the healing process. In 1995, there were more than 130 million people worldwide with diabetes and it is estimated that these figures will increase to 300 million by 2025 (Weiman 1998). Infection, ischaemia and unrelieved pressure, as well as diabetes itself, impede the healing process and can result in a non-healing ulcer that may ultimately lead to amputation. Diabetes care can absorb 4–5 per cent of the National Health Service budget (Laing and Williams 1989). A diabetic patient over 70 years has 70 per cent increased chance of digital gangrene than a non-diabetic patient (Barnett

1992). Hyperglycaemia will impair leucocyte chemotaxis (the summoning of leucocytes to an area of injury).

Pathological changes in diabetes

Non-enzymatic glycation is the mechanism by which proteins, such as collagen, are subject to chronic attack from glucose (Majno and Joris 1996). In wound healing this has huge implications if the blood glucose of the diabetic patient is not stabilized. In diabetes, collagen become increasingly brown and therefore Majno and Joris described the process as the 'browning reaction' and explain it as follows: 'If milk is cooked for a long time, sugar and proteins combine to form a brown and bitter-burnt tasting product called melanoidins. This reaction contributes to the brown colour and toughness of cooked meat. Scientists have found that it is this same reaction involved in diabetes (and ageing).' Accelerated arteriosclerosis, neuropathy and joint stiffness are the results of this 'browning'.

Rheumatoid arthritis

Rheumatoid arthritis will delay healing because the disease also effects the microcirculation within the tissues, lowering the supply of nutrients and oxygen to the wound bed.

Poor circulation such as an arterial component in leg ulcers, will prevent a wound from healing.

The effect of shock on healing

In acute shock, particularly following haemorrhage, the blood supply becomes inadequate to the tissues and leucocytes can become sticky and trapped. The number of leucocytes available is greatly reduced and, therefore, the inflammatory response is depressed. Further complications are vasodilation and lowered blood supply, and these factors open the channels for bacterial invasion and potential for septic shock (Majno and Joris 1996). The result of shock is delayed wound healing, particularly as the lowered inflammatory response reduces the amount of available growth factors required for wound healing.

Any analgesic injection given for pain in this period is likely to be held within the tissues and released once the shock is reduced. The body may then be flooded with the drug.

Stress causes vasoconstriction and the lowered blood delivery can affect the required nutrient supply to the wound bed (Kiecolt-Glaser et al. 1995). Pain causes a stress reaction within the body with resultant vasoconstriction.

Smoking lowers the temperature of the skin. Lock (1979) demonstrated that any drop of temperature in the wound will delay healing for up to four hours. Smoking also causes vasoconstriction and a reduction in fibrolynitic activity with an increase in the viscosity of the blood. Carbon monoxide binds to haemoglobin with an affinity 200 times that of oxygen (Siana et al. 1992). There can be little doubt that the reduction of nutrients and oxygen delays wound healing severely.

Clinical infection will delay the healing process as will anaemia, which reduces oxygen delivery to the wound. Malnourished patients with a wound will almost always have low albumin levels as the protein leaks away in the wound exudate; measurement of serum albumin in 35 patients with pressure sores showed that all had a very low plasma protein level (Lewis 1996). Serum albumin levels are significantly associated with having a pressure sore, with a threefold increase in risk of sore formation, for every gram decrease in serum albumin levels (Lewis 1996). However, it would be difficult to know whether the low albumin was the result of fluid loss or malnutrition. It is known that patients with chronic leg ulcers show diminished levels of vitamin A, vitamin E, carotenes and zinc (Rojas and Phillips 1999). Normal levels of vitamin C and zinc are a necessary part of wound healing.

Age and healing

The ageing process has a detrimental effect on the skin and immunological system and affects the healing process with age-related differences in wound healing. The inflammatory response reduces with age; proliferation, maturation and migration times are also greatly reduced. Nevertheless, although the process is slowed, if all factors leading to good wound healing are in place (nutrients, oxygen, etc.), wounds will heal in the aged.

Structural changes in the skin have been identified by Desia (1997) and include:

- decrease in vascularity, leading to a reduced supply of nutrient and oxygen enriched blood;
- loss of melanocytes and loss of natural protection against ultra-violet rays;
- decreased innervation and lowered tissue responses;
- elastic fibre changes;
- decrease in number and function of sweat glands;
- sebaceous gland hyperplasia and drying of the tissues;
- thinning of the epidermis;
- decrease of type III collagen leading to reduced activity for the collagen matrix and decreased density;
- slower and less intense inflammatory response, therefore slower healing;
- reduction in production of mast cells;
- reduction in fibroblast proliferation leading to a decrease in wound contraction and slower wound healing.

These changes may lead to decreased healing rates and lower immunological responses leading to increased potential of clinical infection. Linked to the fact that the elderly have an increased potential for diabetes, cardiovascular problems and are likely to be taking drugs related to lowered healing, the indications would be an increase in the potential for poor wound healing.

Free radicals

Atoms are small particles that make up all living matter. They have a central nucleus made up of positively charged protons and uncharged neutrons. Around the central nucleus spin negatively charged electrons and it is important to the stability of the atom that a full complement of electrons is in place. An isolated atom is an unstable entity and therefore, atoms form bonds with other atoms through covalent or ionic bonding. When a group of atoms bond together they are called a molecule. Free radicals are molecules without the full complement of electrons making the molecule unstable and reactive. The instability can cause the molecule to react with other molecules in a chain reaction sometimes causing the radicals to attack DNA, which in turn can make the cell division unstable, with potential for forming cancer. Simply put, a free radical is an atom or a group of atoms with an uneven electrical charge. To complete itself, it steals a charged particle (electron) from another cell and this can set up a chain reaction that produces more free radicals which can damage other cells, causing them to misbehave.

Niwa (1987) found that the action of free oxygen radicals causes chronic damage to newly formed tissue in chronic injuries. The cause of the release of free radicals may be traced back to poor circulation. Fresh fruit and vegetables are antioxidants and a daily intake of both is believed to be a protection against free radicals. Vitamin C is also a useful supplement in protection against free radicals.

Oedema

The body of a normal adult contains approximately 40 litres of water with 25 litres in the cells and 12 litres in extracellular spaces. There is a fine fluid balance in the body with potassium and sodium exchange being responsible for keeping that balance. Serum albumin maintains a pressure within the venous system that balances the fluid between the extracellular and venous systems.

Several conditions produce oedema:

- Low serum albumin tends to produce an almost translucent, pale oedema. The tissues are generally soft, swollen and pale yellow. Normal serum albumin is generally 4.5 per cent and oedema will occur if this level drops to 2.5 per cent.
- Venous obstruction: an elastic band tied around a finger would cause local oedema, as would a too tight plaster cast. Venous congestion (leading to ulceration) can be included in this type of oedema. A finger pressed onto the skin will produce a 'pit' that remains for some time.
- Lymphatic obstruction: if the lymphatic system is unable to perform its function, oedema is the result. The oedema is hard to the touch and does not 'pit' when pressed and the skin between the toes cannot be pinched (positive Stermmer's sign).
- Acute inflammatory oedema is accompanied by the signs of infection with pain, redness, heat and swelling. Pitting will be absent because the fibrin network acts as a gel and traps the fluid (Majno and Joris 1996).
- Cardiac oedema is caused by poor cardiac output causing a 'backlog' of fluid. Care should be taken when using compression

bandaging or bed elevation for patients with chronic cardiac failure as the sudden flood of fluid from the compression can cause cardiogenic shock.

- Kidney failure can present a problem for wound healing although oedema is rarely severe unless in the latter stages.

Oxygenation

Oxygen involvement in wound healing can be extrinsic (on the wound bed surface) or intrinsic (cellular requirements). Hypoxia can initially be a potent stimulus for angiogenesis and fibroblast proliferation. However, oxygen is vital for repair of the tissues and, therefore, wound healing will be impaired if hypoxia persists (Stadelmann et al. 1998). Chronic non-healing wounds are frequently hypoxic (Bowler et al. 2001) as a consequence of poor blood perfusion, and host and microbial cell metabolism contribute further to lowering the pO_2. Wound hypoxia predisposes the wound to infection as neutrophils require large amounts of oxygen for phagocytosis and, without oxygen, bacteria could proliferate unchecked. Each individual cell will undertake a metabolic process in reproducing and growing and this metabolism uses oxygen as part of the process. Lack of oxygen will reduce mitotic activity and will also reduce leucocyte activity, thereby increasing the potential for clinical infection. There may be arguments for keeping a wound deprived of surface oxygen as bacteria also require oxygen for respiration. Depriving the wound surface of oxygen may (1) encourage the wound to increase angiogenesis to provide oxygen and (2) reduce bacterial count in the wound because the oxygen requirements for bacterial respiration is deplete. Therefore, providing an oxygen deplete patient with increased oxygen and providing an occlusive dressing for the wound, may decrease the potential for infection whilst increasing angiogenesis.

Although there are bacteria that enjoy a hypoxic environment (anaerobic bacteria) and providing these with an occlusive dressing may increase proliferation, there is no evidence to suggest this. Anaerobic bacteria are found mainly in pressure sores and fungating wounds, particularly necrotic wounds of all types and in diabetic ulcers (Sharp et al. 1978). Oxygen saturation can be increased through administration of fluids through the increase of blood volume and decrease of viscosity (Bryant 1992). There is also a potential for the use of hyperbaric oxygen (see Chapter 3) although the research undertaken by Winter and Perins (1970) demonstrated faster wound epithelialization when patients were placed in a hyperbaric oxygen chamber. This is contra to the writing of Majno and Joris (1996) who state that anoxia is an important element of angiogenesis. Winter and Perins's work may indicate that hyperbaric oxygen is suitable for the very final stages of healing.

Poor cardiac output, peripheral vascular disease, diabetes mellitus, cigarettes and chronic infection will accelerate cellular hypoxia increasing the risk of infection and delayed healing.

Extrinsic factors

Unrelieved pressure, as in pressure ulcers should be avoided; unless that pressure is removed, the wound will not heal (see Chapter 9).

Cold will delay wound healing as any drop in temperature of more than two degrees will delay mitotic activity for up to four hours (Lock 1979). The reduction in heat will also delay entry of macrophages and leucocytes to the wound bed by up to 12 hours. This will increase the risk of clinical infection. Wound temperature of greater than 30°C reduces the tensile strength of wounds through decreased perfusion from vasoconstriction. Poorly applied dressings, too tight compression, no compression when required, dry dressings, dressings that adhere to the wound, antiseptics (Leaper 1987) will all delay wound healing.

Chronic wound exudate has generally been believed not to be a problem. However, research from the USA (Phillips et al. 1998) is now showing that chronic wound exudate can delay wound healing by inhibiting the growth of fibroblasts. Thompson (1998) found the presence of microbial antigens perpetuates the inflammatory process so that the mechanism, which should promote wound repair becomes detrimental and leads to further tissue damage.

Extravasation, or the leakage of solutions into subcutaneous tissues through intravenous administration of drugs or fluids, can cause minor or major life-threatening damage to the tissues. Figure 1.8 shows a 22-year-old woman who had been administered sodium bicarbonate during resuscitation following a car accident. The damage was immense, exposing tendons and amputation was a very real threat. The foot was saved by negative pressure (vacuum-assisted closure).

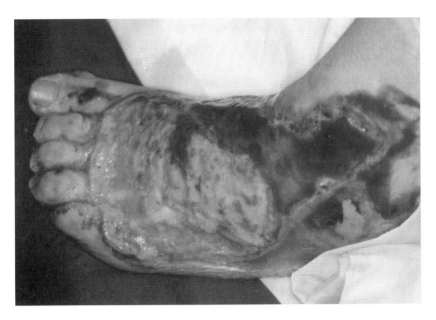

Figure 1.8 Extravasation injury (see Plate 3).

Skin diseases

Eczema and skin sensitization

The literal Greek meaning of eczema is to 'boil over' (Marrs 1990). However, it is sometimes difficult to identify eczema when related to contact dermatitis.

Eczema is multifactorial with endogenous and exogenous factors existing together. All patients with leg ulceration are at risk from skin sensitization because of the number of dressings that are used to treat the ulcer. Many dressings contain allergens or substances that can sensitize and when skin surrounding a wound becomes a concern (such as in contact dermatitis), either the dressing or the exudate should be considered as the possible cause. If the problem is ignored, the tissues can become inflamed and eczema or contact dermatitis can develop.

Injury to the skin is only one area when the protective layer is interrupted. There are over 1000 skin diseases (Williams 1998), which can complicate assessment, particularly as 10–12 per cent of GP consultations concern skin disorders (Dennis 1998). Williams identifies that there are primary lesions present at the onset of the disease and secondary lesions are the results of changes over time, caused by the disease. Williams states that the examiner should be able to distinguish between the two to give an accurate clue to the underlying disease and cause. Of patients referred to a dermatology department 20 per cent have eczema and there has been an increase of atopic eczema since the 1970s (Dennis 1998).

Eczema has a strong association with asthma and is probably largely genetic in origin. There are two main types of eczema: acute, producing blisters and crusts; and chronic, with scaly and thickened appearance of the skin. In eczema, the blood vessels dilate causing erythema and an infiltration of inflammatory cells. These cells cause oedema of the dermis and epidermis, thereby initiating malfunction of epidermal cells. There is a resultant pruritis, excoriation and lichenification. Treatment is emollients and steroid creams. Emollients can be oils applied to the bath water, creams, lotions or ointments. Steroid creams are inadvisable when used for long periods and so treatment is started with a low strength, or with high strength and quickly reduced to a lower strength. An old-fashioned remedy and one that is often sneered at due to lack of clinical evidence is potassium permanganate soaks. However, these are useful in weeping eczema or in weeping oedematous legs, secondary to coronary heart disease.

Contact dermatitis

Patients with venous ulceration are at a higher risk of contact sensitivity due to the sheer amount of dressing material that is applied to their open wounds. About 50–69 per cent of patients with leg ulcers will suffer either single or multiple sensitivity (Cameron 1995). Eczema and dermatitis can be used interchangeably with venous stasis eczema and contact dermatitis mistakenly intermixed in diagnosis. Venous stasis eczema has an endogenous element whereas contact dermatitis is exogenous and due to sensitivity to a dressing or an allergic reaction. Patients with contact dermatitis can be mistakenly prescribed antibiotics for clinical infection as in the case of the patient in Figure 1.9. Dermatitis often has a clear demarcation line, which matches the line of the dressing or bandage. In clinical infection, the erythema is less defined (Figure 1.10) and will extend beyond the line of the dressing and may expand over hours or days.

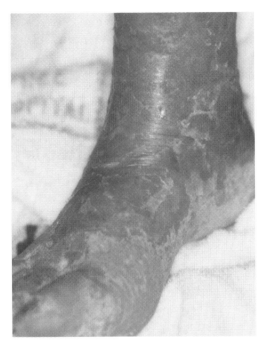

Figure 1.9 Contact dermatitis is frequently mistaken as a clinical infection (See Plate 4).

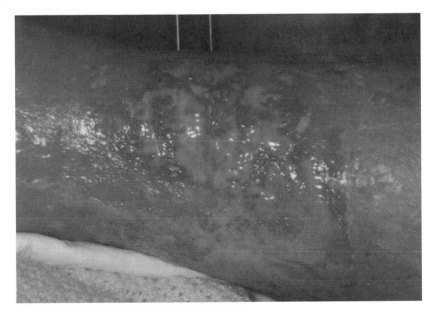

Figure 1.10 The demarcation line of erythema is less defined in clinical infection (see Plate 5).

There are many allergens in dressing materials and any of these may cause a reaction, particularly in patients with leg ulcers. Examples of these are:

1   Lanolin, which is present in many creams, although some manufacturers try to produce hypoallergenic lanolin.
2   Parabens, which are preservatives and are present in some creams. Ointment is unlikely to require preservative additives and is, therefore, safer in leg ulcer patients.
3   Colophony, a product that gives some dressings the 'tackiness' to enable adherence. Hydrocolloids are among these. Hydrocolloid pastes and hydrocolloid fibre dressings do not contain colophony, however, and that explains why hydrocolloid pastes can often be used without causing a reaction when the patient is highly sensitive to hydrocolloid sheets.
4   Gloves that are made of latex or with powder can cause sensitivity reactions. The gloves do not have to come in direct contact with the skin as, if the sensitivity is to powder, the powder can be airborne and will cause a reaction.
5   Topical antibiotics, although these are rarely used today as they may lead to resistance and particularly multi-resistant *Staphylococcus aureas* (MRSA).
6   Alcohol present in Flamazine, E45 and some paste bandages, may cause a reaction.
7   Rubber, which is present in some elasticated bandages and elasticated tubular bandages.
8   Perfume, found in some creams and oils bought over the counter.

Patients should be patch tested prior to application of suspected dressings. However, sensitivities are not easily dealt with, as the patient is unlikely to be sensitive to a product with additives that have never been applied before. The reaction will only occur after the product has been applied on several occasions.

Patch tests can be introduced as a 'battery' of commercially prepared patches with 24 of the most commonly found allergens. However, the nurse on the ward or in the community, needing to use a dressing that has the potential to cause a reaction, can tape a small piece of the dressing to the back or upper thigh. A check on the patch in 24 and 48 hours will establish any problems with sensitivity, as the area under the patch will be red with fairly defined demarcation lines around the area of the dressing.

If a patient is suspected of having contact dermatitis, they should be referred for patch testing at the dermatology clinic so that all sensitive products can be eliminated from dressing regimes. The patient in Figure 1.11 has either multiple sensitivity, or (more likely) is sensitive to her own exudate. The treatment for this particular patient was exposure of the legs to air, bed elevation and daily soaks in potassium permanganate. When any one of these treatments was removed, the ulcers deteriorated. When all three treatment elements were in place the ulcers improved (Figure 1.12). Unfortunately, when the patient returned home from hospital, she was inclined to keep the legs dependent and did not often use leg soaks, common dressings were used to absorb the exudate and the ulcers deteriorated again.

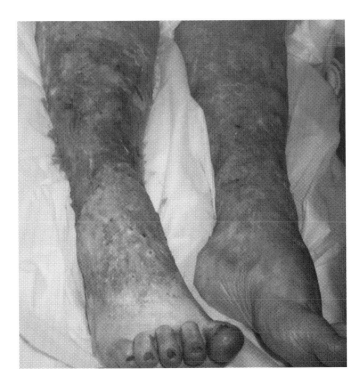

Figure 1.11 This patient has multiple sensitivities, possibly partially due to her own exudate (see Plate 6).

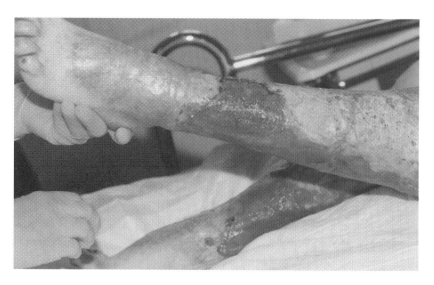

Figure 1.12 The wound following three days of treatment.

Psoriasis

Psoriasis is a chronic, genetically inherited skin problem, which can be distressing for the patient and carers, uncomfortable through itching and can impinge on lifestyles of those patients not wishing to socialize due to embarrassment and self-consciousness. Psoriasis is a common condition, which effects two per cent of the population. If a parent has the condition, the child has a 10 per cent chance of developing the same condition. There are three main types of psoriasis:

1 Plaque psoriasis is usually confined to knees, elbows and the lower back, can be small or large, well defined and pink/red in colour with a covering of silvery scales (Venables 1994).
2 Guttate psoriasis occurs in young adults and is often followed by a streptococci throat infection. It may be chronic or an isolated attack.
3 Pustular psoriasis is a painful condition with pustules on hands and feet.

The cells of the dermis develop and, over a 28-day period, grow, move to the skin surface where they die and become the horny layer of the epidermis. This process is accelerated in psoriasis to only a four-day period, creating an epidermis that is thicker and immature. The immune system is activated and vasodilation and histamine production leads to erythema and inflammation of the tissues.

Sunlight is thought to help reduce psoriasis although advice should be given to the patient, so that burning is avoided. Stress can precede a relapse. Treatment of psoriasis is generally topical steroids, emollients, coal tar solutions, etc., and decisions on the treatment are best left to the dermatologist.

The primary role of the carer/advisor is to keep the tissues viable for as long as possible. When the tissues deteriorate, for whatever reason, it then becomes imperative to ensure that the healing process is maintained through providing an optimum wound healing environment. It is also the role of the carer to ensure that the skin reaction is not a contact dermatitis, which is easily remedied by removing the allergen, such as the dressing.

Pemphigus and pemphigoid

Pemphigus and pemphigoid are similar in appearance but have different outcomes. They are the result of immunologically mediated disorders. Pemphigoid is an autoimmune disorder, occurring between the dermis and the epidermis, causing large blisters that remain firm when pressed by a finger (a negative Nikolsky's sign). The disorder generally recovers eventually although it can persist for some months or years. Treatment may be steroid therapy.

Pemphigus is also an autoimmune disease but is more serious than pemphigoid. The blisters are generally smaller than in pemphigoid and appear softer, particularly when pressed. The fluid in the blister will be seen to spread under the epidermis when firmly pressed and may even disintegrate (a positive Nikolsky's sign). Steroid therapy is the treatment of choice.

Incontinence dermatitis

When skin is overhydrated, its ability to protect underlying structures is compromised and its own integrity is placed at risk. Skin that is damp or wet is more permeable to irritating substances, more readily colonized by microorganisms and will blister easily (Kemp 1994). Leyden et al. (1977) found that skin breakdown associated with urinary incontinence is most likely due to the water content rather than ammonia.

When stools are mixed with urine, there is a rise in pH that, in turn, increases the activity of proteases and lipases. These enzymes will irritate the skin and will increase permeability to irritants (Kemp 1994).

A case study in eczema

A patient with long-term eczema was referred to the authors. This patient had eczema of the hands, feet, legs and over the back and had been visiting dermatology consultants for many years, receiving steroid cream for the lesions. The patient was extremely depressed and his quality of life was affected. The patient's diet was discussed during the assessment, and it became apparent that a large part of the diet was dairy foods, cheese in particular. His love for cheese was so great that the assessor suspected that it may be partially responsible for the skin condition. The assessor requested that he give up dairy products for one month only. If at the end of the month his eczema was no better, he would have lost only one month of his beloved cheese. If, however, his condition had improved, he would then be able to make an informed choice whether to eat cheese or not! He gave up dairy foods for one month and his eczema resolved. For the first time in many years, he was able to hold his hand out for change, without being embarrassed about its cracked and bleeding condition. The only time he experienced any problems during that month, was when he ate an ice cream and within half an hour began to itch. The case study demonstrated the importance of listening to the information supplied by the patient. This particular patient had been using steroids and steroid cream unnecessarily for many years and this may have been avoided had he been holisitically assessed.

Conclusion

When caring for the patient with compromised tissue viability, best practice would include strategies to keep the skin dry but moisturized and free of irritants or prolonged pressure (see Chapter 9). To ensure that best practice is observed the professional must have good basic knowledge of how to care for the skin.

Care of the skin or 'keeping the tissue viable' is vital along with promotion of all the intrinsic and extrinsic factors related to wound healing. The knowledgeable professional can prevent tissue deterioration or promote wound healing and offer cost-effective care, side by side with excellence in quality care. With the acquired knowledge a confident approach to dressing selection will develop and the optimal wound healing environment can be achieved.

Activity

Observe the leg and arm skin of different patients and identify:

- dry skin;
- paper skin;
- steroid skin;
- hardened skin;
- moist skin.

1 Keep a diary for two weeks and decide how each different skin would heal if wounded. What is the physiological reaction preventing or promoting wound healing in each case?
2 What special care would be required for each patient?
3 Complete the diary with a reflective section on the learning achieved through the exercise. Place it in the professional profile.

CHAPTER 2

Holistic wound assessment

Holistic assessment of a patient's wound is possibly the single most important fundamental of healing a wound and will lead to rational decision making. The wound itself, and type of dressing to be used, must be the last consideration with discovery of all factors affecting healing preceding examination of the wound. It is also important to discover, and understand, the patient's own perception of their wound problems, particularly as this is rarely the wound itself. They will identify pain, excessive exudate and malodour as the problems that they wish to have removed from their lives. All of these are in general, easily dealt with if there is holistic assessment and understanding of the processes, intrinsic and extrinsic, that affect wound healing.

Doctors and nurses will all, at some time during their career, be expected to assess and prescribe treatment for wounds. However, few would have received education in the subject and it is left to interested professionals to learn about wound healing in a disjointed way (Davis 1996). Holistic patient assessment by an experienced and knowledgeable practitioner identifies achievable goals. The resultant documentation, related to the assessment, assists the practitioner and others to provide consistent treatment and care, monitor healing, detect complications and assess the effectiveness of the planned and administered care.

Although practitioners can assess wounds using colour grading (Cuzzell 1988), the system is not without faults particularly as the wound should be the last and possibly least important element of wound assessment. An understanding of the processes of wound healing is of primary importance in assessment, leading to appropriate decisions in wound dressings and increased healing rates. Lack of knowledgeable assessment may lead to inappropriate choice of wound dressings and possible deterioration of the wound.

Assessment of the wound begins with sitting with the patient and discovering:

- **Age of the wound** – the age of the wound will have an implication on healing times. A wound that is 50 years old will not heal at the rate of a wound that is 50 weeks old.
- **Medical status of the patient** – rheumatoid arthritis, diabetes, heart disease, multiple sclerosis, chronic obstructive airways disease, athrosclerosis, Buerger's disease (found in young smokers), cancer, venous stasis, arterial disease, immune disorders and anaemia will all have an impact on the status of healing in the wound. Low blood pressure is a predictive factor in pressure ulcer formation (Schubert 1992).
- **Medication that may affect wound healing** – certain medication can have adverse effects, such as chemotherapy, steroid therapy and even simple aspirin. Sometimes the drug may improve the possibility of wound healing, for example, aspirin is thought to prevent micro-thrombi formation.
- **Extrinsic factors** that may affect wound healing include unrelieved pressure, bacterial colonization, dressing sensitivities/allergies and cold. Unless pressure is reduced or relieved the area will continue to deteriorate. Warmth promotes mitosis. Dressing sensitivities can delay wound healing. Therefore, addressing all of these factors must be a prime consideration if wounds are to heal successfully.
- **Dressing selection** – it is the author's experience that wounds are often 'managed' not treated. Increasing the amount of bandages and added wads of Gamgee around a leg ulcer will only manage exudate and placing an ordinary charcoal dressing on the wound may control malodour. Although these dressings are extremely useful, this is merely 'managing' the symptoms rather than 'treating' the problem (see Chapter 3). If these conditions can be therapeutically treated then wound 'management' would possibly be obsolete. Some wound dressings actually impair patient function (Reiber et al. 1998) and this will have an impact on quality of life, healing rates and future mobility.

- **Whether or not the patient smokes** – smoking can have a dramatic effect on wound healing by delaying or impeding improvement in wound status. This is discussed in detail later in this chapter.
- **Nutritional status** – wound healing requires as much as double or triple the normal calorie requirements and this has an implication on serum protein levels (see Chapter 6).
- **Pain and anxiety** – the patient who is in pain or anxious may have delayed wound healing as this has a physiological stress response that can effect delivery of oxygen and nutrients to the wound.
- **Social isolation** – patients may not wish their wounds to improve because healing may lead to social isolation when the district nurse ceases to call. There may be an effect on wound healing through either stress or the psychological need to interfere with the wound to prevent it from healing completely.

The assessment of 12 activities of daily living: their affect on wound healing

Roper et al. (1985) recommended that holistic assessment of the patient should be based on the 12 activities of daily living. The wound should be the last consideration in deciding on treatment as providing the optimum wound healing environment relies on many factors other than the wound's local condition. All other factors should be assessed and addressed where possible before wound healing can commence.

Safety

Immobility can lead to death of tissues where localized pressure prevents blood flow. Any immobile patient must be considered at risk and be supplied with the appropriate pressure-reducing/relieving equipment (see Chapter 9). Support stockings or compression stockings will reduce the risk of developing leg ulceration in people with venous insufficiency but can be dangerous in those with arterial disease.

Necrotic and infected wounds may lead to septicaemia and even death of the patient. Identification of necrotic tissue is simple as non-viable tissue in the wound bed is very visible, black or yellow (Figure 2.1) and, when moist, is usually malodorous because of colonization of aerobic and non-aerobic bacteria. Removal of the necrotic material through use of appropriate dressings or through skilful use of sharp debridement by an experienced practitioner is essential. This last procedure, however, can only follow holistic assessment of the patient and wound for the following reasons.

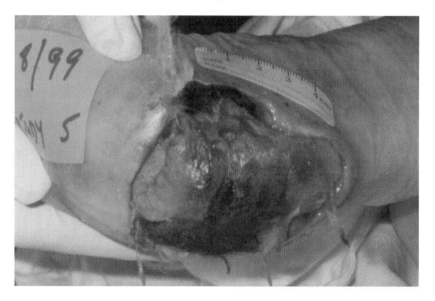

Figure 2.1 Necrotic heel pressure ulcer.

Debridement of a wound can open the tissue to clinical infection and, if prognosis is poor, it would be unacceptable to continue with a procedure that may cause unnecessary pain and suffering to the patient. Poor knowledge of lower structures may lead to severing of tendons, therefore, assessment must include the position of the wound and possible underlying structures. The patient may also experience pain in the wound.

Removing necrotic tissue is acceptable when undertaken by an experienced practitioner (see Chapter 3). Sharp debriding tissue until bleeding is a surgical procedure, which is unacceptable practice for a nurse and should be undertaken by a surgeon. Debridement, in the community especially, can be fraught with dangers, particularly if an artery is accidentally cut, or if a patient has a bleeding condition. Therefore, assessment of a necrotic wound should lead to either a surgical referral or to dressings that will encourage autolysis.

Infection is more difficult to identify (Figure 2.2) as the inflamma-tory stage of healing (identified by heat, pain and swelling) can be mistaken for infection (Hampton 1997b). This may lead to the patient being treated inappropriately with antibiotics, or dressing regimes unnecessarily reviewed, to the detriment of the healing process. Chronic wounds are generally colonized with bacteria (Collier 1994b) causing discharge, often with an offensive odour. These bacteria probably will not invade the host but sit within the wound exudate (Mertz et al. 1994; Flanagan 1997).

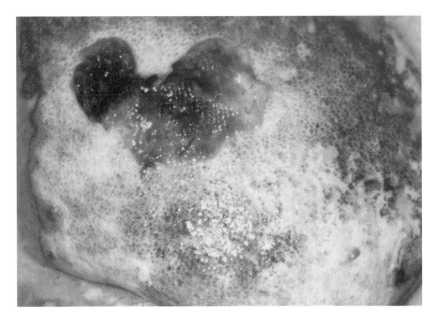

Figure 2.2 A grossly infected pressure ulcer in the sacrum and buttock area.

Latex allergies can raise issues of patient safety and practitioners should be aware of the potential severe reactions that may occur in those sensitive to latex. Keh et al. (2000) studied theatre patients and found that of the 505 patients with latex allergies, four died, 18 devel-oped major anaphylaxes and 483 had minor reactions. During the study, 239 theatre staff also reported latex associated reactions. Unfor-tunately, latex may be a hidden problem with dressing packs contain-ing latex either in the package or in the glue. Some dressings still contain latex although most companies have taken a responsible stand

and are removing it where possible. Adhesive tapes remain a difficult area and, very often, are not latex free. Certain mattresses also contain latex and this is a potential danger to those people with latex allergies.

Communicating

Wound healing can rely on psychological as well as physiological responses in the patient. The 'knitting needle' syndrome is an anecdotal phenomenon known to community nurses who find that some elderly patients, with social isolation, will occasionally interfere with wound healing (Moffatt et al. 1991). This is possibly to ensure continued visits from the nurse (there may be some controversy over this theory) or through lack of understanding of the importance of refraining from scratching an irritating wound. Assessment will help to identify and address the problems of isolation and to offer essential education and information to the patient.

Communication with other professionals is also extremely important to wound assessment. Each dressing change is an opportunity to assess the psychological status of the patient as well as the healing state of the wound and to evaluate care. However, each dressing change may be completed by a different practitioner and lack of documented evidence of the healing condition in previous dressing change would mean that alterations in the wound size, condition or treatment efficacy cannot be critically evaluated. This may lead to difficulties in wound dressing selection and may possibly delay wound healing. Therefore, documentation and/or verbal reports are essential to good practice in wound care.

Care plans are notoriously difficult to complete and can be used to document unnecessary data or may remain incomplete. In the future, integrated care pathways will assist particularly when united with an excellent assessment tool; this would be used as a universal assessment and evaluation document by hospital nurses, community nurses, carers and doctors.

Stress can have a physical reaction that effects wound healing. As adrenaline pumps around the body, vasoconstriction occurs and this reduces the supply of nutrients and oxygen to the wound, slowing the healing process. A confident approach and a positive attitude to the wound will reduce anxiety. Personal stress is often difficult to identify and, without the free co-operation of the patient, may be unsolvable.

Breathing

Tissue repair requires energy which is released during the breakdown of nutrients and oxygen; without oxygen this energy cannot be liberated and wound healing will be delayed. Oxygen is an important substrate of collagen synthesis and any condition that delays transport of oxygen to the wound will therefore affect the healing rate.

Oxygen is required by leucocytes for phagocytosis and without oxygen the destruction of bacteria is greatly reduced, therefore there is a greater potential for infection in the oxygen deplete wound. Holistic assessment would alert the practitioner to the risk hypoxia might pose to the wound. Difficulty with breathing will also reduce the patient's mobility, thereby increasing tissue destruction to any wound caused through pressure.

It is now generally accepted that smoking has a detrimental affect on wound healing (Silverstein 1992; Frick and Seals 1994). Nicotine causes a number of local and systemic responses that inhibit the reparative process (Siana et al. 1992). It is a vasoconstrictor that reduces blood flow to the skin, resulting in a tissue ischaemia, impaired healing and increased platelet adhesiveness, which raises the risk of thrombotic microvascular occlusion and tissue ischaemia (Silverstein 1992). Smoking also lowers the skin temperature and, as Lock's (1979) research demonstrates, any lowering of wound temperature (by as little as two degrees) can halt mitotic activity by up to four hours. At the same time, lowering of temperature will deter leucocytes from the wound, opening the wound bed to potential clinical infection. It is, therefore, helpful if wound assessment includes information on whether the patient is a smoker and treatment includes advice and information on the effect smoking has on delayed healing.

It has been demonstrated in research that intravenous administration of nicotine (Siana et al. 1992):

1 stimulates the autonomous ganglia in low doses;
2 paralyses autonomous ganglia in high doses;
3 leads to vasoconstriction in the hands;
4 leads to a fall in skin temperature of limbs;
5 peripheral blood flow is lowered by 50 per cent for 60 minutes.

Eating and drinking

Large wounds require generous amounts of energy for collagen synthesis, cell replication and angiogenesis to occur (Collett 1994). Phagocytosis also requires energy and without available power for leucocytes to remove bacteria there is greater potential for infection to occur. Assessment of nutritional status may include blood tests for serum albumin levels as hypoproteinaemia leads to oedema and poor wound healing (Wells 1994).

Wound healing is also impaired by vitamin C or zinc deficiencies, as both are required for collagen synthesis. There is some evidence that excessive doses of vitamin C may improve healing (Taylor 1974). Although zinc supplements given to zinc deplete patients have been shown to increase healing rates (Cabak et al. 1963), supplements had little effect when given to patients who were not zinc deplete (Hallbrook and Lanner 1972). Dickerson (1993) writes 'Wounds may fail to heal satisfactorily owing to a general malnutrition as well as a lack of ascorbic acid.' (Nutrition is discussed in detail in Chapter 6.)

Excessive intake of alcohol can lead to anaemia, hypoproteinaemia and liver damage (Cutting 1994) and will delay tissue repair.

Eliminating

Constipation can be indicative of a poor diet and may lead to pain, reduced mobility and vomiting. This will reflect on wound healing and may well delay the healing process.

Incontinence of both faeces and urine may contaminate wounds, increase dressing changes and therefore, delay wound healing. Maceration of the peri-wound areas can occur when tissue is constantly exposed to excessive moisture causing the wound to enlarge.

Personal cleansing and dressing

Assessment of the wound and resultant wound dressing will take into account the personal needs and wishes of the patient. Dressings that show through or under clothes or wound dressings that allow leakage of exudate, can be embarrassing. Personal hygiene may be difficult unless the selected dressing is suitable for individual needs.

As a person ages, there are skin changes that occur. Collagen production is reduced, the skin becomes thinner and drier with a loss of underlying tissue. Washing or bathing with alkaline soap decreases the thickness and number of cell layers in the stratum corneum and excessive use of soap or detergents can interfere with the water-hold capacity of the skin and may lower bacterial resistance (Bryant 1992). Therefore, the patients' hygiene is best achieved with emollients or oils in the water and moisturizing lotions applied to the skin following washing will help to keep the skin moist. Use of talcum powders can clog the pores that produce sebum and may increase skin dryness. The powder can also become united in small clumps, causing soreness and is, therefore, best avoided.

Patients will often experience redness and soreness beneath breasts or in groins. There is a possibility that this may be due to candidiasis (thrush) and application of an antifungal cream (Canneston, Daktarin) will often support healing in these areas. Candidiasis enjoys any warm, dark and moist area in which to grow and it also enjoys the environment provided by antibiotics; hence there is always a possibility that it will occur in patients who are receiving antibiotic therapy. For simple maceration caused through perspiration, Cavilon or SuperSkin film can be painted on the area.

Patients who are not able to care for their own personal hygiene are usually washed and dressed by a carer or a nurse. This is an ideal time to examine skin and to assess the potential for future problems such as leg ulceration or diabetic foot ulceration. Excellence in assessment at this point, revealing potential problems, may well prevent years of misery in the future. A multidisciplinary approach that includes preventive foot care has been reported to reduce the amputation rate by 50 per cent (Apwlqvist 1998) and is, therefore, a prerequisite of assessment.

Controlling body temperature

As already mentioned, any drop in temperature below 37°C leads to a delay in mitosis of up to four hours (Lock 1979), and causes vaso-constriction; a drop in temperature of only two degrees is sufficient to reduce leucocyte activity to zero, thereby increasing the potential of infection (Torrance 1986). Pyrexia will also delay healing (Campbell 1995). Thermal disruption of the wound will be minimized by selection of dressings that can remain in place for several days thereby speeding healing (Torrance 1986). The future of wound healing will lead to warming wounds to promote healing (see Chapter 3).

Mobilizing

Immobilization increases risk of development of pressure sores (see Chapter 9) and, equally, will delay healing of any pre-exisiting pressure sores. Immobilization will also be responsible for a certain amount of haemostasis and can contribute to a lowered delivery of oxygen and nutrients to tissues, increasing the potential of clinical infection and a reduction in wound healing rates.

Working and playing

Dealey (1994a) writes on the fear and anxiety that can accompany a malignant fungating tumour along with the depression and isolation caused by the physical symptoms of the wound. Dealey also discusses the effects on daily activities when bulky dressings, heavy exudate and lymphoedema can make the patient feel isolated from a social life. As stress, caused by life changes, can create delayed wound healing, the patient needs to continue as normal a social and working life as possible and this is often impossible when bulky dressings, malodour or excessive leakage of a wound is apparent. To support the patient's own normal lifestyle it is important to address the problems that may alter that lifestyle.

Expressing sexuality

An important part of wound assessment would include psychological assessment as the position, sight and odour may reflect on body image and be distressing for the patient and/or partner. Dealey (1994a) writes 'A number of patients will deny the problem until it becomes impossible to hide and may see themselves as unclean and not want others to look at it.' Bulky dressings, bandages and malodour may all contribute to a low self-esteem and poor body image.

Sleeping

Studies of nocturnal animals have shown that cell proliferation and protein synthesis peak during the sleep period (Adam and Oswald 1983). Sleep deprivation in rats has certainly been shown to cause widespread deterioration in body tissues, even when food intake is increased (Torrance 1990). Beck et al. (1979) showed that sleep deprivation resulted in a higher secretion of growth hormone when sleep was resumed. Torrance (1990) also writes that 'promoting sleep becomes an essential element in the nursing management of a patient with a wound' and concludes 'it may be that some of the time, meticulous care and attention lavished on the wound would be more beneficial if directed toward the patient!' Therefore, it is beneficial for assessment to include problems of sleeping, working toward promotion of rest to enable restoration of the body's tissues.

Studies on rats have also shown that periods of white-band noise ranging from 2 kHz to 16 kHz reduced healing significantly ($p \leq 0.1$) and the treatment group's weight was lower than the control group ($p \leq 0.1$) although food intake did not vary between the two groups (Wysocki 1996a). In hospital, due to patient admissions, activity during the day and night and necessary medical interventions, there is a possibility that sleep deprivation and noise will occur. Therefore, wound healing may be effected during hospitalization. Conversely, Landis and Whitney (1997) studied sleep deprivation in rats to examine effects of sleep deprivation on cellular and biochemical markers of wound healing. Six rats were deprived of sleep for a 72 hours whilst six control rats remained on usual sleep/wake routines. There was no difference in the numbers of macrophages, granulocytes, fibroblasts, extent of connective tissue present, and total amounts of protein, DNA and hydroxyproline in the implants between sleep-deprived and control rats. Landis and Whitney concluded that there was no evidence from this study that sleep deprivation impairs cellular and biochemical indicators of tissue repair. The results of these two research projects demonstrates that the 'jury is still out' in the case of sleep deprivation and the relationship with reduced wound healing.

Research undertaken at the University of Pennsylvania, testing the effects of sleep deprivation on healthy men and women, found that the subjects have reduced lymphocyte counts and decreases in other immune system cells. This leads to the conclusion that sleep deprivation causes a depressed immune system and that increases the risk factor for clinical infection in wounds (Blakeslee 1993).

Dying

Assessment of a cachexic patient's wounds would require a different assessment criteria and treatment to that of the wound in a healthy patient. Treatment is often palliative rather than aggressive and control of symptoms has a higher importance than providing a healing environment. Pain, control of odour and exudate become the first consideration and removal of necrotic tissue becomes of low priority (unless it affects the systemic condition of the patient); removal of hard eschar can open a wound to clinical infection and often increased pain. It would then be appropriate to leave hard necrotic eschar without rehydration, thereby reducing the potential of infection and unpleasant symptoms.

Dying patients, at risk of pressure ulcer development, must be supplied appropriate pressure-relieving equipment such as dynamic air mattresses. Pressure is removed by these mattresses at regular intervals and the need for patient repositioning is reduced. Any repositioning should be for comfort and daily activities, not for the prevention of pressure sores. However, there will always be patients, who are extremely moribund with total system 'shut-down' and who will develop pressure ulcers even with the most rigorous care and the most expensive preventative equipment.

Wound assessment

Appearance

Black wounds are generally due to necrosis. These necrotic wounds are often filled with hard eschar (dehydrated dead tissue), which will delay healing and may cause septicaemia in the patient (Figure 2.3). Necrotic tissue requires removal in order to provide a healing environment. Debridement can be surgical, biosurgical (larvae therapy), chemical, enzymatic or through autolysis (rehydration of the devitalized tissues). Surgical (or sharp) debridement is the fastest method but requires an experienced practitioner or a surgeon to perform it. Chemical debridement can involve the use of harmful substances such as hypochlorites. Rehydration can be achieved through use of any of the hydrogel products (see Chapter 3), providing there is access for the gel to the lower structure of the tissues. This may be achieved by scoring the hard necrotic tissue.

Yellow wounds are a mixture of rehydrated necrotic tissue, dead bacteria, and dead leucocytes, often with fibrous tissue. This is known as slough (Figure 2.4). Removal of devitalized tissue in wounds is a natural process called autolysis, where tissue is rehydrated and lifts

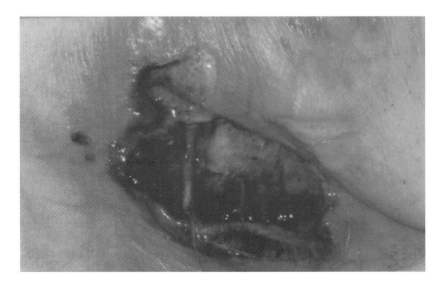

Figure 2.3 Black wound (see Plate 7).

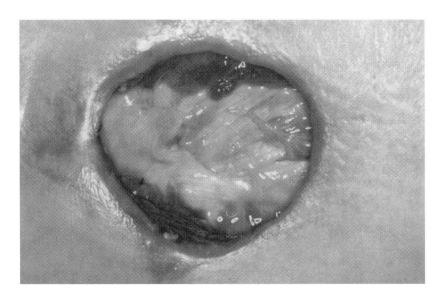

Figure 2.4 Yellow wound (see Plate 8).

free of the wound. Debris and bacteria are then removed through the action of macrophages and neutrophils. When a wound loses the ability to continue the healing process and becomes chronic, autolysis is reduced or ceases and the devitalized tissue remains in the wound bed as slough. Removal of slough is a natural process supported by dressings such as hydrogels. Yellow can also be a sign of newly devitalized tissue, as in Figure 2.5 where the patient was admitted after being found following several hours, unconscious, on the floor and shows the results of urine burns and pressure. This photograph was taken within one hour of admittance to the hospital.

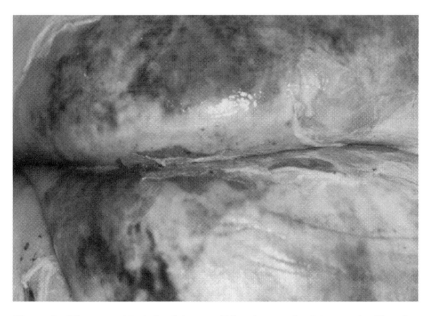

Figure 2.5 The areas of devitalized tissue and blistering can clearly be seen (see Plate 9).

Green wounds indicate the presence of bacteria, particularly *Pseudomonas* (Figure 2.6), which develop into a bright green colour and have a malodorous wound discharge. However, green is not always a sign of clinical infection as bacteria can often colonize a wound without harming the host (Collier 1994b; Flanagan 1997). Nevertheless, some pathogenic organisms may be responsible for delayed healing. Figure 2.6 also shows clinical signs of infection with red friable tissue around the devitalized and green tissue. The colours of discharge from infected wounds can vary according to the invading bacteria and may be yellow, green sludge, red/brown or grey in colour.

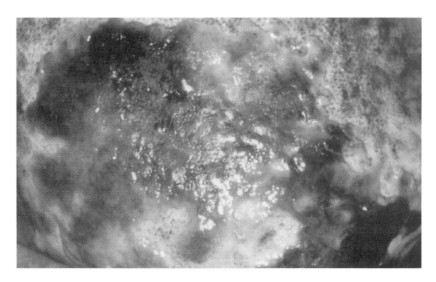

Figure 2.6 A green wound, indicating *Pseudomonas* colonization (see Plate 10).

Red wounds are formed of granulation tissue that is deep pink/red and moist (Figure 2.7). The granular appearance of the wound is the result of the collagen matrix being produced in the wound bed providing a framework for loops of capillaries to force their way through the matrix, producing granule-like lumps. These

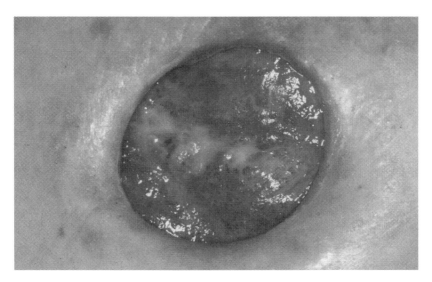

Figure 2.7 A red wound, showing signs of granulation (see Plate 11).

delicate, fragile loops of capillaries are easily damaged and require the least handling possible. It is therefore, important that dressing changes are kept to the minimum and cleansing with water is avoided if possible. This wound is a healthy healing wound and maintaining the optimum wound healing environment is essential, and, unless there is debris to clean out of this wound, cleansing is unnecessary and may be harmful (Hohn et al. 1977). Granulation tissue that becomes 'proud' of the wound is known as overgranulation. Treatment of overgranulation would be application of:

- foam dressings;
- transorb;
- one hydrocolloid dressing placed on top of another and pressed into place;
- a hydrocolloid with a gauze pressure pad over the top to increase pressure;
- double dispersion therapy dressing;
- silver nitrate pencil.

Epithelial tissue cannot migrate across the surface when the granulation tissue extends beyond the surface (overgranulation).

Care should be taken when assessing a red wound as a beefy red, friable wound that is without the noticeable 'granules' of granulation tissue could easily be demonstrating a streptococci clinical infection. The redness may be confusing to the inexperienced eye.

Pink tissue (can be mauve in appearance) is newly forming epithelial tissue which migrates from the edges of the wound and from undamaged hair follicles and moves over the wound surface once the granulation is level with surrounding skin. This requires a moist environment (Winter 1962). Figure 2.8 shows epithelial tissue at the wound margins. The appearance of this tissue along with the clean and granulating appearance of the wound informs the practitioner that this wound is healing successfully.

Assessing wound size

Measurement of a wound has an important place in wound management; without baseline and ongoing wound measurements it is impossible to achieve an objective approach to management and treatment of the wound and to establish the progress of healing. However,

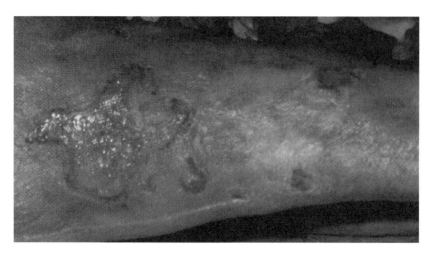

Figure 2.8 An epithelializing wound (see Plate 12).

wounds are three-dimensional structures and require simple methods of calculating the volume of the cavity, which should be achievable by the nurse on the ward or community nurse in the patient's home. Several methods may be used to obtain measurements.

Disposable measures can be used to assess the size of the wound. These can be obtained from manufacturers of some dressings but, as there is not an infinite supply, continued requests may not be supported. An ordinary ruler may be used but should be sterilized after use.

Acetate wound-maps are a useful tool as they are easily compared with earlier maps and changes in the size of the wound are instantly seen. However, unless double acetates are used, the side placed on the wound can become contaminated and difficult to clean. There is also a problem of actually seeing the wound through the acetate as the film mists as soon as it is placed on the warm wound. Two practitioners, asked to outline the same wound, would be unlikely to outline the wound so that the edges of the two assessments match accurately. Nevertheless, this is one of the most useful forms of comparative evaluation. Acetates produced for overhead projector presentations can be used for wound mapping and can be cut in half and placed double on the wound so that the top acetate can be used and the lower, contaminated acetate can be thrown away. This method will not allow the planimetry form of assessing the size of the wound by counting the squares that can be found in the manufacturer-produced wound-mapping systems. Although none of these methods is sterile, bacteria would find it difficult to cling to the surface of the film and, if it is kept clean in a polythene bag, there is little risk of contaminating the wound. Some companies producing film dressings, provide a wound-mapping system as part of the dressing wrapper. However, this can only be utilized if the film dressing is to be used.

Polythene bags are a useful tool for mapping wounds. The polythene is unlikely to become contaminated as bacteria cannot adhere to the smooth surface of the polythene. If the practitioner is concerned, the bag can be turned inside out and then, once the map has been completed, the bag can either be reversed, trapping the 'dirty' side within the bag, or the 'dirty' part of the bag can be cut away. However, this method can look a little 'Heath Robinson' or unprofessional to the patient.

Normal saline can be injected under an adherent film dressing. Once the cavity has been filled, the fluid can be withdrawn and the amount measured and this is probably the most accurate, achievable and inexpensive method of wound measurement for the assessing nurse. However, sacral wounds would be difficult to measure because it would involve the patient being face down and the elderly patients are often unable to reach this position. Nevertheless, dressing removal can cause some discomfort following the measurement and is not advisable in patients with fragile skin. Withdrawal of the saline for measurement can also be painful for the patient.

Dental alginate can be easily placed into the wound to give a three-dimensional view of the cavity. This forms a model of the wound that can be measured, weighed or placed in water to assess the water displacement. This only has uses in research. (This conjures up the mental vision of hundreds of dental alginate moulds, the results of hundreds of wound assessments, sitting on sister's office shelf.)

A wound probe can be placed into the wound cavity and then the depth measured. Useful probes can be a swab, a gloved finger or the probe supplied as part of an alginate ribbon pack (Sorbsan). It should be noted that if the alginate probe is used, it is the rounded end that is placed in the wound. A wound probe is a useful way of discovering the direction and depth of sinus tracts. Reapplication of a probe at each dressing change, will indicate the healing status of the tract.

A sterile 2 ml syringe can be used as a probe and the markers on the syringe used as a comparative tool. However, this is a hard surface, which could easily damage a fragile wound and, therefore, should not be used in a granulating wound.

Photographs taken weekly can be very useful. However, unless a polaroid camera is used, the photograph remains in the camera until the film is complete and this could be even as long as several months. Unfortunately, polaroid pictures do not always provide an ideal picture as the colours of the wound are not always accurately represented by the picture development process. Comparisons are often difficult because it depends greatly on the distance that the camera operator is from the wound (close and the wound will look large, far away and it will appear smaller in the photograph). A linear measure placed on the wound will give a fairly accurate planimetry measurement.

There are new methods being developed as part of photography and wound measurements, including lasers that inform the camera of the distance required from the wound to obtain accurate measurements and new computer programs that will actually measure depth as well as width of wounds. Digital cameras may be the future of assessment as the pictures can be placed directly onto the patient's notes on computer, providing a permanent record of changes. Photographs still remain the principal and favoured assessment tool of those specializing in wound care.

One computer program (BES Rehab) involves placing a small square next to the wound. The picture is then scanned onto the computer and the program can work out the size of the wound from the small square (Figure 2.9). The volume measurement is also achievable with this programme. However, it is an expensive method of measurement and is time consuming. It is unlikely to be used in common practice but will be very useful in research or studies, giving increasingly accurate measurements.

Ultrasonic surface measurements or the use of structured light instruments, are likely to be used only for research unless the future holds a simplified form of producing these measuring devices.

Cavity wounds

There are many ways that cavity wounds will form, for example:

- following surgery when the wound dehisces;
- traumatic injuries;
- pressure damage (often leading to undermining);
- surgical wounds laid open (e.g. pilonidal sinus).

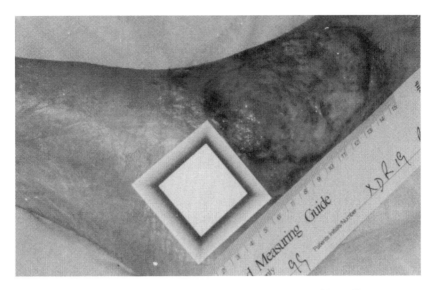

Figure 2.9 Computer tool for measuring wound dimensions (see Plate 13).

These wounds can be treated or managed as follows:

- remove devitalized tissues;
- remove causative factor (i.e. replace high-pressure mattress with pressure-relieving/redistributing mattress);
- review nutritional status;
- assess wound and prescribe dressings and care.

Assessment of pain

Pain is the result of a complex sequence of physiological and psychological events with the release of histamine and prostaglandin playing a large role in the painful outcome. There are different types of fibres and pain receptors: each receptor acts at differing speeds of conduction leading to dissimilar experiences of pain sensation. Burning pain may be the result of polymodal C fibre nociceptor stimulation and pricking pain due to stimulation of Aδ nociceptors.

Melzack and Wall (1984) suggested the 'gate theory' where it was postulated that the potential of large diameter afferents and small diameter afferents are different. The relative amounts of neural activity received by these different neurones, determines the output to higher brain centres. The smaller diameter afferents can increase the perceived pain. However, if activity in the larger diameter afferents is increased, perceived pain is decreased. Therefore, an increase in activity in the larger afferents can 'close the gate' and reduce pain. The use of transcutaneous electrical nerve stimulation (TENS) applies this theory in practice through stimulation of the larger diameter afferents. This explanation gives credence to the 'old wives'' method of dealing with pain: if a child falls and hurts their knee and mother rubs or kisses it better, the pain appears to abate. However, TENS has a greater success rate in reducing neurological pain and may not be of value in painful wounds.

Pain is often ignored in wound healing or passed over as a symptom of the type of wound involved. The result is often erroneous beliefs such as 'venous leg ulcers are never painful' or 'arterial leg ulcers are only painful when the leg is elevated'.

Wounds are often painful for a variety of reasons:

- Leg dependency in venous ulceration may cause pain because hydrostatic pressure increases, the leg becomes increasingly oedematous and potential for pain increases.

Conversely, leg elevation in venous ulceration may increase pain as in the case of the lady in Figure 2.10 when her pain became unbearable at 2am every morning. Suicide was a very real consideration in this case. The treatment of leg elevation and compression also

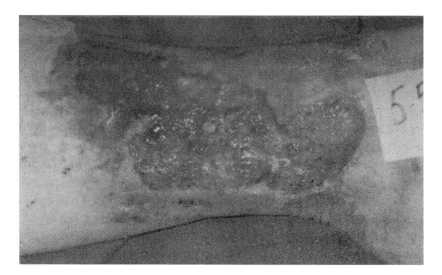

Figure 2.10 Venous ulcers heal faster if legs are elevated.

increased the pain but the use of analgesics as a method of pain control allowed the treatment to continue.

- Ischaemic pain is either acute or chronic and can be incredibly painful. Ischaemia can be a result of intermittent claudication, poor blood delivery in the large arteries or small arterioles or due to unrelieved pressure. Ischaemia can become increasingly painful when the leg is elevated, because blood supply to the feet will be decreased, and can lead to arterial ulcers, which are very painful and difficult to heal. However, some arterial ulcers are not painful and others may increase in pain when legs are dependent. Ischaemia can lead to vasculitic ulceration in patients with rheumatoid arthritis or to foot ulcers in diabetic patients.
- Some ulceration may be due to vasculitis when the blood supply is not reaching the dermis. The pain from vasculitis has been described as 11 on a scale of 1–10 with 10 as the 'worst pain you could suffer'.
- Wounds may be painful because the wound bed is exerting pressure on the wound margins, causing pain in the nerve supply surrounding the wound.
- Dressings can also increase pain in wounds, particularly when a hydrophilic dressing is applied. Alginates, sugar paste, foams, dispersion technology can all increase pain in an already dry and painful wound. A moist dressing would 'bathe' nerve endings to reduce pain. Removal of dressings may cause pain, particularly if the dressing adheres to the wound.
- Soaking wounds in water for a long period may increase pain as osmosis permits the water to be taken on by the cells within the wound. The cells may burst due to the increased pressure of water and this can cause pain and may increase wound size if left unchecked.
- Some bacteria may cause wounds to feel painful. *Pseudomonas aeruginosa* is a difficult pathogen to treat because antibiotics are largely ineffective and the bacterium can be responsible for many deaths in hospitalized patients (Hancock 1997). It can also be the cause of pain as clinical infection will nearly always increase wound pain.
- Atrophy blanche, a particularly painful dermal condition associated with venous ulceration, can be seen as white patches around the ankle and calf (see Chapter 5).

Patients who identify pain related to leg ulcers, when questioned, may report that the pain is in the ulcer, around the ulcer or elsewhere in the leg and, in actual fact, not always related to the ulcer. Leg ulcer pain that is described as 'burning' usually responds well to non-steroidal anti-inflammatory drugs (Emflorgo 1999), although it should be remembered that non-steroidal anti-inflammatory drugs can limit the production of prostaglandins which, in turn, will effect wound healing. If the pain is described as 'throbbing', the patient may require opiates and 'tingling', smarting or 'stinging' pain may require anti-epileptic drugs (Emflorgo 1999). Dressing removal that is painful may require nitrous oxide and oxygen to allow painless dressing changes.

Pain in pressure sores is usually at its height when the sore is grade 1 to grade 2 (EPUAP 2001). When the dermis is lost and muscle is involved it is less likely to be painful and grade 4 (EPUAP 2001) is rarely painful because all nerve tissue has gone. However, these ulcers can be painful if the surrounding viable tissue is involved, either through continued pressure or through dressings or procedures 'pulling' on the peri-wound area.

It is important that any wound assessment includes a tool for assessing pain. A pain visual analogue scale of '1 equals no pain and 5 (or 10) equals worst pain ever' can usually be recognized and used by patients, allowing the assessor to identify alterations in the level of pain. This will lead to optimum selection and evaluation of dressings' performance in reducing pain.

Pain has a physiological response that causes vasoconstriction, reducing blood delivery to the wound bed, increasing pain and delaying wound healing. Therefore, analgesia must be the second consideration and dressings the first consideration in reducing wound pain; in other words, use a dressing that will 'bathe' the painful nerve endings such as hydrocolloids, film dressings or hydrogels. 'Dry' dressings such as alginates, foams and cadexomer pastes, and osmotic dressings such as sugar paste, may increase pain initially when the 'pull' of the new dressing causes the nerve endings to be stimulated. Generally, this initial pain will decrease within half an hour when the dressing becomes moistened.

Substances released following injury (alogens) are associated with both pain and inflammation, and include bradykinin histamine and serotonin (Rice 1994). Prostaglandins are also released during injury and one of the factors related to their production is increased sensation of pain. The effect on pain can be reduced through the use of analgesia that reduces production of prostaglandins (NSAIDs, aspirin, etc.). However, as prostaglandins are promoters of the inflammatory process and influence cell activity by acting as messengers between cells, any reduction in their production can have an adverse effect on healing.

Haines et al. (1997) suggest that chronic pain is a major health problem and produces many demands on health-care resources. Pain has also been a major problem for a long time and, apart from analgesia, wound pain is poorly addressed. Many patients will refuse analgesia because they are concerned about side effects such as feeling less in control. Moist dressings may reduce pain by 'bathing' raw nerve endings. However, to date, there is no dressing available that is designed to deal with wound pain and the chemicals that may assist (lignocaine, etc.) are, unfortunately, not licensed for wound care.

The single most important aspect of pain control is to identify the causative factor and rapid, multidimensional treatment is urgent and vital.

Assessment of factitious wounds

Some patients can be identified as being responsible for the production of their wound or for the failure of a wound to heal, whilst denying the responsibility. This is known as a factitious wound and can be found in patients with an underlying psychological problem. Simple interference with the wound may be enough to prevent healing. However, there is also a potential for patients to inject themselves with substances (such as household cleaning agents) that may result in sterile or infected abscesses. The cause of these are difficult to identify because of the fineness of the needle when the substances are injected.

Factitious wounds are more commonly found in adolescent females who are psychologically immature and have difficulty with personal relationships (Young 2000). Patients, with a considered factitious wound, will need to confront the responsibility of causing the wound (Baragwanath 1994) and this requires the assistance of a professional psychotherapist.

Unfortunately, there is a potential for the young adolescent female to be labelled as self-harming simply because of youth. For example, one young girl was treated for factitious wounds for nearly a year, and accused many times of creating the wounds. It was eventually discovered that she had an immunological problem and the abscesses were formed merely through daily living, when gentle knocks caused slight bruising which deteriorated to sterile abscesses.

Assessment of burns

Until the middle of this century, large burns nearly always had a fatal outcome due to loss of fluid (Settle 1986). Assessment, in the case of large burns, can be life saving:

- Ensure the airway is clear. In severe burns there may be smoke, steam, chemical or flame inhalation and the patient may require emergency endotracheal intubation or emergency tracheotomy.
- Clean the skin of any corrosive chemicals by flushing with water (Settle 1986).
- Replace fluid loss with fluid drip. A fluid replacement requirement relies largely on the extent of the tissue damage and the size of the patient.
- Provide analgesia.

Burns that can be assessed by using the 'rule of nines' to decide the percentage of burns: 9 per cent for each arm, 9 per cent for the head, 18 per cent for each leg, 18 per cent for back of trunk and 18 per cent for front of trunk. Assessment of the depth and severity of the wound may be difficult when the patient is first admitted as the wound will change and develop according to the type of burn. There may be blanched areas due to necrosis and these areas are likely to be quite deep.

The weight of the patient is part of a useful assessment as it would help to determine fluid loss that occurs with large area tissue loss. There are specialist beds that weigh the patient and these are particularly useful when there is difficulty in movement due to pain. Large air fluidized beds support the patient on air and can offer greater comfort to the burn patient.

Depth of the burn is classified as:

- 1st degree burn a superficial layer of skin is affected.
- 2nd degree burn the deep dermis is involved.
- 3rd degree burn is a full thickness burn.

If a deep burn is less than 30 per cent of the total body surface area, excision followed by skin grafting is usually possible (Arturson 1993). If the injury covers a greater area than 30 per cent of the total body surface, or if an associated illness is present, skin grafting is likely to be delayed thereby extending recovery and hospitalization.

Oedema occurs due to:

- vasodilation caused by release of histamine;
- increased extra-vascular osmotic activity pulling fluid into the interstitial spaces;
- increase in microvascular permeability;
- release of mediators from leucocyte infiltration (Petch 1993).

Reduction of heat on the affected area is important. Application of cold water is vastly more important than the removal of clothes, particularly as precious moments can be lost in removing the garments (Petch 1993). Cooling the skin reduces pain and should be continued. However, practitioners should be aware that, in small children, this can result in hypothermia.

Dressings for burns should be non-adherent, highly absorbent and should prevent access of bacteria. The most effective and useful dressings would be non-adherent, could remain on the skin for long periods and would support the use of a secondary dressings that can be changed when required. Mepital, Omiderm, Tegapor and Telfa are dressings that would fit these criteria, allowing fluid to pass through the layer into Gamgee that can be applied as the secondary dressing. The Gamgee can be replaced as often as necessary and the primary dressing can stay *in situ* for as long as required, reducing pain on dressing changes. Paraffin gauze dressings are a popular choice but can adhere to the wound causing pain on removal (Lawrence 1989) (see Chapter 3).

Film dressings, and polythene bags etc can be useful in reducing pain (cling film is particularly useful as a temporary dressing when a wound is new) and creams such as silver sulphadiazine can be applied under the film to reduce colonization and soothe. However, it should be remembered that silver sulphadiazine cream can dissolve some polythene.

Compression garments are ideal for prevention of uneven scarring and silicone gel pads (e.g. Cica-Care) will prevent keloid scars.

Tapeless (Mediplus) products are particularly useful for securing the dressings without adhesive tapes.

Burns over joints and flexor surfaces are prone to contracture, so particular care must be exercised (Lawrence 1989). De-roofing blisters may be harmful and can open the wound to clinical infection. The fluid can be withdrawn using a fine needle. Larger blisters, involving necrotic tissue, must be debrided. However, patients with large burns, requiring hospitalization, are very likely to be admitted to specialist units with expertise in caring for extensive burns.

Foot assessment

The condition of the feet can provide an enormous amount of information about the patient. Foot ulceration should lead to blood glucose tests to ensure the patient is not diabetic. Nails that are flaky and misshapen are possibly a fungal infection and require the attentions of a podiatrist. Small sore areas between the toes may be fungal infections and require treatment with antifungal cream or powder. Charcot joint would lead to glucose tests, X-rays to establish the condition of the joint and a plan for protecting the joint from ulceration. Any ulceration, particularly in the diabetic patient, could have covert tracking which could travel as deep as to bone. If this is the case, there is a potential for osteomylitis. Thick and flaky skin is possibly due to lack of cleansing. Soaking in a bucket or bowl (lined with a clean polythene bag) of tap water and an emollient will clean and moisturize the skin.

Assessment of factors that delay healing

Maceration

Maceration continues to be a difficulty in wound healing and few studies have addressed the problem (Hampton 1997a, 1998b). Wound exudate and 'wet' dressings such as hydrogels, can exacerbate the problem. When assessment indicates that a 'wet' dressing is required to facilitate wound healing, should this decision be reversed when maceration occurs? The treatment of the wound should be appropriate and if this is changed to an inappropriate dressing to suit the peri-wound area then deterioration in the wound could be expected.

Maceration occurs when the tissues are kept over-moist for long periods of time. The cells become 'waterlogged', softened, fragile and easily damaged (Figure 2.11) and this can lead to excoriation. The tissues have the appearance of white or pink, softened skin. There are significant differences in structure and characteristics of skin of various people of all ages. Skin that is oily, dry, moist, papery or normal will react differently to any mechanical insult applied to it. Therefore, patients' wounds may be treated in identical ways with one having a successful outcome and another's healing delayed by complications. Maceration is one of the complications that can occur, caused possibly by a wet discharge from the wound or wound dressing such as hydrocolloids or hydrogels, which moisten the viable tissue surrounding the wound. Tissues softened in this way become easily damaged and have the potential for grazing to occur, offering an entry for infection. Maceration can occur around a wound or stoma or can be a direct result of faecal or urinary incontinence. Injury caused to tissues from faecal fluid incontinence is particularly difficult to treat as dressings may constantly require removal following each bout of diarrhoea, the nature of the fluid increases risk of contamination and the continual insult to the tissues causes damage. Maceration can delay or increase the size of the wound and should be prevented where possible. Protection with creams, lotions or painless liquid film dressings (see Chapter 3) are vital.

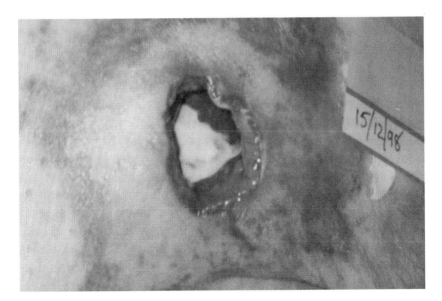

Figure 2.11 Tissue maceration (see Plate 14).

Dressing suitability

All dry dressings have the ability to adhere to a low exudating wound. It is important to assess the wound for the potential of adherence prior to selecting the dressing. If it is suspected that adherence may occur, a film dressing over the primary dressing will reduce the potential. However, the primary dressing should be of high absorbency to prevent leakage of the dressings. Any dressing that sticks to an individual wound should not be used on that same wound again as newly forming tissues may well be torn when the dressing is removed.

However, the vacuum-assisted closure (VAC) (see Chapter 3) will almost always leave a wound bed bleeding following removal of the sponge and this does not appear to delay healing.

Excoriation

Excoriation over peri-wound areas can be caused by:

- aggressive removal of tapes from fragile skin;
- irritation from exudate and wet dressings;
- sensitivity to dressings;
- friction from the dressings or from changing position and dragging the skin.

Excoriation may be defined as an area of skin that is superficially broken in multiple places and has inflammation present.

Exudate

Exudate is a shared problem between nurse and patient. It is particularly problematic when the peri-wound areas deteriorate because of exudate 'over-spill'. It is important to understand exudate so that treatment for the wound and peri-wound area is appropriate (see Chapter 1).

Wound exudate is a generic term given to fluid produced from chronic wounds, fistulae or acute injuries once haemostasis has been achieved (Thomas 1997b). Exudate is blood from which red cells and platelets have been filtered out as it passes through the walls of capillaries (Thomas 1997b). The vessel walls dilate in injury due to the production of histamine and exudate increases. However, bacteria can also influence the production of exudate by causing an increase in capillary permeability. There are several other factors involved in production of exudate (Thomas 1997b):

- hydrostatic pressure;
- wound infection;
- wound colonization;
- temperature;
- wound type;
- type of dressing.

Exudate in a wound can be an excellent indicator of what is happening within the wound and is, therefore, valuable to assessment. The volume, consistency, and particularly odour and colour will inform the practitioner of bacterial contamination, infection (see Chapter 4) and stage of healing. The optimal level of wound exudate required to facilitate healing has not yet been determined (Cutting 1999). It remains unclear whether moisture is actually a prerequisite to wound healing as Winter's work (1962) on the moist wound was performed on epithelializing tissue, not on a full thickness, highly exuding wound. Indeed, there has never been a definition to qualify a moist wound and there is little information available on how much fluid should be in the wound bed to be able to call the wound moist. It may well be that the fluid produced, moment by moment, within the wound bed and soaked into the dressing, is sufficient to promote wound healing and the term 'dry dressing' may be a misnomer when this fluid exchange is constantly occurring.

Exudate is thought to have many purposes and effects:

- metalloproteinases found in exudate break down collagens and help to remodel the extracellular matrix in healing (Vickery 1997);
- a moist wound environment promotes healing (Winter 1962);
- fibroblasts grow faster in exudate (Vickery 1997);
- exudate contains growth factors that promote tissue regeneration (Kreig and Eming 1997);
- exudate facilitates the migration of cells involved in tissue repair;
- exudate acts as a transport medium for white cells;
- Staphylococci easily replicate in exudate (Vickery 1997);
- high exudate production can equal low serum proteins;

- patients may consider exudate 'dirty' or the odour may be offensive and it may limit social life;
- exudate requires a large amount of nurses' time for changing dressings;
- exudate is associated with maceration of skin (Kreig and Eming 1997);
- bacteria in the exudate can be proteolytic, which delays healing and damages peri-wound areas;
- exudate assists in the process of autolysis (Dealey 1997);
- exudate contains neutrophils and is, therefore, anti-bacterial in nature.

Potential problems caused by exudate include:

- exacerbation of skin damage through irritation (Cameron and Powell 1996);
- bacteria can have proteolytic enzymes which delay healing and damage peri-wound areas (Phillips et al. 1998);
- copious exudate requires a large amount of nurses' time in changing dressings;
- high exudate production can equal low serum proteins;
- Staphylococci easily replicate in exudate (Vickery 1997).

The colour of exudate is altered by the presence of chemicals or bacteria such as *Pseudomonas aeruginosa*, which produces a pigment that turns the exudate bright green (Thomas 1997a). At the same time, bacterial by-products (proteolytic enzymes) and dead white cells increase the viscosity of exudate and create a characteristic odour (Bowler et al. 1999) that causes distress for both patient and carer. For instance, *Pseudomonas aeruginosa* creates a strong, sweet, musty odour that can be detected by others even when the sufferer is not in close proximity. The presence of large numbers of bacteria can increase capillary permeability thereby increasing exudate production. Therefore, bacteria may be largely responsible for copious, malodorous exudate found in colonized wounds (Thomas 1997a).

Phillips et al. (1998) reported that chronic wound fluid has a negative effect on wound healing, which is thought to be due to the selective effect it has on fast-proliferating stem-cell-like fibroblasts. It follows that removal or reduction of exudate would potentially increase healing rates by removal of the negative effect on fibroblast activity. Therefore, observation of the wound should involve information on the changing status of wound exudate.

Assessment and communication

Working in a multidisciplinary team

Involvement of the multidisciplinary team in assessment and treatment is prerequisite. Nutrition, mobility, infection and treatment require knowledge and experience of all those involved in patient care. Figure 2.12 shows a laser being used by a physiotherapist to successfully treat the wound. This wound healed well following assessment, provision of a pressure-redistributing air mattress, treatment for pain, sharp debridement of the devitalized tissue, administration of antibiotics, liaison with the dietician and end-stage laser treatment by the physiotherapist. Healing time was 10 weeks from admittance to hospital to discharge of the patient with a healed wound.

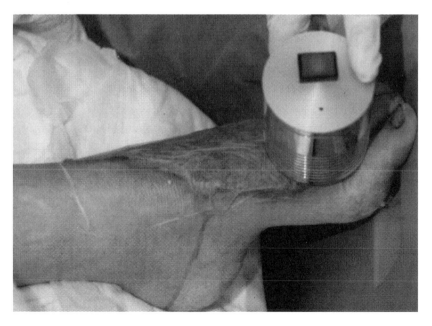

Figure 2.12 Laser treatment.

Quality of life

The patient's quality of life can be easily affected by the development of a wound. It is rarely the wound itself that is the problem, but pain, exudate, malodour and finally scarring can have a huge impact on socialization and body image. Quality of life can also be effected conversely when a wound is healing and the patient sees that they may soon lose a valuable outside contact when the wound heals and the nurse is no longer required to visit. Assessment should include the physiological and psychological effects on the patient's quality of life. These issues should then be addressed and evaluated to ensure a successful conclusion.

Optimal wound care management can improve mobilization and quality of life by promoting wound healing, reducing discomfort, pain, leakage and malodour from dressings, enabling the patient to continue personal relationships and social/leisure activities (Wollina 1997).

Some quality of life issues may effect wound healing. For instance, the patient who enjoys smoking may be reluctant to give up, even though aware that not giving up may have dire consequences on wound healing, potentially leading to amputation. This patient would see giving up smoking as a reduction in quality of life.

When being cared for, patients are often placed in the 'patient role' and there is a potential for them to feel 'out of control' with doctors and/or nurses 'in control'. This may cause a resentment and/or non-concordance with treatment and may lead to poor outcomes in healing and feelings of low self-worth. To promote a feeling of being 'in control' the patient (and possibly their loved ones) should be involved in all decisions of wound care. If they are unhappy with a therapy, the consequences should be explained, the regimen withdrawn and replaced with a more acceptable treatment. The nurse or doctor does not have the right to impose treatment on a patient as in the following case of Miss X.

Miss X is a lady of 72 years, living in a warden-assisted flat. She is a bright and intelligent lady with a previously active social life (prior to leg ulceration). Dopplers were performed by the vascular surgeon and treatment of short-stretch compression bandages were prescribed. Miss X is visited, twice weekly, by district nurses, a G-grade sister, two staff nurses and, sometimes, a bank nurse.

As soon as Miss X has identified the day's visiting nurse, she is able to say whether she will be in pain for several days, will be comfortable or will have a copiously oozing leg ulcer. Each nurse bandages the leg with different sub-bandage compression and there are also differences in the amount of padding that is placed under the bandage. One nurse bandages so tightly that Miss X knows she will be in discomfort for four days. The nurse refuses to listen when Miss X asks for the bandage to be slightly looser as 'The bandage must be tight or it will not work'. The nurse has never appreciated that she is wasting her time as the patient will quickly loosen the bandage when the nurse leaves the flat. Before she loosens the bandage, Miss X is often distressed and often cries. When the G-grade sister bandages the leg, Miss X knows that she will be comfortable for the next four days.

In such cases, it would be important to listen to the patient, to explain the consequences of lower sub-bandage pressures, but to comply with the patient's wishes. If this is not acted on, the quality of the patient's life may well be affected – as in the case of Miss X, and the nurse may well be puzzled with the lack of healing when the patient interferes with the bandage.

Documentation guidelines

Documentation of the future will be easier to achieve with increased guidelines and integrated care pathways to follow rather than writing reams of care plans. Nevertheless, the practitioner following those guidelines will require a deeper knowledge of wound healing to be able to place the wound treatment on the correct pathway. Photographs will become an increasingly important way of demonstrating wound changes. The introduction of digital cameras will provide a permanent record of changes.

Critical care pathways

The future of documentation and assessment will almost certainly lie with 'critical care pathways', which detail the anticipated flow of

care for the patient with a specific diagnosis and involve a multidisciplinary approach. The care pathway document is pre-printed and is
used by each member of the team who ticks or signs for interventions. Care pathways will reduce the amount of paperwork
commonly experienced by nurses, will unite the care given by all
members of the team and will use resources more efficiently. Care
pathways have the potential to reduce hospital stay and to offer
uniformity of care universally as each hospital could use the same
care pathway.

Wound healing is a complex process and involves critical thinking
skills to identify the causes of individual wounds and to make decisions on treatment. Evaluation of underlying pathology and of
outcomes in wound healing will lead practitioners to care for the
wound in the most appropriate way and will inform and support
other practitioners caring for the same wound. In a court of law, if
the care is not documented, it is not thought to have been given. In
the modern climate of litigation (see Chapter 12), documentation is
the practitioner's own protective armour and it is important that the
armour is applied daily. Documenting care need not involve reams
of paper and hours of time. A simple tick-box system, or integrated
care pathways, and a signature may suffice to say that the care has
been given. Prescription of care is a little more complex, however.
Core care plans do not always allow the individualization of holistic
care and, therefore, it may be necessary to spend time writing or
typing on the computer to enable the next practitioner to follow the
prescribed care.

Today we have a better understanding of wound healing and the
requirements of an optimal wound healing environment. We know that
exposure of the wound will drop the temperature, delay mitotic activity
and increase the possibility of clinical infection. Wounds are now left for
as long as possible without being disturbed. However, when planning
care, it is difficult to provide accurate plans on how often the dressing
should be changed. Each wound is individual and the dressing must be
changed when necessary. The wound condition will largely dictate its
own needs with 'strike-through' of exudate when the dressing requires
changing. Documentation of recommendations and changes in wound
condition is vital for continuation of quality care.

Conclusion

Warmth and non-adherence are important in granulating wounds, and, if the wound is healing, the dressing should only be changed when necessary. Weekly is ideal in some instances, e.g. with paste bandages. Other dressings are probably best changed every 3–4 days. Nevertheless, there are anecdotal instances of tramps, having wounds dressed and then not returning for the wound to be redressed for weeks. The wounds are usually without problems and have healed fairly well in the time. Doctors and nurses, traditionally, used observation as the finest form of assessment (Bryant 1992). Therefore, documentation of each wound must be individual to that wound.

Use of a holistic model of assessment when evaluating wounds can help to focus attention on the intrinsic and extrinsic factors that can delay healing and, where possible, problems corrected so that consideration can then be given to assessment of the wound and to dressing selection.

The development of chronic wounds, and the failure to heal, is multifactorial. Therefore, treatment of chronic wounds relies on an excellent and knowledgeable assessment with treatment directed toward correcting contributing factors. Examination of the wound and choice of an appropriate dressing is the final (and possibly the least important) component leading to provision of an optimum wound healing environment.

Activity

Select a patient with a chronic wound; assess using the activities of daily living (Roper et al. 1985) as set out above. Identify and address the problems related to wound healing delay. Write a 500 word evaluation of the effect the interventions have made and what has been learned from the exercise. This can be used for the professional profile folder.

CHAPTER 3
Dressings and treatments

Nurses play a vital role in wound healing as they hold responsibility for monitoring surgical and chronic wounds, setting standards in wound management and giving hands-on care. However, although nurses stand on the threshold of a new era in wound care, with treatments becoming increasingly scientific, not all nurses have followed developments and may miss the opportunity to be knowledgeable or leaders in wound care. An overwhelming variety of dressing choices can only add to potential confusion. O'Connor (1993) found that there is a gap between theory and practice, with a lack of sound in-depth knowledge among nurses. Practice is often based on tradition and there are difficulties in applying knowledge to practice. However, changing wound care practice is often difficult and the enthusiasm of some nurses may not always lead to quality care; Flanagan (1992b) found that nurses often have problems selecting appropriate care due to the resistance of some colleagues to change rather than a lack of knowledge. Emmott (1992) found that nurses had great difficulty in associating wound non-healing with the patients' other physical problems and this was also the experience of Wilkes et al. (1996) in Australia.

Bryant (1992) writes, 'Nursing interventions can either enhance or delay wound-healing; thus nurses must be knowledgeable regarding the wound-healing process and the implications for wound management'. No longer can professionals select wound dressings on personal preference; nor will the future relationship between suppliers and nurses or purchasers be able to influence the purchase of dressings (Rainey 1996). The advent of clinical governance will ensure that dressing selection is founded on research-based principles and care will not be given unless evidence based. However, Bryant (1992) also writes, 'The longer and more intently one cares for wounds, the more complex the concept "wound" becomes'. This statement is very true. Wound care knowledge is a 'bottomless pit' and the deeper one goes in learning the concepts, the more one realizes how much there is to learn. Therefore, there may be some justification for those practitioners, GPs and nurses, deciding on a dressing as a 'favourite' and remaining faithful to that one dressing for every wound. Nevertheless, in the future, there will be no justifiable circumstances where that can happen; wounds must be treated, not managed!

Wounds have historically been treated by bizarre methods. Lizard's dung, pigeon's blood, cobwebs, boiling oil and hot irons are a few of the oddest treatments (Bibbings 1986). In AD129–200, Galen considered pus 'laudable' (Naylor 1999), and for many centuries it was considered efficacious for a wound to produce pus; those wounds that remained clean would have pus (from another's wound) introduced to stimulate production. Today, there is an increase in the scientific approach to healing with 'old' treatments now rationalized and shown effective before they are used (larvae therapy, sugar, leeches, tea tree oil, etc.). However, the oddest dressings, still in use today, are hypochlorite solutions (Edinburgh Solution of Lime (EUSOL) and Milton), which are essentially toilet cleaner solutions (these are discussed later in this chapter).

There are abundant dressings on the market and selection for all professionals is difficult. However, dressings do not contain miracle substances that 'heal' wounds and those manufacturers who claim their dressings can are bending the truth. Dressings can only provide optimum wound healing environments as the wound is responsible for its own healing and the practitioners selection of dressing will provide the environment in which the body can heal itself. Galen said, 'For the treatment of every sore there are four things which should be considered. The first and main one is God, the second the surgeon, the third is the medicine and the fourth is the patient. Should any of these fail then the sore shall never be healed' (Naylor 1999).

Dressing selection must rely entirely on the practitioner's knowledge of how to provide an optimum wound healing environment (Table 3.1) or how to prepare a wound bed that is not healing, through use of modern interactive dressings, thereby, controlling the microenvironment of the wound. 'Blanket' treatment of wounds such as potassium permanganate soaks or the use of hypochlorites for every leg ulcer is no longer acceptable; each individual wound has different requirements for provision of an optimum healing environment and skilled assessment of the wound will lead to informed decisions in wound care.

Use of a variety of dressings to treat one wound is not acceptable. Lidowski and Patterson (1985, quoted in Young 1997b) wrote 'One of the greatest detriments to wound healing is to have many methods and products used on a wound'. However, the practitioner must be able to identify when the wound has entered the next stage of healing and no longer requires the dressing that suited the previous stage of healing. This takes skill, knowledge and experience and is the art and science of nursing.

This chapter looks at how dressings might be selected for the individual patient, and assists the nurse or carer to provide the optimum wound healing environment and to understand how dressings work.

Dressing selection

Wound bed preparation (the removal of deterrents to healing) is a vital component of wound healing as stimulating regeneration in humans by altering the wound-healing environment has been the most successful approach since the 1950s (Carlson 1998). There are no magical properties in dressings to heal wounds and wounds will heal only if the optimum wound healing environment is provided. Therefore, dressing selection relies on the skilful observation of the assessing nurse or GP and appropriate choice will lead to provision of the optimum wound healing environment. Different dressings have a part to play in the healing or non-healing wound and depend on the status of healing (Table 3.1, p. 80).

Selection of a dressing for a wound relies entirely on the individual assessment of the patient. However, this also relies on in-depth knowledge of the selected dressing and this knowledge is often difficult to obtain. Restrictions of the drug tariff or hospital formularies will limit the potential for comparing dressing types and new dressings.

The plethora of dressing products has resulted in the nurse often using a combination of products (Young 1997b). This not only has a high cost implication, but also is a potential problem if the dressings interact. Scientists have not yet evaluated the mix of dressings such as silver sulphadiazine cream and iodine and the potential for an adverse reaction is high.

Cost-effectiveness of a dressing must be an important consideration in dressing selection. However, the actual price of the dressing is not necessarily related to the cost-effectiveness status. An expensive dressing that promotes wound healing and rapidly leads to the desired clinical conclusion can be judged as cost-effective.

Dressings generally fall naturally into three categories:

1 Passive dressings: including gauze, paraffin gauze, non-adherent dressings (NAs), absorbent dressings, foams and semi-permeable films. These dressings are inactive within the wound and play a passive role in the provision of an ideal wound healing environment. They would not be expected to debride or deslough a wound.
2 Active dressings: hydrocolloids, alginates, dispersion therapy, hydrofibres, hyaluronic acid dressings, iodine, silver, charcoal dressings and medicated bandages can all be considered to play an active role in the provision of an ideal wound healing environment and will promote debridement and desloughing within the wound.
3 Mechanical: warm-up dressing and vacuum-assisted closure would be considered within this category.

Treatment of wounds

Rapid rehydration of eschar and removal of hard, devitalized tissue can be achieved by a combination of methods:

- surgical/sharp debridement;
- enzymatic;
- autolysis;
- biosurgical;
- chemical;
- mechanical.

Wound debridement

Taken from the French débridement, or débrider to remove adhesions, literally, to unbridle, from Middle French desbrider, the surgical removal of lacerated, devitalized, or contaminated tissue, the

Table 3.1 Selection of dressings according to wound assessment findings

Wound colour	Aims	Treatment
BLACK	Soften hard eschar Remove rehydrated/moist necrotic tissue. Wound will show signs of granulation tissue within one week.	Varidase + hydrogel + hydrocolloid for 48 hours Then: hydrogel OR: Iodine cadexomer for 1 to 2 weeks. OR: Hydrocolloid paste + hydrocolloid. Dispersion therapy dressing + film.
SOFT BLACK YELLOW	Removal	Hydrogel Hydrocolloid Hydrocolloid paste VAC Dispersion therapy Aquacel Alginate Combiderm
BLACK HEEL (HARD)	Remove pressure Rehydration Debridement	Air mattress Air cushion for heel if supported during the day Dressings as above for black wound If ABPI is >0.8 consider compression bandage to redistribute pressure and then a back slab POP
BLACK HEEL BLISTER	Protection – bursting the blister will encourage infection	Air mattress Air cushion for heel if supported during the day Tulle dressing Foam dressing If ABPI is >0.8 consider compression bandage to redistribute pressure and then back slab POP

Wound appearance	Aims	Dressings
BLACK TOES	Prevent trauma Keep dry Refer for surgery	Dry dressings only Protect with dry bandages Pain control
BROWN (blood red) DISCHARGE (May have the odour of old blood – possible *Staphylococcus aureus* colonization)	Observe for signs of clinical infection (as above) Remove colonization Wound will show signs of granulation within one week	Iodine cadexomer OR: Drawtex OR: Negative pressure therapy OR: Actisorb plus OR: Sugar paste
BRIGHT RED WOUND (Friable, has appearance of old beef – possible *Streptococci* infection)	Take a swab Antibiotics if required Protect Wound will show signs of granulation in two weeks	Treat with gentle wound care product until infection subsides e.g. Alginate OR: Drawtex OR: Hydrocolloid/hydrocolloid paste OR: Hydrofibre OR: Hydrogel OR: Hydrogel sheet with glycerine
CELLULITIS AROUND THE WOUND Increased in size Patient pyrexial Offensive	Take a swab Antibiotic cover Defer wound treatment decision until infection is controlled	Povidone-iodine (Inadine) change dressing 1 to 2 times daily Cadexomer iodine (Iodoflex, Iodosorb) change dressing every 2–3 days (PRN) Sugar paste VAC
DEEP PINK WITH DEEP RED RAISED SPOTS (Granulation tissue)	Protect Provide warmth Provide moist environment Leave undisturbed as long as possible	Hydrocolloid OR: Hydrofibre OR: Foam dressing
PALE PINK/MAUVE EPITHELIAL TISSUE Pink wound with white edges – contracting in	Protect	Simple dressing only if required Foam dressing Hydrocolloid thin Film dressing

Table 3.1 Continued

Wound colour	Aims	Treatment
PRESSURE ULCER with hard, swollen edges to the wound (induration)	Prevent further tissue damage Heal the wound	Air mattress and cushion VAC Dressing selection according to wound colour
VENOUS ULCER (ABPI > 0.8)	Assessment of healing status of the wound Address pain	Compression bandage Intermittent compression therapy Dressing according to the colour of the wound Soak in bucket of water for 5 minutes at each dressing change Paste bandage (ensure patient is not sensitive to paste bandage) N/A ultra

ARTERIAL ULCER (ABPI > 0.8)	This ulcer may not heal
	Treat symptoms
	Support any healing
	Address pain
		Sometimes helped by potassium permanganate soaks
		Dressing according to symptoms i.e.
		   Paste bandage
		   Hydrocolloid
		   Hydrocolloid paste
		   Hydrogel
		   Foam

BLISTERS FROM CFF Fracture	DO NOT USE Adhesive dressings Keep dry	Sometimes helped by potassium permanganate soaks Non-adherent silicone dressing Tulle dressing of any type Non-adherent dressing of any type
HAEMATOMA	Reduction of the haematoma before deterioration of the tissues occur	Leech therapy Lasonil

BURNS	Prevention of infection Pain free removal of dressings	Sheet gels Silver sulphadiazine cream Several layers of tulle (may still adhere) Meptil Non-adherent dressing (may still adhere)
SKIN GRAFT	Protection	VAC Sheet gel Tulle dressing (may adhere) N/A ultra Meptil
BLISTERS FOLLOWING ORTHOPAEDIC SURGERY	Prevention	Change adhesive securing dressing

modern definition is removal of lacerated, devitalized or contaminated tissue by various means.

Hardened eschar is a product of the coagulum in non-occlusive treated wounds (Lydon et al. 1990). It is not an amorphous mass but consists of structural elements in the form of collagen I, II, III, IV, V and chondroitin sulphate, fibronectin, fibrinogen and elastin (Thomas 1999). Thomas noted that the structural composition of eschar appears to vary between patients.

Necrotic tissue can be life-threatening, can prevent wounds from healing and can prevent removal of devitalized tissue, particulate matter, or foreign materials from a wound. Debridement is therefore the first goal of wound care (Fowler and van Rijswijk 1995). Toxins from the necrotic tissue and infected wound can contribute to cardiac problems. Nevertheless, there is controversy over whether nurses should be surgically debriding wounds, particularly when other effective methods of debridement are available and nurses knowledge of wound debridement still seems to be based mainly on empirical and practical principles (Mekkes 1998) rather than formed through education.

Sharp debridement

The most rapid and effective method of debridement is sharp or surgical debridement when necrotic tissue is dissected from viable tissue by use of sterile scissors or scalpel and may be performed at the bedside by an experienced practitioner (Hoffman 1996; Hampton 1997a). Sharp debridement of non-viable tissue not only exposes the healthy, perfused tissue required to initiate wound healing but also effectively removes the majority of microbial contaminants and any associated malodour, thus reducing the potential for clinical infection (Bowler et al. 2001). Sharp debridement, performed by inexperienced hands, could be dangerous practice as fibrous tissue can have the appearance of slough and there is a potential for ligaments to be accidentally severed (Hampton 1997a). It could also be a dangerous practice if small arteries are severed or patients with a medical condition leading to bleeding are accidentally cut. This is particularly dangerous if carried out by a practitioner in the community when the medical services are not immediately available if required in an emergency.

Sharp debridement should not be carried out when there are signs of clinical infection or in wounds where there is a potential for bleeding, e.g. malignant wounds. Enormous care must also be shown in the case of diabetic foot ulceration and it is often wisest to leave (diabetic) debridement to podiatrists or to surgeons.

The UKCC has given guidance for nurses who wish to take on new practices such as sharp debridement and state 'Each nurse shall acknowledge any limitations in knowledge or competence and decline any duties unless able to perform them in a safe and skilled manner.' Surgical debridement is a skill that requires knowledge of underlying structures, an understanding of wound assessment and the experience to decide when debridement should not be performed. The inexperienced nurse would require the support and guidance of a more experienced practitioner. However, finding a practitioner experienced in surgical debridement may prove difficult and, as doctors are often less experienced than nurses in wound care (Hampton 1997a), finding a mentor may be difficult.

Surgical consultants may advocate cutting the necrotic tissue until bleeding tissue is exposed. This is accepted practice for a surgeon because, by initiating the clotting cascade (by injuring capillaries), the wound will become inflamed and it is this inflammation that will 'kick-start' the wound to heal. This is supported by Steed (1998), who recommends sharp debridement down to healthy viable tissue to initiate bleeding. Steed identifies that platelets, activated to control the haemorrhage, will release growth factors that 'kick-start' the healing process.

However, all practitioners undertaking this task as a role development, should be fully aware of the consequences. Bleeding can lead to clinical infection or haemorrhage or there is a potential for severing tendons and, as viable tissue is being excised, this is a surgical procedure and as such should be performed by a surgeon. The experienced practitioner would be advised to remove only the necrotic tissue leaving the small edges of non-viable tissue to be removed through autolysis. In the future, there will be nurse practitioners that have been trained to perform surgical debridement. Nurses must question their own competency before undertaking what could be thought of as a doctor's duty (Rieu 1994).

Certain necrotic wounds should not be sharp debrided. For instance, ischaemic toes must be referred to a surgeon and, if surgery is not an option, the toes should be left to dry and to demarcate. Allowing dry gangerene toes to become wet through debridement will open the necrotic tissue to aerobic and anaerobic pathogens.

Malignant wounds may have the inclination to bleed and debriding such wounds surgically could be dangerous, particularly when debriding in the community when the emergency department is a distance away.

Wounds may have other structures close to the surface (Figure 3.1) and these could be accidentally severed, particularly as tendons can mimic slough. Should this occur, the patient could potentially lose the use of an arm or foot.

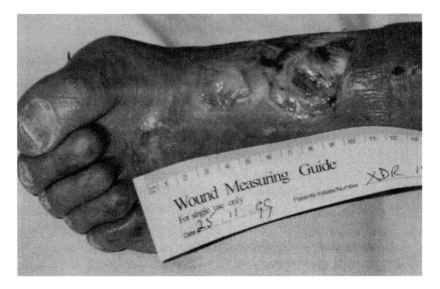

Figure 3.1 Tendons exposed as a result of poor bandaging techniques in mixed aetiology leg ulcers (see Plate 15).

Hard eschar (Figure 3.2) requires softening, before surgical debridement can be performed. This can be achieved by rehydration over 24–48 hours by the use of enzymes or by the use of hydrocolloid or hydrogel. After softening, the eschar will often lift at the edges allowing the experienced practitioner to hold the necrotic tissue with a scalpel (Figure 3.3) and dissect it, using scissors or scalpel.

There is unlikely to be pain from the procedure as the tissue being removed is necrotic and without a viable nerve supply. However, healthy tissues surrounding the cavity may be sensitive, or positioning may lead the patient to experience pain or discomfort. Pain, experienced in the wound bed or surrounding tissues, may be

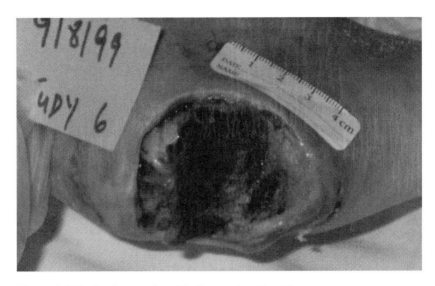

Figure 3.2 Hard eschar requires debridement (see Plate 16).

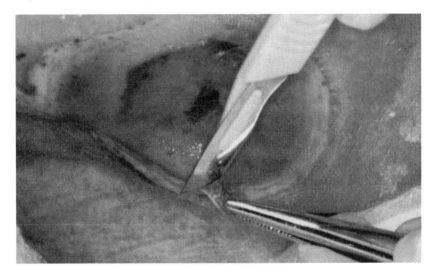

Figure 3.3 Sharp debridement (see Plate 17).

reduced by the use of analgesia or injection of local anaesthetic (Hansson et al. 1993). Kristofferson (1998) found that pain intensity during debridement decreased significantly with increasing duration with EMLA cream (eutectic mixture of local anaesthetics) application and this was confirmed in a study by Rosenthal et al. (2001).

However, it should be noted that topical anaesthetics used in wound care have not yet been licensed for such use within the UK, although they are widely used in Europe. Drucker et al. (1998) found that the use of Lidocaine in wounds does not substantially alter wound healing and Rosenthal et al. (2001) had similar results with EMLA cream in a study of painless wound debridement.

Entinox is always useful when dressing painful wounds. When the devitalized tissue is lifted free, the process of autolysis may treat any remaining slough supported by dressings that promote this natural action.

Enzymatic debridement

The problem of hard eschar can be partly addressed by scoring the leathery surface with a scalpel, exposing the softer tissue beneath. Common practice is to inject Varidase (streptokinase and streptodornase) beneath the surface of the eschar and this can have a rapid effect (Morison 1993). The practitioner, however, must ensure that the fluid is actually being placed in devitalized tissue as streptokinase can cause sensitivities and produce a reaction if another injection is given within six months (Green 1993; Bux et al. 1997). The *British National Formulary* does not list this method as a recommended procedure. Streptokinase and streptodornase are two enzymes traditionally used to promote debridement of necrotic wounds. Streptokinase is a thrombolytic, which acts directly on a substrate of fibrin by activating a fibrinolytic enzyme in human serum breaking up thrombi (Martin 1996). Commonly used in the treatment of myocardial infarction and often referred to as the 'clot buster', the enzyme dissolves clots in the arteries and reduces the damage within the heart muscle. Streptodornase liquefies the viscous nucleoprotein of dead cells or pus. The joint action of the two enzymes rehydrates the hard necrotic material in a wound and allows the secondary dressing and/or irrigation to remove the liquefied material.

The recommendation of the *British National Formulary* is that Varidase should be applied as a wet dressing and changed once or twice daily. However, mixed with a hydrogel (Granugel, Intrasite gel, Sterigel, Aquaform) and placed under a hydrocolloid (Granuflex, Comfeel, Tegasorb, etc), the effect can be extended for 24–48 hours. There is, however, little evidence to support the use of enzymatic debridement, and Martin (1996) found that a hydrogel (Ky Jelly) was as useful in rehydrating wounds; nevertheless, this result was from one small study and it would be difficult to place credence without further studies. Some of the problems that may be associated with the use of enzymes are listed below:

- Varidase 'poured' directly onto a wound is unlikely to remain in the required position.
- Changing dressings twice daily is difficult to achieve on very busy wards often without enough qualified nurses to undertake that workload.
- The cost of Varidase, particularly if used twice daily, is prohibitive, especially when there is a lack of evidence (Martin 1996) to say that it is more effective than other debriding agents.
- Varidase is often soaked into gauze and placed on eschar. This probably treats the gauze very well but is unlikely to benefit the wound!
- It is not successful on dehydrated and hard eschar (Flanagan 1997).

Rutter et al. (2000) offered the following guideline for using Varidase:

- Contents of the vial should be gently mixed (not shaken) with 20mls of saline.
- Varidase can be applied by soaking gauze with the solution, applying the gauze and then occluding with a film dressing but this raises an uncertainty as the action of debridement may be achieved through the moisture applied to the wound.
- It can also be mixed with a hydrogel but hydrogels can successfully debride wounds and, therefore, it is not fully known whether it would be the enzyme that is debriding or the hydrogel. Varidase can be injected under the hard eschar that has been scored although there is a potential for a reaction to the enzymes (Green 1993) and accidental injection into viable tissue may cause anaphylaxis.

The enzyme mixture is best applied to a wound by mixing the powder with 5 mls of sterile water then uniting the mixture with a hydrogel. This is then placed on a wound with an occlusive dressing as cover to keep the area as moist as possible. This can be left for 48 hours. However, it is uncertain how much of the enzyme actually comes into contact with the tissue requiring treatment when mixed with another substance such as hydrogels or which is responsible for the debridement, hydrogel or enzyme.

Autolysis

Autolysis is the body's natural capacity for removing necrotic tissue as it uses it's own enzymes to lyze, or breakdown, devitalized tissue (Bale 1997). There are many modern dressings that support the body with autolysis and any wet dressings will support this process and assist with liquefaction of eschar and removal of waste products. For example:

- hydrogels;
- hydrocolloids;
- cadexomer iodine;
- film dressings;
- tenderwet.

The eschar is rehydrated and then the body begins to destroy and remove the dead tissue. However, eschar that is exposed to air or dressed with a dry dressing, remains hard and autolysis is impossible. Therefore, to enable autolysis to occur, the eschar should be covered with a 'wet' dressing such as a hydrogel or hydrocolloid. These dressings will rehydrate the eschar and allow the body to remove the necrotic material. There are occasions when (generally in the USA) wet gauze is placed on the wound, deliberately allowed to dry and then pulled away to debride the wound (see 'wet to dry' later in this chapter).

There are occasions when wounds are best left undebrided. Superficial heel wounds will heal effectively without removal of the necrotic tissue when the edges of the necrotic tissue lift, exposing pink epithelial tissue underneath. However, it requires an experienced practitioner to decide whether the necrotic tissue is superficial or deeply set and possibly dangerous.

Hardened or mummified necrotic areas, caused by ischaemia, will potentially become colonized or infected if rehydrated. Healing will be low in these instances and must be balanced by the potential of clinical infection and distressing malodour.

The wound in Figure 3.3 was rehydrated by the use of hydrocolloid hydrogel (Granugel) covered with a secondary dressing of hydrocolloid (Granuflex) for 48 hours. The treatment continued to break down the necrotic tissue through autolysis following sharp debridement of the surface necrosis. This debridement can involve cutting away the top area or scoring the surface to allow entry of moisture and so speed up the process of natural autolysis.

Biosurgery

Natural myiasis (the infection of wounds with larvae) is seen commonly in hot climates, occasionally in this country and is often greeted with horror when the dressing is removed to expose the infestation (Flanagan 1997). Nevertheless, maggot therapy has been used for many centuries as a natural debrider of wounds and there is evidence that the benefits of maggots were noted in 1557 (Morgan 1997a) and during the American Civil war (Thomas et al. 1996a). Morgan (1997a) relates anecdotal reports of Malay Indians using maggots to remove superficial malignancies. Stanton Livingston studied maggot therapy and found it the most effective means of promoting wound healing (Graner 1997). Recently, there has been an increased interest in maggot therapy with many articles written on the benefits (Stoddard et al. 1995; Boon et al. 1996; Thomas et al. 1996b; Jones and Thomas 1997). The wound cleansing has been successful in a supporting treatment of necrotizing fasciitis (Thomas et al. 1996a).

One fear of nurses may be that the maggots will disappear in sinuses. This fear is unfounded as maggots will struggle to leave the wound on the fourth or fifth day. Wherever they are within the wound they will return to the surface to prepare to leave to pupate. There may be less maggots leaving the wound than were supplied and this is because they either die naturally and are removed by the body or they are eaten by the other, stronger maggots when the food supply becomes short.

The most commonly used fly in biosurgery is *Lucilia sericata* or greenbottle fly (Thomas et al. 1996b).

Maggots can be obtained in gauze bags to remove the dislike or distrust that nurses often have. The fact that they are contained within a bag would make it a little easier and more acceptable when placing them on the wound. How the maggots are able to interact with the wound when inside the bag is a moot point. They would be able to live on wound exudate but could not stimulate the wound bed in the way that free maggots possibly can.

Maggots are applied as follows:

- A hydrocolloid sheet is cut with a hole the shape of the wound and covers the peri-wound area.
- The maggots are placed in the centre of the wound.
- A fine mesh (supplied with the maggots) is placed over the wound and the hydrocolloid.
- Sleek is placed as a seal around the mesh edge and extends over the hydrocolloid.
- A dressing is placed on the top to soak up exudate.
- The maggots are left *in situ* for 3–5 days (any longer and the maggots will be trying to escape to find a place to pupate).
- The maggots are rinsed from the wound in saline.
- A second or third application is used if required.

Maggots will not pupate in the wound and so the patient, doctor and nurse can be assured that the dressing will not be removed to find flies. Following use, the maggots must be destroyed by incineration as disposal via sluice or any other means can lead to resistant bacteria entering the food chain.

This method of debridement is increasing in popularity, and for difficult wounds requiring palliative management such as gangrenous feet (Figure 3.4) or fungating tumours, as a reduction of odour and exudate can be achieved by the treatment (Thomas et al. 1996a, 1996b). However, maggots should not be used on wounds that bleed easily, and they are extremely fussy about the type of dressing used prior to their application. They are particularly unhappy about hydrogels apart from Purilon, which does not contain propylene glycol (Andrews et al. 1998).

Chemical debridement

For many years, it was the practice to use chemicals, such hydrogen peroxide or hypochlorites (EUSOL, Milton, etc.) to debride wounds. Research has shown that there are some hazards in using chemicals in wounds and, even though the research is inconclusive and sometimes flawed, it is generally accepted that the use of chemicals such as hypochlorites is unnecessary if not dangerous. Sleigh and Linter (1985) refer to two cases where the use of hydrogen peroxide led to one case of surgical emphysema and one case of oxygen embolus. Irrigation under

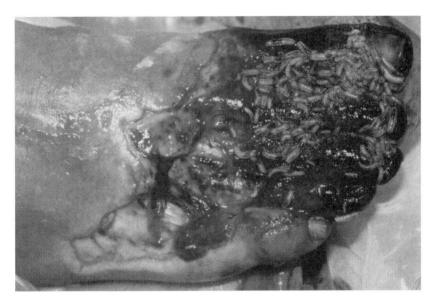

Figure 3.4 Maggots being used to debride gangrenous tissue (see Plate 18).

pressure into enclosed cavities can lead to the enzyme catalase causing a rapid decomposing and the effervescent action (due to the liberation of water and oxygen) of the hydrogen peroxide may force the oxygen into the tissues, forming an oxygen embolus (Bassan et al. 1982).

Modern dressings debride successfully, without side effects and without the pain associated with some chemicals. There is evidence that bacteria (e.g. MRSA) will become resistant to antiseptics (Cookson et al. 1991; Leelaporn et al. 1994; Irizarry et al. 1996) giving greater importance to the avoidance of using such chemicals in wound care. Older products, such as Aserbine, have been successfully used in debridement although it can harm healthy peri-wound areas (Morison 1992).

There is still a body of medical opinion that supports the use of hypochlorites (Flanagan 1997) and many nurses may be forced into using the substance against their own judgement. The UKCC document *Exercising Accountability* (UKCC 1989) guides nurses to give an explanation of why they do not wish to use the product and to invite the doctor/sister to administer the treatment themselves.

Fear of the consequences of refusal could lead to nurses using another product without informing the doctor that the prescribed dressing was not used. This not only can have serious consequences for the nurse when the deception is exposed, but can also reinforce the doctor's belief that the prescription is favourable, when it may well be the nurse's own prescription that is cleansing the wound.

Documentation is crucial when a doubtful situation arises and it is important for the nurse to seek the advice of the first line manager, particularly when researched evidence leads the nurse to question the recommendations of the doctor. Refusal to give care prescribed by the doctor is permissible providing the nurse is convinced that the treatment will cause harm. However, refusal must be based on evidence and fact, not on research that has been used and adapted according to the person telling the story (anecdotal evidence).

Use of hypochlorites may be an example of how research can be taken out of proportion. The work was completed on a granulating wound, produced in a rabbit's ear chamber (Leaper and Simpson 1986) when the product was found to have a marked effect on the microcirculation causing shut down of capillaries and local capillary death. The wound was clean and granulating, not a sloughy, infected and necrotic wound for which hypochlorites were generally used. Following their research, Leaper and Simpson (1986) recommended that hypochlorites should be used with caution, they did not say they should never be used and Lawrence (1996) doubt that they should be banned as they are inexpensive to use and effective in cleaning wounds. This leads to the question, should a nurse refuse to use hypochlorites? If the nurse refuses and the wound deteriorates, the prescribing doctor may claim that it is the consequence of not following the prescription (even if untrue) and will be able to produce evidence that hypochlorites clean sloughy wounds. Fotherby et al. (1991) found no significant difference in healing rates between hypochlorite solution application and the use of a hydrocolloid or saline soaked gauze.

Wound care is a science and much of the evidence against the use of hypochlorites does not meet the strict scientific criteria that we should apply to wound care substances used in wound care today (Peel 1993). This scenario is not set to frighten nurses into applying hypochlorites as the product can be very painful (Bloomfield 1985) and other products are kinder with possibly greater effectiveness. There can be no question that hypochlorites are toxic to local tissues (Bloomfield 1985) although the tissues that are involved must be viable to enable them to be harmed. The types of wounds where hypochlorites are used are generally packed with devitalized tissue.

Nurses should be fully cognizant with the product, and be able to critically analyse the research before making the decision to refuse to apply dressings according to the prescribing doctor's instructions. The decision is then based on clinical evidence and the nurse can offer an argument that 'harm to the patient is foreseeable' and that the professional code of practice supports refusal to apply any substance that is thought to be harmful to the patient.

Wet to dry debridement

The 'wet to dry' method is commonly used in America as a method of wound debridement. Gauze, soaked in saline, is placed in the wound, allowed to dry and then torn away, removing any necrotic material that has become attached to the dried gauze. This method of debridement is described and recommended by Steed (1998) as effective and simple, but it may be painful. Mulder (1995) found that wet to dry debridement was only minimally lower cost than the use of hydrogel and foam. Nevertheless, this method is cheap, rapid, simple, clinically proven and potentially extremely painful for the patient. However, it is not used or recommended in the UK where painless and effective methods are preferred.

Although debridement is often viewed separately from other wound management techniques, particularly when managing patients with chronic wounds, it should never be viewed in isolation. Rather it is one aspect of patient care (Fowler and van Rijswijk 1995).

Overgranulation

Overgranulation or hypergranulation poses a problem for the practitioner in wound healing. Modern wound healing has become extremely sophisticated and it may be this very sophistication that is increasing the problem of hypergranulation. Use of occlusive dressing (Ashurst 1975), and other products, possibly over-promote angiogenesis leading to overgranulation (Van Luyn et al. 1992). An extended period of inflammatory response, possibly linked to chronic infection can lead to granulation tissue with the appearance of a soft gelatinous lump protruding over the level of the surrounding tissue. Traditionally, silver nitrate pencils or topical steroids have been used to reduce overgranulation. However, both are thought to delay healing (Young 1997a) and are largely unused today. Products thought to reduce overgranulation are:

- foam dressings (Young 1995; Williams 1996);
- doubled hydrocolloids;
- hydrocolloid with a gauze pad used for pressure over the dressing;
- double dispersion therapy dressings;
- silver nitrate pencil;
- corticosteroid cream (this should only be done under medical supervision as a last resort).

Use of non-traumatic dressings to reduce hypergranulation should be the recommended first choice. However, the use of silver nitrate pencil in some cases provides a faster dressing route to healing. Although foam dressings and pressure dressings do achieve eventual success, it is slow, whereas silver nitrate pencil rapidly destroys the overgranulated tissue, leaving a flat bed of tissue that will support epithelial migration. It must be emphasized, however, that this is the authors' own opinion and is unresearched and unsupported.

Morison (1991) found silver nitrate to be caustic and with a potential to initiate methaemoglobinaemia and metabolic disturbances. Silver nitrate is, therefore, a treatment for very short-term use only. When used, the wound will immediately turn white as the blood vessels constrict, and then will become necrotic. The tissue dies and falls away leaving a clean, healthy wound bed.

Blisters

Blisters occur when separation between the dermis and epidermis occurs. The area is filled with fluid and the thin raised epidermis discloses the blister fluid beneath the surface. Blisters occur, generally, because the skin surface has rubbed against a harder surface, such as a shoe or a bed. If the blister surface is damaged, the lower dermis is exposed and this opens the area to potential of clinical infection and further tissue deterioration.

Blisters should be protected by the dressing that is used to cover them and adhesive dressings such as film dressings or hydrocolloids should be avoided at all costs as these will tear the blister roof as they are removed. Fluid can be removed through the use of a syringe if necessary. Otherwise, the blister can be left intact and covered with a dry dressing that will offer some pressure relief.

Orthopaedic patients often develop blisters post surgery and this problem is addressed in Chapter 7. Burn blisters are discussed in Chapter 2.

Pretibial lacerations and general skin tears (degloving injury)

The treatment for skin tears relies greatly on the condition of the skin concerned. Steroid type skin, fragile and papery, should not be treated in the same way as the skin of a healthy subject. The skin loss may be superficial or full thickness and there may be a haematoma formation.

Once the laceration is noted, it is helpful, if possible, to bring the edges into apposition with the use of steri-strips or wound glue such as Dermabond or Histoacryl blue. Sutures are associated with a significant increase in necrosis and slow healing (Bradley 2001). Once in position, the skin should then be kept *in situ* for as long as possible. A deeper laceration would require removal of any haematoma and any devitalized tissue. Healthy subjects can be supplied with a film dressing or hydrocolloid and this can be left *in situ* for a week. However, those patients with fragile skin should have a slightly moist non-adherent dressing to hold the strips in place. Either a dressing, such as Mepital or several layers of paraffin gauze is ideal for the purpose. Should paraffin gauze adhere (several layers will help to prevent adherence), hydrogel such as Ky jelly, gently massaged into the surface of the gauze, will help to lift it away from the wound. Paraffin gauze is hydrophobic and water will not remove it once it has adhered. A bandage can then be used to retain the treatment in place for up to a week. The steroidal skin is less likely to heal and may become an ulcer. Depending on how the trauma occurred, skin tears have the potential to become clinically infected. The treatment would then change and antibiotic cover would be of prime importance.

Angiogenesis and negative pressure

A wound bed is a war zone with bacteria and white cells fighting for supremacy. Each uses up large amounts of oxygen in bursts of energy, with white cells calling on the microcirculation for their

requirements and the bacteria calling on the wound environment for
their own supply. The tissues also require oxygen for energy in
regeneration and it is therefore, oxygen vital for rapid repair.

Fibroblasts appear to have a finite life and if wound healing is
delayed, fibroblasts can stop production and wound healing
altogether. Therefore, it is important to heal a wound as rapidly as
possible. Negative pressure creates a hypoxic environment within the
wound bed in which aerobic bacteria cannot survive and thereby
reduces the bacterial count by 1000 times in four days (Collier 1997).
This hypoxic environment forces the microcirculation to regenerate
rapidly and produce a large amount of capillaries.

At the same time, the negative pressure forces blood into the
wound bed, which brings growth factors and macrophages to an
area that is deplete in bacterial contamination. This possibly releases
large reserves of oxygen as energy for tissue regeneration. The
suction also removes any slough or loose necrotic material from the
wound leaving it clean and with an excellent blood supply. Therefore, negative pressure promotes faster granulation and moist wound
healing. Early work showed that negative pressure reduces local
tissue oedema, increases local blood supply, reduces bacterial colonization, mechanically closes the wound and removes wound
exudate (Banwell et al. 1998).

Negative pressure is an excellent treatment for pressure ulcers, even
grade 4 (EPUAP 2001) wounds heal rapidly. Large grade 4 ulcers
(exposing bone) tend to heal in an average of five weeks. There are two
types of machines available, at present, for negative pressure. The
VAC (vacuum-assisted closure), a static model that can only be
successfully used on immobile or low mobility patients, and a new
model, an ambulatory VAC that can be used in the community. The
cost is prohibitive, although it could be argued that faster healing rates
easily offset the cost. The VAC involves subatmospheric pressure,
reduces interstitial pressure, restores blood flow and removes cell-
inhibitory factors within chronic wound fluid (Bowler et al. 2001).

Negative pressure can be used on:

- pressure ulcers;
- dehisced wounds (providing the wound does not lead to a body
  cavity);
- leg ulcers;

- surgical wounds;
- difficult wounds;
- diabetic wounds.

Negative pressure has been found to be useful in diabetic foot ulcers when the microcirculatory system is compromized. A large ulcer over a charcot joint had been proving difficult to heal with the patient hospitalized for nine weeks. Negative pressure was applied and the wound granulated to the surface in two weeks and epithelial-ization occurred very soon after.

Using dressings to treat symptoms

Pain

Wounds that are painful (see Chapter 2) need dressings that will gently 'bathe' nerve endings. Hydrogels, hydrocolloids, hydrocolloid pastes, sheet gels will all support this. Venous ulcers will often be painful until compression is applied, then pain usually disappears within the first few hours post dressing. Analgesia is an option that should be considered if the pain cannot be controlled through the dressing and is sometimes required as a short-term method of reduc-ing the pain whilst the dressing completes it's role in pain control.

Any dressing that exerts an osmotic 'pull' on the wound bed will increase pain. This is any hydrophilic dressing such as:

- alginates;
- sugar paste;
- cadexomers;
- foams;
- hydrofibres;
- dispersion technology;
- the vacuum-assisted closure (VAC).

Some dressings can cause intense pain on removal and may require Entinox. If this is the case, the practitioner should question why the dressing has been selected in this instance. A study undertaken by Martini et al. (1999) found patients reported intense pain on removal of paraffin gauze and no or slight pain on removal of the trial dress-ing (Allevyn).

A new method of controlling pain is warm-up wound therapy. The dressing causes vasodilation, is soothing and has been shown to reduce pain (Vosskuhler 1999). If the principle of this is to cause vasodilation through warmth, then there is an argument for washing venous ulcers in water that is warmer than blood and for wrapping the wound up in several layers of dressings or bandages. However, although this may help, there is no evidence to say that this aids healing as the shorter period of time, and the cooling of the water may negate the effect that is seen in warm-up wound therapy, which maintains a set warmth.

Malodour

The odour in a wound is an indication of the type of bacteria colonizing the wound. Reduce the colonization and the odour will generally disappear. Soaking in a bucket of tap water and emollient for five minutes daily for three days often helps leg ulcers and appears to reduce colonization. However, consideration should be given to osmosis as the cells within the tissues may absorb non-isotonic water (water not in balance with body fluid), swell and burst, causing pain and possible increase in wound size. Dressings during this time depend on the type of bacteria in the wound.

Gram-negative bacteria, such as *Pseudomonas*, can be very malodorous; for example, has a musty, sweet smell and can be detected on entry to any room containing the afflicted patient. The malodour and discharge can be distressing for the patient and carers. Treatment over 1–3 days with silver sulphadiazine cream (Flamazine) can reduce colonization dramatically and will benefit the patient as well as reducing the amount of dressing changes required. Silver is a relatively inert metal that interacts with wound fluids and becomes active in the wound bed where it binds to tissue proteins and causes structural changes in the bacterial cell wall. Silver binds to and denatures bacterial DNA and RNA, thereby inhibiting replication (Lansdown 2002).

If silver sulphadiazine is used over long periods, the Pseudomonal colonization will return. Kucan et al. (1981) found silver sulphadiazine a successful way to decrease contamination. Regular use of silver sulphadiazine can cause neutropenia (Fowler and Norberg 1994), which may account for why low-grade colonization returns. Use of a carbon and silver ions dressing (Actisorb Silver 220) will also reduce colonization and malodour. In 1993 a study by Davis (1998) was unable to identify any silver resistant strains of MRSA. Arglaes film dressing contains silver and is excellent when used for grazes and superficial wounds. The manufacturers claim that the silver can be transported through a primary dressing when Arglaes is used as a secondary dressing. Acticoat is a foam dressing containing silver which will both absorb exudate and reduce contamination.

Cadexomer iodine has been widely researched for its effect on the microbiological content of a wound and can as effectively reduce malodour particularly in Gram-positive colonization such as *Staphylococcus aureas*.

Honey has been shown to reduce *Pseudomonas* in wounds (Cooper and Molan 1999) and has antiseptic properties, possibly with the same osmotic action as sugar. Oryan and Zaker (1998) found that honey, placed cutaneously on wounds, accelerates the healing process. Sugar has a strong osmotic effect on the bacterial cell and is bactericidal. However, sugar paste is messy and can be difficult to manage.

A glycerine dressing (Novogel) may be a useful alternative. The glycerine is set in a firm absorbent gel that absorbs exudate whilst destroying bacteria.

Carbon dressings absorb odours but only one dressing contains silver ions (Actisorb Silver 220). This dressing also contains carbon to reduce odour in a wound and is used as a primary dressing although it is often used mistakenly as a secondary dressing; this is a waste of expensive silver.

Any dressing that is likely to reduce bacterial colonization will reduce odour and discharge from the wound. It is likely that dispersion therapy has a similar effect, reducing colonization and cleansing the wound.

When a wound is offensive, there will be bacteria present and a necrotic wound, in the process of natural debridement, will almost certainly contain anaerobic bacteria producing an evil malodour. Antibacterial dressings will remove the bacteria and appropriate dressings will continue debriding the wound. Iodine cadexomer (Iodoflex, Iodosorb) is a useful dressing for this purpose. Iodine is an antiseptic that bacteria have not yet learned to resist (Leelaporn et al. 1994; Hampton 1998a). Goldheim (1993a) reports that povidone-iodine is possibly less injurious to wounds than water and would not affect wound healing adversely (Goldheim 1993a; Mertz et al. 1994).

Nevertheless, iodine is rapidly deactivated in the presence of pus (Leaper 1988; Van den Broek 1982) and may, therefore, have limited use as a cleanser. However, iodine cadexomer dressings (Iodoflex, Iodosorb) have the ability to absorb exudate in exchange for iodine over a 72-hour period. This allows the iodine to be slowly released into the wound during this period, extending the activity of the antiseptic properties. Iodine is also absorbed into the tissues and converted to iodide. When leucocytes ingest bacteria, they degranulate and a burst of oxygen consumption follows, exposing bacteria to antibacterial enzymes including myloperoxidase (Hunt 1995). Myloperoxidase requires iodide and so it could be said that iodine ultimately works in unison with the body to reduce infection/colonization and promote healing. As the wound is cleaned of necrotic material, the healthy cells are exposed to iodine and the slight aggravation of the tissues can set up inflammation, initiating the wound healing process. Mertz et al. (1994) found that cadexomer iodine is a low-level iodine and has no deleterious effect on epithelialization and, in fact, accelerates it. Therefore, iodine cadexomer can be a very useful addition to chronic wound treatment.

Iodine is absorbed and becomes attached to tyrosine residues in serum albumin (Alexander and Nishimoto 1981). Nevertheless, absorbed iodine is quickly excreted provided renal function is unimpaired. Once the malodour has disappeared, the iodine should be discontinued, to prevent any destructive element from reversing the process and thereby eliminating healing.

Metronidazole gel (or oral Metronidazole) is useful in anaerobic bacterial colonization when the malodorous nature of the wound can be distressing for patients and for those caring for them. The malodour is due to volatile fatty acids that are the products of bacterial metabolism and, possibly putrecine and cadaverine, both of which are formed in necrotic tissue. Metronidazole enters the cell and binds to deoxyribonucleic acid and interferes with reproduction. Malodour can be reduced within seven days with use of Metronidazole (Hampton 1996).

There are machines called aroma detectors (Greenwood et al. 1997b) that can identify bacteria by odour. An experienced practitioner would be able to detect bacteria by odour without the support of a machine and the future may well dictate that bacterial colonization is identified, by experienced people, using colour and odour.

This would save a great deal of expense in unnecessary swabs, which, at the time of writing, cost between £19 and £21 per swab. The method of identifying colour and odour would not identify all the bacteria in a wound but would select the highest bacterial colonization, whether a Gram-negative or positive and will lead to selection of a dressing to reduce the bacterial count in the wound.

Exudate

The first consideration in the control of exudate should not be how to manage the exudate but how to reduce exudate production by eliminating the cause (antibacterials and/or compression), the second consideration should be which dressing can absorb exudate. There are many dressings that absorb sufficiently well, foams, cadexomers, alginates, hydrofibres, however, this is managing the wound, not treating the symptoms. Therefore, the dressing should only be selected for control, once the wound has been treated and exudate reduced.

A general rule of thumb in selecting a dressing is to keep wet wounds dry and dry wounds wet. This is not to promote a dry wound bed, which should always be kept moist (Winter 1962), but to promote an environment that is not 'wet' through too much exudate being encouraged by the use of 'wet' dressings.

Exudate may be the patient's main problem. Malodour, colour, maceration of peri-wound areas and the volume of discharge may all lead to distress. However, exudate contains growth factors, which promote tissue regeneration (Kreig and Eming 1997) and the dressing should support natural exudate. Nevertheless, several factors can combine to increase the amount of exudate (Thomas 1997a):

• hydrostatic pressure;
• wound infection;
• wound colonization;
• temperature;
• wound type;
• type of dressing.

The most likely of these causes would be bacterial colonization.

The reduction of colonization generally leads to a decrease in exudate along with malodour and sometimes pain. Hydrostatic pressure is also an important element in exudate production in venous leg ulcers and the provision of pressure, within a wound bed, equal to that of capillary pressure will reduce exudate. This can be seen in the use of compression bandages (Thomas 1997b) or with a dressing that forms a seal around the wound such as a hydrocolloid (Thomas and Loveless 1991). There is some evidence that use of the warm-up dressing may increase exudate due to the increased vasodilation. However, it may also be argued that the vasodilation will increase blood supply to the wound bed, bringing chemical mediators, nutrients and oxygen to the area.

Another useful way of keeping the wound moist but free from harmful exudate is through negative pressure. Negative pressure is a new, exciting and progressive method of wound healing. The proliferative phase (see Chapter 1) has obvious angiogenesis occurring with the capillary buds appearing as red 'bumps' in the wound bed surrounded by pink, healthy tissue. This stage is called 'granulation' because the capillary buds appear to be 'granule' like in appearance. This is the stage of wound healing that all dressings should try to achieve. With the use of the negative pressure this stage occurs more rapidly.

A simpler dressing that appears to be having similar results is the hydrophilic dressing used in dispersion therapy. This dressing is not only highly absorbent but also rapidly transports the exudate away from the wound, which appears to provide a negative pressure on the wound face. The results on the wound bed are often similar in appearance to the VAC with a bright red and moist wound. This may reduce bacterial colonization, and resultant excessive exudate, by absorbing the organisms and removing them from the wound bed.

The wound easily bleeds

Patients with fungating wounds will often find that the wound bleeds easily. This is due to an increased vascularity of the wound. Alginates have haemostatic properties and exchange calcium ions for sodium ions in the wound bed. Calcium initiates the clotting cascade and, therefore, alginates are a useful dressing in wounds that bleed easily. Kaltostat is the only alginate that has ever carried a licence as a haemostat although all alginates will promote the clotting cascade.

Occasionally, certain clinical infections (such as haemolytic strep-tococci) will cause a wound to bleed. These wounds are often a dark beefy red in colour. The correct treatment would be to identify the pathogen (see Chapter 4) and to commence antibiotic therapy. Dressings will not assist in clinical infection.

The use of antibacterials in wound care

Silver

Silver has been used for medicinal purposes for thousands of years and the arrival of MRSA has led to a reintroduction of silver as an alternative to antibiotic therapy.

Bacteria have not yet produced a resistance to silver and Thurman and Gerba (1989) attributed the action to three mechanisms:

* interference with electron transportation;
* silver binding to the DNA of bacteria;
* cell membrane interactions causing structural damage.

Lansdown et al. (1997) found that silver enhanced wound healing, possibly because of the trace elements zinc and calcium. Calcium also has an effect on haemostasis within a wound as calcium ions are required to initiate the clotting cascade. Several dressings contain silver and probably the most widely used of these is silver sulphadi-azine cream (Flamazine). This cream is a chemotherapeutic agent with a wide spectrum of activity and no emergent resistant strains. Particularly useful in Gram-negative infections such as *Pseudomonas*. The use of silver should be avoided in pregnancy and in babies under two months of age.

Iodine and other antiseptics

Antiseptics, such as iodine, are known to damage healthy tissues (Leaper 1988; Archer et al. 1990). However, consideration should be given to the fact that a necrotic, long-standing wound is not a healing wound and, therefore, antiseptics are unlikely to find any healing cells to damage. It is well established that iodine has a high bacterial kill rate (McLure and Gordon 1992). Goldheim (1993a) reports that povidone-iodine is possibly less injurious to wounds than water and would not adversely affect wound healing. Nevertheless, iodine is deactivated in the presence of pus (Leaper 1987) and so use of iodine as an antiseptic in wound care may be effective as a short-term measure but the reduced antiseptic effect may negate its use in long-term wound care. Bacteria have not been shown to develop resistance to iodine and, therefore, if the half-life of iodine can be extended, its use in wound care would be justified. Iodine cadexomer (Iodoflex) is a modified hydrophilic starch powder to which elemental iodine is bound. It absorbs wound exudate and will simultaneously release iodine in a controlled manner; the amount of iodine released is proportional to the amount of exudate absorbed (Danielsen et al. 1997). Therefore, iodine cadexomer paste is designed to absorb exudate, to extend the half-life of the iodine and to be bactericidal. The benefits of the iodine cadexomer and rate of kill can last up to 72 hours following application depending on the amount of exudate/pus in the wound.

The outcome of this is that (apart from iodine cadexomers and silver) antiseptics are of little value in wounds unless dressings are changed several times a day. This is not acceptable practice in wound healing as any drop in temperature will delay wound healing by up to four hours (Lock 1979) and the tensile strength of the wound will be reduced. Therefore, dressings should remain *in situ* for as long as possible. However, cadexomer iodine is designed to slowly release iodine in exchange for wound fluid at the wound surface (Mertz et al. 1994) and can be left *in situ*, with the iodine effective, for up to 72 hours.

It is possible that debridement of the wound with iodine cadexomers will initially damage newly exposed tissues during the debridement process and may have a 'kick start effect' on healing. Surgeons, however, when surgically debriding a wound, will cut back until the wound has a healthy, bleeding bed of tissue (Goldheim 1993a). This brings a wound back to the inflammatory phase of healing, which is one of the most important phases when macrophages and mast cells introduce chemicals that initiate healing. Therefore, the slight damage caused by the iodine cadexomer may well have the same effect 'kick-starting' a previously non-healing wound. It would be unwise, however, to continue using the dressing for long periods of time because, eventually, it may have an adverse effect and slow the healing down. Up to a two-week treatment of iodine cadexomer is recommended for a colonized wound.

Staphylococcus aureus often has an 'old blood' odour, which is not as strong as *Pseudomonas* but is generally more detectable when dressings are removed. Patients often believe their wounds have bled when they see and smell the bacterial contamination.

If bacteria have a negative effect on wound healing and antibiotics and general antiseptics have limited value in wound care, alternative methods of reducing bacterial colonization must be found to increase wound-healing rates.

A new dressing is a glycerine hydrogel (Novogel), which is a bacteriostatic and fungistatic sheet gel. This product can be useful in reducing pressure, particularly in the diabetic foot, whilst cleansing the wound.

Use of antiseptics is not generally considered good practice and their damaging effects are well known (Leaper 1988). However, chlorhexidine is considered by some (Hedin and Hambraeus 1993) to prevent colonization, whilst Brennan et al. (1985) found chlorhexidine to be as innocuous as normal saline. It is up to the assessing practitioner to decide whether the negative effects outweigh the positive ones. It should be noted that, in a sloughy and contaminated wound, there is unlikely to be healing due possibly to a low ability of the wound to absorb chemicals.

Sugar paste and honey

One, little used, method of reducing odour and bacterial colonization is through the use of old remedies such as sugar paste and honey. Sugar is used by cooks to 'pickle' fruit as the sugar's osmotic action pulls fluid from bacterial cells, thereby destroying the bacteria and preserving the fruit. Although sugar is a very effective method of cleansing and deodorizing a wound (due to reduction of bacterial colonization), it is messy and difficult to apply. One problem associated with the use of sugar paste is the osmotic effect on the microcellular environment of the wound. Pain may be experienced as fluid is drawn from cells, particularly in already painful wounds.

Sugar paste has been developed at Northwick Park Hospital with the ingredients shown in Table 3.3 (Morgan 1997b).

Sugar is non-toxic, even in wounds of diabetic patients, although it should be used with caution in renal disease (Topham 2000).

Honey has excellent antibacterial properties (Surguna et al. 1993) and it is an excellent wound cleanser, although quite messy. Honey contains

Table 3.3 Sugar paste

Ingredient	Thin paste	Thick paste
caster sugar	1200 g	1200 g
icing sugar (additive free, powdered sucrose)	1800 g	1800 g
polyethylene glycol 400	1416 ml	686 ml
hydrogen peroxide	23.1 ml	19ml

hydrogen peroxide, which is produced by enzymes secreted by the bees and is partly responsible for the antibacterial performance. Also, the high osmolarity of honey deprives bacteria of the water required to reproduce, which, partnered with the 'withdrawing' of fluid from within the bacterial cells, provides a strong antibacterial action. Honey has recently received increased attention and a resurgence of interest. Dunford (2000) reports that honey is thought to resolve infection, reduce odour, promote debridement and stimulate tissue regeneration.

Dry dressings

Wood (1976) found that cotton gauze rapidly disintegrates when wound exudate is absorbed and that cotton fibres could be found in 10 per cent of the wounds (a focus for infection) following removal of a cotton gauze dressing. However, Lawrence (1997) and Thomas (1997c) critiqued this research and found no evidence to suggest that fibres within the wound actually cause infection. Wood had confused the materials used in the research and it is possible that the warp fibres of the dressing were in fact rayon/viscose.

Dry dressings also permit the wound to dry out very quickly, leaving the surface of the wound dry and forcing epithelial cells to migrate through the deeper dermal tissue, so delaying wound healing (Winter 1962). The cotton gauze also allows angiogenesis to take place through the holes of the gauze, so that removal of the dressing tears the newly formed capillaries and causes bleeding. Any adherence of dressings should inform the practitioner not to use that same dressing again on that individual patient.

Although Winter's work (see Chapter 1) has probably become the most quoted research, it should be noted here that his work looked at epithelialization as the end product of healing. He found that the epithelial tissue did not migrate easily across dry granulation tissue and this slowed the final healing. His work did not show what happens when a dry dressing is used on a very wet and sloughy wound.

Nevertheless, dry dressings, of any kind, can adhere to a low exudate wound surface. This is due to the exudate forming a 'glue like' material as it dries (Thomas 1994) and causing the adherence. Thomas points out another problem when a dressing is left undisturbed for a while; small capillary loops may penetrate the structure of the dressing effectively incorporating it into the newly formed tissue. These loops will be torn away when the dressing is removed and will cause pain and bleeding within the wound bed.

Protection against overhydrated skin

Overhydrated skin can be found in incontinence, around stomas, around peri-wound areas and between toes. Wet or damp skin is not an immediate problem but prolonged moisture can increase tissue permeability, which increases potential for bacterial or fungal colonization and will increase potential for maceration and excoriation. Skin breakdown associated with incontinence is a complex cascade of interacting events that weaken the skin and make it vulnerable to further damage, particularly from clothing, bed-linen and poorly designed body-worn underpads (Jeter and Lutz 1996).

The elderly are particularly at risk of contact dermatitis as loss of skin turger and minute cracks in the dry skin increase the potential of colonization of microorganisms. Protection from overhydration of the skin must also include moisturization of the tissues to promote the balance between cell formation and desquamation.

Tissue must be kept free from prolonged contact with moisture and irritants. Body shaped underpads can be used which often contain a wicking gel to ensure the skin is kept dry. The large non-body-worn pads, can 'pill' (roll into small lumps within the pad), reflect urine onto the skin and crease, causing 'hot-spots' of pressure under the patient. It is advisable to use these pads for procedures only and to assess the patient's individual needs for provision of body-worn pads. It is unknown whether the use of creams affects the surface of body-worn underpads although work suggests that it may have an effect if applied liberally. There are moves to provide washable/reusable cloth pads for incontinent patients as this reduces cost and supports the ecological concerns associated with disposal of paper pads.

There are certain manufacturers that provide pads designed for males with 'dribble' incontinence problems. These pads fit around the penis and provide a sense of security. An alternative to pads could be urinary sheaths, which are available for men and urinary pouches, available for women. The urinary pouches are difficult to apply and retain but offer incontinent women some security.

To provide high-quality care, incontinent patients must receive good holistic assessment to ensure their full potential of continence is evaluated, with advice and education given as a priority.

There is a possibility that pelvic floor exercises and losing weight may have a significant effect on the problem.

Creams can successfully protect the skin against overhydration. However, care should be taken to choose creams that are without lanolin or that contain hypoallergenic lanolin. Creams may contain preservatives such as parabens, which often cause sensitivities or allergic skin reactions.

Pastes are created by adding powder to ointment and this creates a thick, visible covering for the skin. However, pastes may be difficult to remove and vigorous cleansing may reduce the positive effects of the paste. To remove zinc-oxide paste, a mineral oil should be used rather than soap and water (Kemp 1994).

Ointments are an excellent way of protecting the skin because there is less potential for contact dermatitis. If creams or ointments are easily removed from the skin, they are unlikely to be durable in the presence of faeces or urine. The skin should never be washed with soap and water. Aqueous cream/emollients should be the cleanser of choice. When choosing products to clean or protect the skin, consideration should be given to ensuring the pH level of the product is within the desirable range (4–7) (Fiers 1996).

An excellent product produced for skin protection is liquid film (Cavilon, SuperSkin). These can be painted onto the skin and, when dry, will protect the tissues against incontinence or maceration. Catheterization must be the last choice in prevention of overhydration of the skin as use of catheters may lead to urinary tract infection. Peri-wound areas are particularly difficult to treat as the required adherence of dressings limits the use of creams and ointments. Cavilon film dressing and Super-Skin are both liquid, non-sting films that, when dry, present a surface that will protect the lower tissues whilst allowing the dressing to adhere.

There is an added benefit that these films may protect the skin against contact dermatitis or allergic reactions to the dressings.

Protection for dry skin

Legs are often found to have dry skin, particularly under bandages when legs have not been washed in a bucket of water. It is important to cleanse the tissues surrounding the wound rather than the wound itself. This will offer some protection to the undamaged skin and prevent further breakdown. Emollients added to tap water, in a polythene bag-lined bucket, will reduce the potential for skin cracks and will restore lipids between the cells of the horny layer.

Emollients are useful as the liquid can replace soap during washing patients' 'at risk' areas such as perineum, sacrum and legs. The different brands of emollients have differing consistencies of oil. The emollient is added to water and application to skin forms a barrier over the surface of the stratum corneum, trapping water underneath it. This build-up of water then passes back into the stratum corneum, reducing further cracking (Burr 1999). Legs can often benefit from application of paste or ointment bandages (e.g. zinc paste bandages or zipzoc).

Use of miscellaneous dressings

Occasionally, products can be sold by the manufacturer with the recommendation to use them together; gels and foams used in unison are unlikely to cause a problem within the wound. However, medical and nursing staff need to be aware that treating a pharmaceutical product in a way not recommended by the manufacturer could result in the user having to bear liability should a problem occur (Thomas 1990). Uniting one manufacturer's product with a different manufacturer's product could be seen as a product alteration at ward level and this alone could make the user liable in a court of law.

Products requested by the patient

The patient has a right to be responsible for decisions in their own wound treatment and the practitioner should listen and respect those decisions. If the treatment is considered unsuitable for the wound, then the practitioner should put the case for not using the product. Refusal to use it would lead to potential litigation should the wound deteriorate with use of the practitioner's choice of dressing. Although a court of law is likely to uphold the practitioner's decision, it would be an unpleasant experience for both patient and practitioner and would lead to resentment and a strong belief that, should the practitioner have used the patient's own dressing, the wound would have improved. Should a practitioner decide to use the patient's own requested dressings, it would be wise to keep a complete record of all that had been said and done.

One example of this was a patient who requested a mudpack on the wound. The immediate reaction was 'absolutely not'! On reflection, the patient had the right to request her specific treatment, the mudpack was recommended for wound treatment by the manufacturer and it had the potential to provide moisture, warmth and occlusion, thereby promoting an optimum healing environment. The mudpack (Moor-Life) was used under a semi-permeable film covering and the wound healed in eight weeks (Figures 3.5a and b). It would be difficult to say categorically what the healing influence had been in this wound as an air-mattress (Pegasus airwave) and the semi-permeable film would have both had an effect on the healing rate. However, the wound healed well and there were no detrimental effects from using the patient's own prescription. Indeed, the effects of the mudpack may well have been extremely beneficial to the wound.

When patients' own medicines have been administered, to allow full compliance with Consumer Protection regulations, it is required to generally retain records for 13 years (Thomas 1990).

Removal of dressings

Dressing removal is usually only a problem if dry dressings are used on a fairly dry wound. Trauma to the wound must be minimized and the following suggestions will facilitate easy removal:

- thoroughly soak the dressing with saline or tap water;
- leg ulcers can be thoroughly soaked in a plastic bag-lined bucket with tap water and added oil (with Oilatum, olive oil, arachis oil, etc. care must be taken to ensure there are no previous allergies to nuts, etc.);
- the dressing can be 'rolled' off the wound by using a downward pull;
- the patient can remove it (this generally causes less pain because the patient is in control);

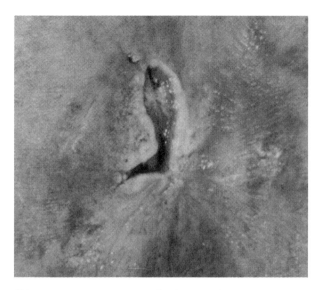

Figure 3.5a Wound prior to mudpack application (see Plate 19).

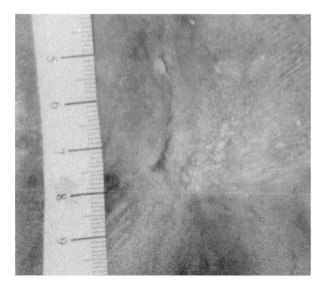

Figure 3.5b Healed wound after five weeks following regular mud applications (see Plate 20).

- a low-adherent dressing can be used beneath the dry dressing. (Telfa, Mepital, NA Ultra, Tegasorb, Omiderm). It should be noted that use of these dressings under interactive dressings such as the VAC may decrease the healing time.

Hyperbaric oxygen

Appropriate levels and delivery of oxygen is essential to wound healing and prevention of clinical infection. The process of healing demands a dramatic metabolic response and will utilize, and potentially deplete, oxygen reserves. The demand for energy could outstrip the supply and reduce available oxygen available to leucocytes for phagocytosis. Hyperbaric oxygen therapy is a non-invasive therapy. The patient breathes in 100 per cent oxygen whilst in a chamber which is pressurized to greater than normal atmospheric pressure (Senior 2000). Hyperbaric oxygen works by elevating the plasma oxygen level in proportion to the partial pressure of inspired oxygen. The involved process enables the oxygen to be delivered to the cells even in absence of haemoglobin (Senior 2000), ensuring the oxygen supply is rich for wound repair and leucocyte activity.

Wounds often fail to heal because the tissue is ischaemic and consequently starved of oxygen, nutrients and host defence cells that are essential to the healing process (Bowler et al. 2001). Oxygen tension variations are thought to increase healing (Hunt and Pai 1975). Hunt and Pai found that fibroblasts synthesize the molecules that comprise the extracellular matrix; increase of oxygen tension in the wound increases collagen synthesis by the fibroblasts. Wounds may suffer hypoxia for various reasons. Airways disease, anaemia or ischaemia, and some of the causes will not be affected by increased oxygen presentation (for example anaemia when there is no iron carrier). Hyperbaric oxygen refers to a deliberately elevated partial pressure of oxygen delivered through a whole body oxygen chamber or through topical hyperbaric therapy. Whole body chambers are relatively rare, are available only in specialist centres and may be potentially dangerous (Bale 1992). Topical hyperbaric oxygen is relatively safe and can be performed in any hospital. However, topical hyperbaric oxygen only penetrates wounds to a depth of 70 microns and, therefore, will not be as effective as systemic hyperbaric oxygen.

High partial pressures of oxygen are useful in the treatment of anaerobic bacteria, such as gas gangrene and in necrotizing soft tissue infections (Neal 1994). In gas gangrene the main affect of hyperbaric oxygen is to stem the production of toxins from the bacteria, the most significant of which is Alpha toxin (Neal 1994). Alpha toxin is necro-toxic and cardiotoxic, resulting in cardiac instability (Neal 1994).

Fibroblast proliferation and angiogenesis are encouraged by a hypoxic environment (Moffatt 1992b) coupled with adequate oxygenation in the tissues. A suggestion for a future study may be to look at the results of providing hyperbaric oxygen whilst providing a hypoxic wound bed environment with negative pressure. If negative pressure offers increased angiogenesis and hyperbaric oxygen offers greater delivery of oxygen to the tissues, the two methods may well complement each other to increase healing and reduce bacterial contamination and infection.

Laser therapy

Low-power laser therapy is the application of light energy waves over a wound to stimulate the healing process. It is thought to increase cell proliferation, respiration, motility and the immune response. Low-level laser therapy is used at approximately 10 Joules cm^2 with powers of 50 mW (Flemming et al. 1999). Results of such studies show no significant improvement in healing rates when lasers are used although the studies were based on small sample numbers (Flemming et al. 1999).

The type of laser therapy used for wound treatment is photo-chemical, not thermal. The low-energy light triggers normal cellular function (Thor International 1993). Photons are absorbed in cytochromes and porphyrins within the mitochondria and at the cell membrane, with the visible red light absorbed within the mitochondria and the infrared light absorbed at the cell membrane. This creates changes in the cell membrane permeability, increase levels of adenosine triphosphate (ATP) levels and effects deoxyribonucleic acid production (DNA), all of which cause physiological changes within the wound (Thor International 1993). Physiological changes will involve the following:

- bradykinin;
- serotonin;
- macrophages;
- fibroblasts;

- keratinocytes;
- reduction in pain;
- reduction in inflammation.

Heparin

Heparin is an anticoagulant that prevents the uptake of vitamin K in the gut. Vitamin K is essential for the clotting process and, therefore, heparin acts as a useful anticoagulant in the treatment of cardiac patients and as a short-term treatment for those patients with deep vein thrombosis. The role of heparin in wound healing has been demonstrated *in vitro* and *in vivo* studies and is associated with rapid and effective endothelial cell repair (Galvan 1996). Patients with burns and diabetic foot ulcers showed an increase in capillary circulation and a decreased healing time (Galvan 1996).

The wound

The final problem, and often the patient's least worry, is the wound itself. When the patient's identified problems (pain, malodour, discharge) have been addressed and the wound is in a healing state, then provision of the optimum wound healing environment is essential (Table 1.1). It is at this point that the skill of the assessing nurse can be vital as selection of an inappropriate dressing may delay wound healing.

Hyaluronic acid dressings

It is thought that the presence of hyaluronic acid in the foetus is the reason for scarless healing, allowing regeneration rather than fibrosis (Devlin 1994). Iocono et al. (1998) found that chronic addition of hyaluronic acid to wounds of mice appeared to mimic the foetal dermal connective tissue. Dressings are now being designed and used to incorporate this feature and hyaluron is thought to cleanse a wound and promote healing.

Hyalofil is a dressing that is in the form of a non-woven material almost entirely composed of Hyaff – a 60 per cent esterified derivative of hyaluronic acid. Hyalofill is used to prepare wounds for treatment with cultured keratinocytes or to treat poorly healing wounds. When Hyalofill is in contact with serum or wound exudate, a hydrophilic gel is produced which creates a hyaluronic acid-rich environment. This provides the optimum wound healing environment.

Leeches

Leeches are an ancient treatment of disease and are known to have been used 2500 years ago (Cmiel 1990, cited by Coull 1993). The leech is a 32-segmented invertebrate, with each segment containing an elementary brain (Peel 1993b). The leech will seek its prey and fasten to the victim's surface by use of posterior suckers. The anterior sucker, which contains the mouth, then searches for an area to attach the three ridges of small sharp teeth, which saw into the host's skin. The leech then injects an analgesic substance into the tissues and the victim may report a slight burning as the leech attaches but that disappears quickly. The salivary glands of the leech produce an anticoagulant, hirudin, which enables the leech to feed without problems of clotting occurring.

Leeches are used to:

• reduce haemotomas;
• in plastic surgery to reduce venous congestion;
• to encourage blood flow into poorly perfused areas (see Cases 1 and 2).

Leeches will not attach to necrotic tissue or if the arterial supply is unsatisfactory. Therefore, leech rejection indicates a poor prognosis (Coull 1993).

In areas of bruising or micro-thrombi, the leech will suck out the congested blood causing prolonged bleeding up to 12 hours or more. The injection of hirudin, an anticoagulant, will inhibit blood clotting creating further bleeding which is further encouraged by the introduction of orgelase, an enzyme that increases blood flow.

Removing hungry leeches from their container of gel can be interesting. The author's (SH) first experience was to lift a leech with a gloved hand, using two fingers around the back of the leech's 'head'. The author found that the leech can mimic an elastic band, stretching and spinning to attach to the finger that was holding it. It was quickly dropped before it could attach to the gloved finger. The easiest methods of introducing leeches to tissue are:

1 Take the gel-bag to the patient and allow the leech to find the required area.
2 Lift the leech out of the container with a 'lollypop' stick and place on the area.

3   Using blunt forceps to lift the leech from the pot. If this method is
    used, the handling should be gentle.

If the leech refuses to attach, it can be encouraged by the application
of 5 per cent glucose solution to the area where the leech is required.
However, it is the author's opinion that this is not often successful
and probably not worth the effort of trying.

Once attached, the leech will feed for approximately 20 minutes
although this can be longer or shorter. The leech should be observed
during this period to ensure that is does not 'wander' to another area
on the patient or fall off and disappear. When feeding is complete,
the bite marks should be wiped free of clots to ensure that the wound
continues bleeding to enhance the beneficial effects of micro-
thrombi removal and blood supply stimulation. As bleeding is the
primary reason for applying leeches, consideration for the patient's
haemoglobin is important, particularly when more than one application of leeches is used.

The use of leeches in plastic surgery is specialized and likely to be
fairly common within that speciality. The use is less common in
general hospitals but is, nevertheless, useful when the occasion arises.

Case 1

An elderly lady with a haematoma that had caused her problems for two weeks (Figure 3.6). The haematoma circum-
vented the leg and was extremely painful. Excision was not
possible because of the size of the haematoma and the gel-like
substance of the clot. Leeches were suggested.

   The lady was not worried about having leeches applied,
she said she had 'seen worse in the war'. Three leeches were
applied, Larry, Garry and George (named by the ward nurses).
The suckers attached and then the heads came around so that
the leeches formed a letter C. The leeches then fed for approximately 20 minutes, and, as they fed, they pulsated and grew in
size. Once they had fed, they dropped away from the leg and
were easily picked up and placed in saline. The relief of pain

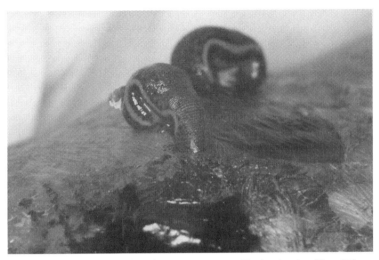

Figure 3.6 Elderly lady with a haematoma treated by leeches (see Plate 21).

was almost instant. The wounds continued to bleed for 12 hours and the haematoma had largely reduced by the morning. The wounds were encouraged to bleed by wiping away any crusts that formed over the bite areas.

One note of caution learned from this case was never to manhandle the leech when unfed. The author (SH) believed they could not expect an old lady to accept the leeches unless they were able to handle them when applying them. The leech was taken by the neck and lifted, with gloved fingers, free from the pot. The leech was able to extend and elongate its body so that it could turn and grasp a finger. The result was an undignified mess with the leech dropped. The author was terrified, the photographer was beside himself with laughter and the old lady looked heavenward at the stupidity of it all.

Three more leeches were applied 48 hours later. Following the use of leeches, the pain had gone, the tissues recovered and healed well.

Case 2

A young man presented with a large bruised area caused by a
fall from a ladder. The consultant wished the bruise to reduce
prior to discharge and requested leech therapy. The young
man was in a ward of other young men, all with something to
say about how he would feel when the leeches were applied.
He was determined to be outwardly brave about the procedure but appeared most uncomfortable with the idea when the
leeches appeared. The leeches were offered to the bruised area
and, apart from a slight burning sensation as they were
applied, he said he felt little. He became instantly worried
when he felt some of the liquid the leeches had been kept in,
running down his side and thought it was an escapee! A doctor
named the leeches Botham and Goff (obviously a cricket fan!).

The patient named one leech as David, as his brother was
David and the patient had always 'felt he was a bit of a leech'.
The leeches were attached for 30 minutes and the sites bled for
approximately 14 hours following leech removal. The success
of the mission can be seen in Figures 3.7a and 3.7b.

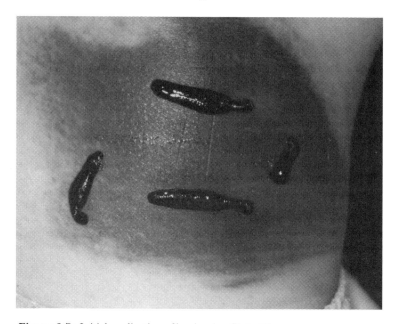

Figure 3.7a Initial application of leeches (see Plate 22).

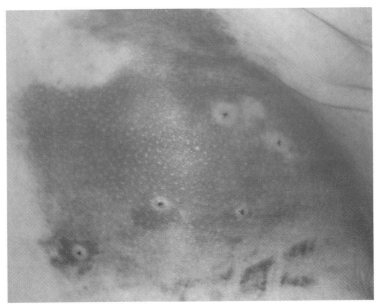

Figure 3.7b Twenty-four hours post leech application (see Plate 23).

Useful information

Leeches must be sterile and previously unfed although they can be kept unfed for six months. They will generally attach to the area that is presented to it. Therefore, placing the leech container in the area where the bite is required usually ensures the leech attaches to the correct site. Any wandering leech should be quickly brought back to the required area before it attaches in the wrong place. Once attached, removal is difficult because the teeth can be torn away if removal is attempted. Leech wounds will continue to bleed for 12–48 hours. This can be encouraged by cleaning the bite wounds to remove any clots that may form during this time.

They can be reapplied to the same patient, providing they have disgorged the blood. This can be messy as it is done through either placing the leech in five per cent saline solution for one minute or by squeezing the blood out by rolling the leech like a tube of toothpaste. The leeches are often reluctant to feed the second time and this has been likened to having a curry on a Saturday night, being ill and then being expected to eat another meal!

Leeches are cannibalistic and, if placed with unfed leeches, will be drained of the blood they have engorged. Once fed, they then contain blood products and must be destroyed by placing them in five per cent alcohol for a few minutes then into 95 per cent alcohol. They can then be disposed of through incineration.

Leeches cost £9 each at the time of writing.

Infrared treatment for wounds

Infrared treatment for wounds is undergoing a revival. Infrared stimulates the production of nitrous oxide in the deep dermis. Nitrous oxide was once called the endothelial cell derived relaxing factor and has been shown to have a vital role in promoting normal blood flow (Bliss 1998). Therefore, nitrous oxide causes vasodilation and offers increased exchange of oxygen and nutrients to the area where the collagen matrix is being built.

The infrared light is placed on the wound for half an hour either daily or three times per week. The wound seems to have a reduced exudate production and can appear dry although the healing rate appears to markedly increase.

Alternative therapy in wound care

The use of alternative therapy in wound care is undergoing a process of change. There are groups who strongly believe in the benefits, groups who do not believe and groups with little opinion either way. Whatever the belief of the practitioner, unlicensed alternative medicines cannot be used in patient care without a doctor's prescription or the agreement of the trust or employer. When the use of an alternative medical product is agreed by the employer, medical prescriber and/or ethics committee, the practitioner deciding on the product should be qualified in the use of alternative medicines. Anything less would be a disservice to the patient.

There are some dressings, however, whose use is not advised in wound care (Morgan 1997b):

• Fucidin Intertulle (antibiotic, can be responsible for bacterial resistance);

- Sofra-Tulle (antibiotic, can be responsible for bacterial resistance);
- Cicatrin (antibiotic, can be responsible for bacterial resistance);
- Topical antibiotics (can be responsible for bacterial resistance);
- Chlorinated solutions.

Dressing sensitivities

Allergy is often used interchangeably with hypersensitivity (Fox 1996) and refers to an abnormal response to allergens. Immediate hypersensitivity can form a dramatic reaction to a dressing with atopic dermatitis and other symptoms. This is the result of antibodies of the IgE class. Delayed hypersensitivity can take hours or days to develop and are a cell-mediated T lymphocyte response (Fox 1996). If a dressing is causing the sensitivity, there will be a distinct and dusky red mark in the shape of the dressing around the wound area. The symptoms are pain, itching, stinging and burning and signs can vary from erythema to frank eczema (Cameron and Powell 1996). Treatment would be discontinuation of the dressing and possibly antihistamines and/or short-term topical corticosteroid therapy.

Sometimes, the peri-wound area will appear to have an allergic reaction when it is actually due to the exudate from the wound. Dressings sometimes do not absorb or have absorbed all the fluid of which they are capable and then holds the exudate under the dressing and against the wound. This macerates or possibly 'burns' the good tissue, leaving either a dusky red or bright red mark in the shape of the dressing. It is, therefore, often difficult to distinguish whether the area is due to hypersensitivity to the dressing or exudate. The wise decision would be to select an alternative and more absorbent dressing. In either case, use of a skin barrier film, such as Cavilon or Super-Skin, would protect the delicate peri-wound area.

A problem may be lack of professional understanding or lack of skill in defining wound infection, dressing sensitivity or natural discolouration of the tissues. A sensitivity to dressings will nearly always have clear demarcation lines to the redness that follows the shape of the dressing (Figure 3.8). The treatment is to remove the dressing and never use it on that patient again. However, patients with long-standing leg ulcers are often hypersensitive to many dressings, making dressing selection and treatment difficult.

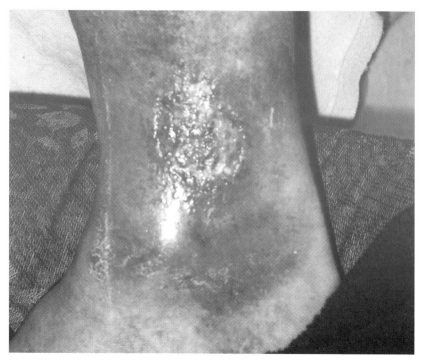

Figure 3.8 A clear demarcation line created by an inappropriate dressing (see Plate 24).

Iodine in wound management

Neutrophils discharge the enzyme myloperoxidase – catalysing the conversion of acids which are potent oxidants. In addition, to myloperoxidase, the neutrophil granules contain two metallopro-teinases that attack proteases. Myloperoxidase utilizes iodide and, together with the metalloproteinases, the enzymes form a killing zone around the activated neutrophil (Ganong 1995).

Myloperoxidase has an affinity for iodide, which is possibly remarkable for wound care. The body absorbs iodine from iodine dressings, and converts it to iodide a form that myloperoxidase can utilize in its performance as a 'killing machine'. At the same time, iodine has a high kill rate of its own. Goldheim (1993b) and McLure and Gordon (1992) found that povidone-iodine achieved a full kill rate with all 33 strains of clinical isolates whereas chlorhexidine elim-inated only three of the 33 strains (P value of <0.001). Therefore, it is possible that iodine dressings may increase healing rates, protect against bacterial colonization/ infection by reducing bacterial contamination (using the internal mechanism of myloperoxidase) and at the same time, killing bacteria in the wound bed itself, by the antiseptic action.

Alginate dressings

Alginate dressings are made from seaweed, create a hydrophilic gel in the presence of exudate and have a high content of calcium. A large number of reactions in mitochondria are calcium-dependent and calcium can thus be regarded as an intracellular messenger by which particular reactions are speeded up whilst others are slowed. The transport of calcium across the mitochondrial membrane can be seen as an important cellular control mechanism. Some alginates are high in mannuronic acid (MA) whilst others are high in galuronic acid (GA). MA and GA are obtained from different parts of the seaweed plant. Otterlei et al. (1991) reported that MA alginates were ten times more potent in inducing cytokine production than the GA alginates, although these findings were disputed by Klock et al. (1994).

Morgan (1996) writes:

> A reverse action occurs when calcium alginate fibres are placed in a solution containing an excess of sodium ions: calcium ions on the fibre are replaced by sodium and the material becomes soluble. Thus when in contact with serum or wound exudate, the insoluble calcium alginate is partially converted to the soluble sodium salt. A hydrophilic gel is produced over the wound providing an ideal moist wound-healing environment and pain-free dressing changes.

When a blood vessel is damaged, a mixture of clotting factors utilizes calcium to initiate the clotting cascade; therefore, calcium is an important part of stabilizing the wound. Alginate dressings are used to stem the flow of haemorrhage (or simple bleeding wounds) because of the dressing's content of calcium and the resultant haemostatic properties. The alginate absorbs exudate, releases calcium into the wound in exchange for sodium. This initiates the clotting cascade, thereby speeding up wound repair. However, *in vivo*, a plasma calcium level low enough to interfere with blood clotting, is incompatible with life (Ganong 1995).

Hydrocolloids

Hydrocolloids provide an ideal wound healing environment (Table 3.4) with one of the most important features being occlusion and protection against bacteria contamination (particularly MRSA). It takes an average of 8.5 days, *in vitro*, for bacteria to penetrate the hydrocolloid (Dunn and Wilson 1990).

Table 3.4 Dressings to promote autolysis

Hydrogels
Hydrocolloids
Cadexomer iodine
Film dressings
Tenderwet
Any wet dressings will promote autolysis

Hydrocolloids generally have an outer protective layer that, not only prevents bacterial contamination, but also prevents exudate 'strike through'. The inner adhesive layer contains hydrophilic particles surrounded by a hydrophobic polymer. The hydrophilic particles absorb exudate and swell into a gel, which moulds into the wound keeping the wound moist but not wet. The adhesive layer often contains colophony, a substance that is tacky to the touch and gives the dressing it's ability to adhere but may be allergenic. The hydrocolloid pastes do not contain colophony and, therefore, are less likely to cause allergic reactions; the patient can bath or shower with the dressing *in situ*. However, some hydrocolloid dressings have a distinctive malodour, which can be distressing for some patients. The anaerobic condition provided by the hypoxic environment encourages angiogenesis.

Hydrogels

Amorphous hydrogels are water donating and have water as the main dressing constituent. The high water content (70–90 per cent water) keeps the wound moist, reduces pain by 'bathing' nerve endings and aids debridement of necrotic tissue (Table 3.5). The gel can increase the potential for maceration in heavily exuding wounds. The type of secondary dressing used can influence the bacterial and fluid permeability of the hydrocolloid (Choucair and Phillips 1998).

Table 3.5 Factors that positively influence exudate production

Hydrostatic pressure
Wound infection
Wound colonization
Temperature
Wound type
Type of dressing

(Thomas, 1997)

Silicone-gel sheets have a stable, cross-linked macrostructure and retain their physical form as they absorb fluid (Jones and Milton 2000). They are being used successfully in clinical investigations to reduce the severity of hypertrophic scarring in burn rehabilitation and on grafts. A result of a study completed by Torres et al. (1998) showed there was a better hydration of the epidermis and a defined improvement of skin quality. The conclusion of the study is that silicon-gel sheets are a good alternative to pressure garments for the reduction of scarring.

Regenerative biological engineering or 'artificial skin'

Tissue engineering or construction of tissues outside the human body represents a valuable alternative to the management of tissue replacement (Abatangelo 1998). In cultures *in vitro* it is impossible to achieve the three-dimensional structure found *in vivo*. Therefore, a scaffold or dermal-like supports must be produced to provide cells with an appropriate environment to grow (Abatangelo 1998). Therefore, cultured dermis consists of neonatal dermal fibroblasts cultured *in vitro* on a biosorbable polyglactin (Vicryl) mesh (Grey et al. 1998). This cultured tissue is thought to replace damaged tissue with living healthy dermal tissue consisting of collagen, fibronectin, glycosaminoglycans and growth factors (Grey et al. 1998).

Stocum (1998) writes:

> Biodegradable artificial matrixes can induce dermal regeneration in excisional skin wounds, although the regeneration is imperfect. The matrixes consist of collagen or gelatin sponges to which other components such as chindroitin 6-sulfate or elastin are added. Fibroblasts migrate from the surrounding dermis into the matrix, altering the matrix dermis to a more normal construction.

Apligraft is the first full thickness, living bilayered allogenic human skin equivalent consisting of keratinocytes and fibroblasts from neonatal foreskins and type 1 bovine collagen (Falanga 1998). It is an active material, capable of responding to different environments and wound types (Parenteau et al. 1998). Falanga's (1998) work showed that healing with Apligraft plus compression was almost three times faster than use of compression alone. A bacterial load of $>10^5$ adversely effects Apligraft take and, therefore, the bacterial load should be assessed prior to applying the dressing (Raman and Sibbald 1998).

Dermagraft is a dermo-replacement containing human skin fibroblasts and naturally occurring extracellular matrix proteins (Martin et al. 1998). Martin et al. found that Dermagraft enhances angiogenesis.

Oasis is a tissue derived extracellular matrix that promotes tissue-specific growth and differentation of cells *in vitro*.

Integra is a dermal regeneration template that is a bilayer skin replacement system designed to provide immediate wound closure and permanent regeneration of dermis. The lower layer consists of collagen/glycosaminoglycan and is a 3-dimensional matrix of cross-linked collagen and glycosaminoglycan.

Growth factors

Platelet-derived growth factor (PDGF) (see Chapter 1) is the most highly researched factor with some evidence that it increases wound healing and is largely used in diabetic ulceration. Growth factors are found in the alpha granules of platelets and can be released using thrombin. An obtainable growth factor dressing is 0.01 per cent becaplermin gel (Regranex). It is hoped that application of growth factors in a non-healing wound will correct the body's natural growth factor deficiencies. However, not all growth factors are responsible for healing and some will 'switch off' the healing process. The restorative process of wound healing is often considered to be a biological default mechanism in the event that regeneration does not take place (Carlson 1998). Most cells will not survive if separated from a direct blood supply of more than a few microns. Therefore, vascularization of engineered tissues is encouraged by use of very thin layers so that cells can survive by diffusion until vascular sprouts can grow in them (Carlson 1998).

Alternative therapy dressing

Aloa vera

Aloe vera has potential in wound care as it's healing properties have been known for thousands of years; it belongs to the lily family and is related to the onion, garlic and asparagus (Atherton 1998). The aloe plant is 99–99.5 per cent water with an average pH of 4.5, and 75 other ingredients including vitamins, minerals, enzymes, sugars, sterols, amino acids and salicylic acid (Atherton 1998).

Aloe vera appears to speed up healing through:

- providing essential micronutrients;
- providing an anti-inflammatory effect;
- providing an anti-microbial effect;
- the stimulation of skin fibroblasts (Atherton 1998).

Tea tree oil

Tea tree oil is derived from the Australian tea tree *Melaleuca alternifolia* and is thought to possess antimicrobial properties. Faoagali et al. (1997) identified its usefulness in *Staphylococcus aureas* but concluded from the study that the cytotoxicity in wounds may lead to increased scarring and delayed healing. There may be value in using tea tree oil as an environmental protection against *Staphylococcus aureas* and MRSA.

Propolis

Propolis is a resinous material produced by bees from the leaf buds and bark of trees (Trevelyan 1997). The bees prevent their beehive from invasion by sealing all openings with propolis and coat any intruders with the substance to prevent the rotting bodies from causing a threat (Trevelyan 1997). Trevelyan describes propolis as having 'Greater antibacterial activity than that of penicillin and other antibiotic drugs' and 'Propolis raises the body's natural resistance to infection through stimulation of the immune system' (Tyler 1987, cited by Trevelyan 1997). Work completed at Oxford University Biochemistry department, indicates that propolis has definite bacterial action against some types of bacteria and may increase the effect of antibiotics in removing bacteria.

Psychological aspect of wound healing

The practice of healing is often more art than science. Medical standards insist that all practice should be evidence based. Very little is written on the difference that the mind can make on wound healing. There is, of course, a physiological background to healing; stress has a chemical and physical response, with vasoconstriction being one of these responses. Stress and resultant vasoconstriction will undoubtedly delay healing. The patient may present with a malodorous and painful wound and is fearful that the practitioner will be unable to assist with the problem. The practitioner shakes his or her head when seeing the wound and the patient's fear immediately escalates.

Helpful in these situations is a 'magic wave of the hand', which goes with the expression 'I can sort that for you'. The patient becomes relaxed and feels confident that their problems will be dealt with. Vasodilation occurs and a greater exchange of oxygen and nutrients will be supported at the wound site. This 'magic wave' is probably 80 per cent of the healing accomplished. However, this has to be tempered with facts. If presented with an arterial ulcer or fungating tumour, healing may not be an option; reduction of pain and malodour may well be within the skills of the practitioner and may well be the solution for the patient.

Conclusion

Selection of an appropriate dressing is a skill that is achieved partly through obtaining knowledge and partly through 'hands-on' experience. Wound care cannot be learned from journals without the reflective experience of practically applying the knowledge that has been gained. Once the art of providing an ideal environment is achieved, then wound care becomes common sense. There has never been a magical dressing to heal all wounds although some dressings are more likely to achieve the ideal environment in certain wounds.

Chronic wounds inflict a huge cost on society and this requires attention. However, the cost of wound care cannot be addressed through use of inexpensive dressings, particularly if those dressings are inappropriate for the individual wound. Cost-effective wound care takes into account the length of time of healing as well as the individual cost of the dressings.

Wound care stands on the edge of a new era in wound healing. Growth factors, dispersion therapy, negative pressure, maintenance/ increasing wound bed temperature are all leading practitioners to a unique opportunity of healing wounds using pure science. Wounds will no longer be managed but will be treated with the most appropriate methods, selected through holistic assessment. Holistic assessment is vital because, unless the underlying pathology that is responsible for the delayed healing is addressed, the wound will not heal despite the application of resourceful and unique dressings. Clarifying the mechanisms by which wounds heal is vitally important and the future will rely on patient treatment not wound management.

Appendix 1 lists some of available dressings and describes how these dressings might be used.

Activity

When assessing a wound and deciding on a dressing, consider the optimum wound healing environment: what does this particular wound require to bring it to a healing state? Make notes of your conclusions and write down the aims. Decide what you would like to see happen to this wound over the next three dressing changes. Photograph the wound (with the patient's permission) at each dressing change three times. Take a wound map at each dressing change. Compare the three wound maps and photographs. Has the dressing you selected achieved your aim? If not, what might have happened to prevent the aim being achieved?

CHAPTER 4

Wound infection and colonization

There is a fine balance between environmental flora and skin flora and this balance maintains an equilibrium, determined by conditions such as skin moisture and pH balance (Thompson 1998) until there is a break in the human protective layer – the skin (Heggers 1998a). When a wound becomes 'chronic' (of longer duration than six weeks) then contamination or colonization, particularly through skin flora, is an almost certain consequence. Wounds generally harbour mixed flora of Gram-negative and Gram-positive aerobic or anaerobic organisms (Thompson 1998). The quantity of bacteria in a wound creates a potential for wound infection (Krizek and Robson 1975), which can lead to sepsis and death (Thompson 1998). Robson (1988) writes, 'Infection in a wound is a manifestation of a disturbed host-bacteria equilibrium in favour of the bacteria. This not only elicits a systemic response but actually inhibits the processes involved in wound healing'. Therefore, reduction in colonization must be an important consideration in wound healing. Harding (1996) states that 'work cited as long ago as 1970 suggests that optimal wound healing cannot be achieved unless bacteria are eliminated from wounds'. Danielsen et al. (1997) suggests that extracellular toxins produced by bacteria might interfere with the healing process with the responsible bacterial enzymes and metalloproteinases degrading fibrin and wound growth factors.

There are three main routes for the acquisition of bacteria by skin wounds:

1 Self-contamination by scratching, direct from the surrounding skin flora or gastrointestinal tract (often faecal organisms).

132

2 Airborne contamination through dust, skin squames or water droplets.
3 Contact contamination from unwashed hands, clothing, equipment or contact with the skin of carers.

Two major factors determine whether a wound will become infected:

1 Microorganic contamination of the wound.
2 The patient's resistance to that contamination (Kingsley 1992).

Many papers describe bacterial colonization/infection in wounds and the effect on delayed healing (Liedberg et al. 1955; Bendy et al. 1964; Harding 1996; Danielsen et al. 1997), but these generally look to antibiotics or antiseptics to reduce bacterial count. The nature of certain wounds will prevent the effectiveness of antibiotics, particularly in ischaemia, and antiseptics can be damaging to healing wound tissues (Leaper and Simpson 1986; Ferguson 1993). Indiscriminate use of antiseptics and antibiotics can lead to introduction of new resistant strains of bacteria such as methicillin-resistant *Staphylococcus aureus* (MRSA). MRSA is now endemic in hospitals and is the cause of life-threatening infection in patients. Antibiotics are now used with caution with antiseptics becoming more widely used in hospitals in the control of infection (Irizarry et al. 1996). However, the law of 'survival of the fittest' means that there may only be limited time before bacteria mutate and become antiseptic/disinfectant resistant.

Bacteria are some of the most abundant life forms on earth. Each bacterium is a single cell without nucleus and contains a single DNA chromosome carrying between 1000 and 5000 genes. Bacteria can reproduce every 20 minutes and, under some conditions, can produce millions of new cells every day; they can also mutate (Hampton 1997a). Bacteria are classically divided into Gram-positive and Gram-negative organisms depending on the reaction to gram staining (Lehninger 1975). Gram-negative cell walls are rich in lipids; Gram-positive cell walls contain very little lipid.

A wound bed will present with a slimy covering consisting of bacteria and dozens of cells. This slimy coating allows the bacteria to bury themselves where it is partially protected from phagocytes, lymphocytes, antibodies and (most importantly) antibiotics.

Patients with pressure sores are 49 per cent likely to also have bacteraemia with mortality rates of about 55 per cent (Bryan et al. 1983). Sugarman et al. (1983) found that nine out of 28 patients with a non-healing pressure sore had osteomylitis as a contributing factor.

Definitions

There is sometimes confusion between infected, colonized and contaminated wounds. The following is a working definition.

Infected wounds

Infected wounds are caused by microorganisms that evade the victim's immunological defences, enter and establish themselves within tissues of the potential host and multiply successfully (Gould 1994). A meeting of the European Tissue Repair Society and European Wound Management Society reached a consensus on the definition of an infected wound as follows (Leaper 1998):

- suppuration;
- cellulitis;
- lymphangitis;
- sepsis;
- bacteraemia;
- pyrexia;
- tachycardia;
- tachypnoea;
- raised white cell count.

An infected wound, therefore, will generally have positive clinical signs. Increased pain, copious exudate, malodour, cellulitis, pyrexia, abscess, increase in size of the wound and unwellness could all suggest clinical infection, which generally can be confirmed by swab results. The patient should be considered for antibiotics. Exudate may increase and the wound may enlarge. It will certainly be delayed in healing. Difficulty in identifying infection arises in patients who are immunologically compromised or elderly, who possibly may have subclinical infection with minimal symptoms. Swabs results are unreliable as they only take up surface bacteria and do not always expose the type of bacteria that is established within the tissues (discussed later in this chapter). The only reasonably accurate way of identifying clinical infection is through biopsy from the wound bed and this is not an acceptable option as it may increase risk of clinical infection. The professional should rely on host reaction to indicate clinical infection and, preferably, take a pus sample to identify the bacteria causing the infection. Dressings will not be effective whilst the clinical infection remains and selection should rely on supporting the symptoms of the infection (pain, discharge and odour) until the cellulitis subsides. The dressing selection can then be appropriate for a healing wound.

Colonized wounds

Multiplication of organisms without host reaction can be found in colonized wounds (Davis 1998). Signs of colonization can be increased pain, copious exudate and malodour linked with lack of cellulitis, pyrexia and malaise could suggest colonization. This can be confirmed by swab results ($<10^5$). Antibiotics are unnecessary in colonized wounds. Colonization may be reduced through use of dressings such as:

- slow release iodine cadexomer dressings, such as Iodoflex (Mertz et al. 1994);
- dressings containing silver such as Flamazine, Arglaes, Actisorb plus;
- dressings that remove bacteria by immobilizing bacteria within the matrix such as Algosteril (Bowler et al. 1999) and Aquacel.

Bacteria will nearly always be found in chronic wounds but are usually simple skin flora or faecal organisms. In colonized wounds, the bacteria sit within the wound exudate and multiply without invading the tissues. Antibiotics are unnecessary.

Contamination

Wound contamination occurs when organisms are present (within wound exudate) but not multiplying or clinically affecting the host (can be demonstrated by swab cultures). Antibiotics are unnecessary (Gould 1994).

Exogenous bacteria

These are present in the environment, on curtains, hands, floors, doctors' and nurses' hands and clothes. Wounds provide a poor environment for many microbial species to multiply and there is low risk of clinical wound infection from exogenous bacteria although acute wounds remain at risk (Cooper 1996b). To protect the wound from exogenous bacteria, wound dressing changes should not be undertaken during floor cleaning or when electric fans are being used to cool the room.

Endogenous bacteria

These bacteria survive on or within the host. It is endogenous bacteria that are likely to cause clinical infection post-operatively, particularly through dehiscence (Cutting 1998). Endogenous bacteria are generally harmless until the skin loses the protective layer and a wound has formed.

Identification of infected wounds

Undiagnosed clinically infected wounds can pose a problem as the wound may not heal or will be slow to heal. Infected wounds will also have increased exudate and malodour from the bacteria, and this can be distressful for the patient. Equally, the patient with a colonized wound is likely to be swabbed, which may result in inappropriate administration of antibiotics; this would be unwise. The over-prescribing of antibiotics has resulted in the emergence of MRSA (Davis 1998) and, as colonizing bacteria are in the wound exudate, not infecting the host, prescribing antibiotics will have minimal effect.

Erythema around the wound, plus pyrexia, are the obvious signs of clinical infection but patients who have diabetes or rheumatoid arthritis or who are elderly may present with subclinical infections. Subclinical infection should be suspected in a non-healing wound that is steadily increasing in size or one that is beefy red and easily bleeds. These symptoms may lead the practitioner to swab the wound. Swab results, demonstrating a bacterial count greater than 10^5 will indicate possible clinical infection or increased potential for infection.

Bacteria normally inhabit skin and the intestinal tract, and host and microbes generally live in harmony. Indeed, microbial communities often establish a relatively stable but interactive relationship with their human host without causing damage (Cooper 1996b). Microbial pathogens would need to compete with the normal inhabitants to establish themselves (Cutting 1998) and, therefore, it is the normal skin flora that is likely to colonize wounds. There is some evidence that bacterial contamination/colonization will not slow healing rates (Hutchinson 1992). However, Gilliand et al. (1988) and Schreibman (1990) disagree and claim that *Staphylococcus aureus*, *Pseudomonas* and β-haemolytic streptococci may have a detrimental affect on healing rates. Danielsen et al. (1997) also claim that wounds with *Pseudomonas aeruginosa* sometimes enlarge, despite compression therapy. Tengrove et al. (1996) found that the number of types (i.e. four or more types) of bacteria present affected wound healing rather than the specific type of bacteria.

Culture and sensitivity: swabbing technique

A chronic wound will nearly always test positive to bacteria as colonization will be almost a certainty. If colonization is more likely than clinical infection and given that granulating or epithelializing wounds are placed at risk when swabbed due to trauma of the new tissues (Towler 2001), then wounds should not be swabbed unnecessarily. However, when infection is suspected and if a swab is considered necessary, the technique should be precise although a gold standard for wound swabbing has never been identified. Donovan (1998) looked at nurses swabbing techniques and found that only one nurse had been taught a technique for swabbing wounds. Donovan suggests that, although surface swabs are the most common method, this only reflects colonization within the wound and will not identify the microbes that have invaded the host tissues. As the bacterial content of wound exudate may be different to those trapped in deeper tissues, true reflection of a clinical infection would rely on a tissue biopsy from the within the wound; however, this is likely to be too painful for the patient. Gilchrist (1994) points out that chronic wounds have a concentration gradient with a decreasing number of bacteria toward the wound surface. This indicates that biopsy would be the only accurate means of assessing quantities of bacterial contamination or infection.

Several authors have suggested various ways of obtaining a swab. Each author appears to recommend a different method and it is uncertain whether wounds should be cleaned prior to swabbing (Cooper and Lawrence 1996) or not cleaned prior to swabbing (Gilchrist and Reed 1989). There is also debate on the method of swabbing with Cooper and Lawrence (1996) and Donovan (1998) suggesting a zigzag motion with simultaneous twirling and sampling small areas (probably more commonly used in general practice).

Donovan recommends the following method of swabbing:

1 Initiate swabbing prior to the administration of antibiotics.
2 Irrigate the wound with warm normal saline to remove surface contamination.
3 Moisten the swab with saline or transport medium.
4 Use a zigzag motion across the wound, rotating the swab between the fingers.
5 Sample the whole wound surface area.
6 Place the swab immediately in the transport medium.
7 Ensure rapid delivery of the swab to the laboratory.

If the wound has undermining, the swab procedure should include insertion into the enclosed cavity.

There is also the difficulty associated with obtaining accurate results through wound swabbing. As swabbing will only identify bacteria in wound exudate and not the bacteria causing a host reaction, there is a strong argument for not swabbing wounds unless there is identifiable host reaction (redness, swelling, pain). Results should also be reviewed with caution, understanding that the results may not reflect what is actually occurring in the wound tissues.

Bacterial types, their affect on wound healing, identification and prevention of infection

Staphylococcus aureus

Nearly all chronic wounds will be colonized with bacteria. The commonest bacteria is *Staphylococcus aureus*, a Gram-positive and generally a non-pathogenic organism. It is spherical in shape approximately 1 micron in diameter and clusters together in groups that appear grape-like (Figure 4.1). In fact, staphyle is Latin for a ' bunch of grapes'. *Staphylococcus aureus* is non-motile and an opportunistic pathogen with a cell wall that has rigid structure, consisting of parallel polysaccharide chains covalently cross-linked by peptide chains. It destroys tissues when it forms an abscess and can be found in 30 per cent of the population (Parker 1979), possibly within the nasal passage with little, or more likely, no effects from the colonization. Various strains of this species produce toxins including those that cause food poisoning and toxic shock syndrome. When cultured on agar, *Staphylococcus* produces white, yellow or orange coloured colonies. When colonizing a wound, it produces distinctive golden-yellow pus.

Problems occur when patients have a wound that is contaminated by *Staphylococcus aureus* or MRSA as this will potentially slow down the healing process, possibly increasing the hospital stay. There is always a potential for moribund patients to succumb to clinical infection following MRSA colonization, and morbidity can be increased (Esuvaranathan et al. 1992). Therefore, MRSA can have a cost implication for the hospital as well as the distress experienced by the patient. The delay in wound healing and the potential for clinical infection can be life-threatening to moribund patients.

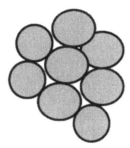

Figure 4.1*Staphylococcus aureas* appears to cluster like bunches of grapes.

Staphylococcus aureus has the ability to produce the enzyme coagulase. This enzyme will clot plasma and protect the bacteria against host defence mechanisms (Griffiths-Jones 1995).

Streptococcus

Streptococcus is a Gram-positive bacteria, oval in shape and unites together like strings of beads. Some kinds of streptococci discolour or destroy red blood cells and are called haemolytic streptococci. A wound infected by streptococci is likely to be beefy red in colour, possibly painful and friable. It is the second most common bacteria found in wounds. Oedema counteracts the skin's defences against β-haemolytic streptococci, the organism localizes in oedematous tissues (Heggers 1998a).

Pseudomonas aeruginosa

Pseudomonas aeruginosa is a rod shaped, Gram-negative, opportunistic bacterium that is notoriously resistant to antimicrobial therapy due to the presence of a relatively impermeable outer membrane layer (Cooper and Molan 1999). Cooper and Molan believe that the effect of *Pseudomonas aeruginosa* on wound healing has been underestimated; it may have a greater significance in wound healing than previously thought and may delay healing considerably. This is also the belief of Daltrey et al. (1981). Experience of colonization of *Pseudomonas* suggests that it not only delays healing but also increases the potential for pain. If *Pseudomonas* is reduced, pain often decreases in the wound.

Pseudomonas is a motile rod that will rapidly colonize humidifiers, sinks, flower vases and buckets of water, even when those buckets contain disinfectants. It can also grow in sterile solutions and can contaminate ointments (Gibson 1979). Wounds colonized by *Pseudomonas aeruginosa* are likely to have (sometimes almost fluorescent) green exudate (Figure 2.6) due to two coloured pigments: pyocyanin, which produces blue pigments, and fluorescein, which produces a yellow-red colour. *Pseudomonas aeruginosa* has a musty and almost sweet odour that can be detected by nurses even when they are many meters away from the colonized wound. There may be increased pain and there will certainly be an increase in exudate production. Patients with *Pseudomonas* often arrive at hospital with several layers of Gamgee over their dressings to soak up the exudate. *Pseudomonas* responds well to silver sulphadiazine, providing it is not applied over a long period of time (one to two applications only). If the silver sulpha-diazine is continuously used, it appears to lower the local immunity and *Pseudomonas* returns with low-grade contamination.

Necrotizing fasciitis

Necrotizing fasciitis is an uncommon complication in the UK, although it is more common in poorer countries, such as Bulgaria, where surgeons can expect to treat at least four patients with necro-tizing fasciitis, at any one time. Nevertheless, there may be confusion over the definition of the disease as there have been a variety of terms used to describe the infection (Douglas 1996):

• hospital gangrene;
• suppurative fasciitis;

- necrotizing erysipeles;
- acute dermal gangrene;
- acute infective gangrene;
- haemolytic *Streptococcus* gangrene.

The infection is a serious bacterial infection and is usually due to *Streptococcus pyogenes* but can sometimes be caused by *Staphylococcus aureus*. 'The affected area is initially red, hot, swollen and painful and the inflammation spreads rapidly. Dusky purple patches occur over the inflamed area and this is the pathogenic sign' (Laing 1998). The dark patches progress to gangrene and this can spread rapidly.

Treatment for necrotizing fasciitis is early diagnosis, surgical debridement and early administration of broad spectrum antibiotics (Douglas 1996).

Asepsis

Aseptic technique is designed to prevent bacteria from reaching vulnerable sites. The method of achieving asepsis relies on excellent hand-washing techniques, use of sterile equipment and a non-touch technique when caring for patient's wounds or catheterizations.

Historically, there have been many interesting techniques for ensuring that pathogens are not introduced to vulnerable areas and knowledge of these techniques was mostly passed from nurse to nurse and, as in Chinese whispers, the methods can alter as the whisper is passed along. However, asepsis has never been fully researched and there are still rumours and beliefs about the 'right' way to apply asepsis. Work completed by Kelso (1989) demonstrated that aseptic technique using two forceps, was complex and nurses often failed asepsis without knowing that they had done so. When excellence of hand washing was used together with a simple procedure, nurses were less likely to make a mistake and the simplified technique was as microbiologically safe as the non-touch technique using forceps. Forceps may also cause mechanical damage to the wound bed and, therefore, it is advisable to use a gloved hand in place of forceps. Thomlinson (1987) looked at three techniques of wound cleansing, forceps, gloved hand or bare hand washed in Hibsol. This study found that none had a clear advantage and that all methods, instead of removing bacteria, simply redistributed them around the wound. Healthy wounds also contain essential growth factors and defence cells and, therefore, cleansing the wound with saline may be detrimental to healing (Oliver 1997).

The patient should be protected against clinical infection at all costs and excellence of hand washing is the single most important part of that prevention. It is advisable to use unsterile gloves on chronic wounds and never to cleanse wounds unnecessarily (leg ulcers are nearly always soaked in a bucket of tap water to treat the whole leg).

Patients with pressure ulcers may develop infections as part of the process of tissue damage. When tissues are deprived of blood, the inflammatory process begins and bacteria are attracted to the damaged tissues. The tissue deterioration, from redness to skin loss, occurs rapidly and is thought (in part) to be due to the bacteria within the local tissues (Robson and Heggers 1969). Heggers (1998b) cited work completed by Robson, which demonstrated that pressure ulcers might have microbial proliferation that is 100 times greater than other wounds.

Some bacteria are dependent on oxygen for growth and these are called aerobic bacteria. Others are anaerobic and can be found buried beneath necrotic tissue and are partly responsible for the malodour in pressure ulcers. There is a third type of bacteria that can exist in both an oxygenated and a hypoxic environment. These are facultative anaerobes and high-pressure oxygen inhibits their growth with a kill rate that equals antibiotic therapy (Donlin and Bryson 1995).

Antibiotics

Antibiotics were used widely during the 1960s and 1970s with disastrous consequences for today.

Sir Alexander Fleming discovered penicillin in mould in 1928 and led the way to production of antibiotic drugs and the belief that these may eradicate infectious disease. However, bacteria are an example of Darwin's theory of 'survival of the fittest' and in 1961, following over-enthusiastic administration of antibiotics worldwide, methicillin-resistant *Staphylococcus aureus* (MRSA) was reported for the first time (Taylor 1990). We are now aware that antibiotics are creating a new species of super-resistant microbials and this limits the use of prophylactic antibiotics.

In 1976, a new gentamicin-resistant strain emerged (Duckworth et al. 1988), which was found to be more difficult to control as it spread despite precautions of patient isolation (Simpson 1992). Simpson writes 'In 1983 only one regional health authority reported no evidence of MRSA and from 1980 Epidemic MRSA became the most common reported strain of MRSA in Britain'.

MRSA is now endemic in hospitals and is the cause of life-threatening infections in patients (Irizarry et al. 1996). Antibiotics are used with caution now and antiseptics and disinfectants are becoming more widely used in hospitals in the control of infection (Irizarry et al. 1996). However, the law of 'survival of the fittest' means that there may only be limited time before bacteria mutate and become antiseptic/disinfectant resistant.

Penicillins and cephalosporins target most Gram-positive bacterial (and some Gram-negative) cell walls and interfere with the cells' osmotic pressure. This ensures that the cells cannot function, collapse occurs and the cells die. Gram-negative bacteria are usually resistant to antibiotics with this mode of action.

Topical antibiotics are to be avoided as resistant strains often emerge from their use (Cooper 1996b).

With the emergence of resistant strains of bacteria such as MRSA, the use of antibiotics is decreasing. Antibiotics must only be prescribed in wound care when there is clinical evidence of an infection and, even then, the prescription should rely on the swab results, which identify any sensitivities. Sensitivity is ascertained through use of bacteria containing culture plates. Some of the plates also contain antibiotics of differing types. The plates are left to culture for some hours and then measurement of the inhibited areas of bacteria will give an indication of sensitivities.

Clinically infected wounds should always be treated systemically (Gilchrist 1994) and choice of dressing is almost irrelevant until cellulitis is under control. Infected wounds will not heal, even with the most advanced of dressings, therefore, use of expensive dressings are pointless and inexpensive but absorbent dressings are a reasonable option at this time. The selected dressing should rapidly remove bacteria from the surface of the wound. This may be done through the use of hydrophilic dressings (Johnson 1987) which absorb high amounts of exudates and bacteria.

Antibiotic types

- **Penicillin** is a bactericide, destroying the bacteria by interfering with the synthesis of the bacterial cell wall. Useful in *streptococci* and *Staphylococci aureus* infections.
- **Cephalosporins** have a similar bactericidal to penicillin. They are rarely used but can be useful in Gram-positive and some Gram-negative bacterial infections.
- **Metronidazole** is bactericidal and used against anaerobic infections. Often used to eliminate malodour in wounds in the form of oral or intravenous medication or through topical gel application. (Malodour can be caused by colonization of anaerobic bacteria.)
- **Erythromycin** is bacteriostatic and works by blocking protein-synthesis. This will prevent the reproduction of bacteria, causing the microbes to remain 'static'.

Cleansing wounds

Nurses were traditionally taught to always clean a wound with sterile saline or antiseptics. Today, research has shown that cleansing wounds may actually be harmful, and in some instances, use of saline unnecessary and use of antiseptics inadvisable (Morgan 1993). Bacteria can also rapidly become resistant to antiseptics and, in the future, antiseptic use will be as limited as antibiotics are today (Hampton 1997a). Therefore, before cleaning a wound it is important to ask the question 'does the wound require cleaning?' Wound cleansing must have a rationale, and the fact that it makes the practitioner feel better to have performed a certain ritualistic task is not enough (Flanagan 1997).

Cleansing a wound is a controversial issue. Great store is placed on always maintaining warmth in the wound, with justification because lowering temperature will delay healing. However, chronic wounds are frequently filled with necrotic and colonized tissue and are in a non-healing state and changes in temperature will not reduce the length of time to healing. Nevertheless, application of cold fluid to a wound bed may increase pain for the patient and, therefore, fluids should be applied warm.

Leaper (1998) found that, when antiseptics were used, the benefits of cleansing wounds were outweighed by the detrimental effect of the antiseptic. As stated above, research has shown that cleansing wounds may actually be harmful and bacteria can become resistant to antiseptics and so, in the future, the use of antiseptic will be limited. Nevertheless, the emergence of methicillin-resistant bacteria has led to an increased use of antibacterial agents such as chlorhexidine and iodine in an effort to stem the tide of resistance. The potential question of antiseptic resistance that arises from this increased use is discussed later in this chapter.

Necrotic and sloughy wounds often contain anaerobes, which create an unpleasant odour that cleansing alone will not remove. Fibrous, devitalized tissue will generally be firmly attached to the wound surface and the anaerobes will site themselves beneath this layer. Therefore, a second question to ask is 'does the wound require debridement rather than cleaning?' Necrotic tissue and slough has detrimental effects on wound healing and can actually be life threatening (Hampton, 1997b). It is therefore, prerequisite that harmful tissue is removed from a wound through surgical debridement or through autolysis.

Traditionally, asepsis has been an important part of wound care. More recently, researchers have begun to identify that 'clean and dirty' procedures, when two forceps are used interchangeably ('dirty' forceps disposed of in favour of a sterile pair), do not protect wounds from contamination (Kelso 1989). The research has now moved on from there and suggests that forceps should not be used at all as they are clumsy and cumbersome, can damage the delicate granulation tissue in a wound and may cause the patient pain (Wells 1984). Indeed there is evidence to show that it is safe to clean superficial wounds with bare hands providing the hands are clean (Thomlinson 1987). There is even some evidence that superficial acute wounds can be cleaned safely using ungloved fingertips, providing the hand has been well washed. However, it would be wise to wear gloves when caring for many patients although the gloves do not need to be sterile in the case of chronic wounds. Care must be taken when latex gloves are worn to care for patients with known latex sensitivity or patients with leg ulcers and contact dermatitis. It is now considered advisable to wear powder-free vinyl gloves although these do not feel as natural to use as the latex type.

The use of cotton wool for cleaning a wound should be discontinued as cotton gauze swabbing redistributes bacteria within the wound, does not remove them from the wound bed and can actually drive cotton fibres into the tissues where they can act as foci for infection (Wood 1976). There is little to be gained from following this practice and use of cotton, of any type, in wound care should be discouraged. It is unfortunate, that at the time of writing this book, the Department of Health insists that any sterile dressing packs used in the community must include cotton wool balls.

Irrigation and wound cleansing

When cleansing a wound is unavoidable due to gross contamination, irrigation with 30 ml syringe and 18-20 gauge needle is now the recommended method of choice (Chisholm et al. 1992). However, Stephenson et al. (1976) recommended that irrigation should be applied at a pressure of 7 pounds per square inch (psi) whereas Barr (1995) recommends 8–15psi. It was believed that lower pressures would merely redistribute the bacteria and debris and greater pressures may drive the bacteria into tissues, thereby causing clinical infection. However, the practitioner would find difficulty in judging how hard to press the syringe to deliver the recommended amount of pressure and Singer et al. (1994) found that in fact, 25–40 psi could be obtained using this method. There is also a possibility that irrigation may force the bacteria into the tissues, creating a potential for clinical infection.

If irrigation is unavoidable, a pressurized canister of saline (Iriclense) is obtainable and this offers the required amount of pressure (Lawrence 1994). The canister can be placed in warm water to guard against dropping the temperature of the wound during cleaning and this has the effect of increasing the pressure delivered from the canister (>6.88 psi). Given that lowering wound temperature delays mitotic cell division (Lock 1979), to prevent this hindrance to wound healing, the fluid in a pressurized can (used to cleanse the wound), should be warmed prior to application by inserting the can into warmed water for five minutes.

Tap water and wound cleansing

Although tap water is becoming quite acceptable in wound management, the osmotic affect of water on the wound surface is unknown. There is a possibility that cells may absorb water through the osmotic effect causing the cells to swell and burst. This may well cause pain. Therefore, long periods of soaking are inadvisable. However, soaking leg ulcers in tap water has a psychological benefit to the patient, as well as soothing and cleansing the foot and good skin (Figure 4.2a). Figure 4.2b demonstrates the effect of soaking in tap water and emollient three times daily for five minutes with oil applied to the good skin before dressing the wound. The gentleman's legs were then soaked at each dressing change and this wound went on to heal without further difficulties.

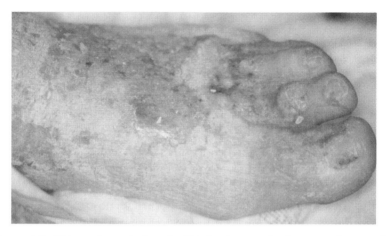

Figure 4.2a This gentleman had not had his feet in water for three years because the nurse believed the ulcer should not be wet (see Plate 25).

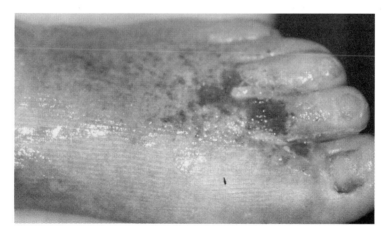

Figure 4.2b The same gentleman after soaking the foot for five minutes a day for three days (see Plate 26).

Patients arrive at clinics with anecdotes of how their feet have not been placed in water for years because a professional has told them 'not to get their leg ulcer wet' and yet these same professionals are happy to squirt saline at the wound – thereby 'wetting' the ulcer. Many progressive clinics now hold buckets for the purpose of soaking the patient's leg ulcers. The buckets are lined with bin-bags and filled with tap water. Ryat and Quinton (1997) examined tap water in an Accident and Emergency (A&E) Department and found no pathogenic bacteria. Hall Angeras et al. (1992) reached the same conclusion, that tap water was safe to use in their A&E department and found that there was lower infection rates in wounds cleaned with tap water than in those cleaned with sterile saline. Patients within hospitals have baths in spite of having wounds and do not appear to suffer ill effects. This leads us to assume that water from home taps must be superior and safe to use for soaking leg ulcers and tap water within hospitals may be safe to use in this instance. However, it should be noted that only mains water should be used for cleansing wounds. Water from basin taps may be directed from a static tank and it is not possible to see whether the tank is free from contamination.

Use of tap water cannot be transferred to a ward setting without further investigation because of the nature of nosocomial bacteria. Nevertheless, the author (Hampton) has been soaking leg ulcers in buckets of tap water, in the ward environment, for four years without one case of clinical infection occurring in that time. Certainly, following surgical procedures, the wound will be ready to accept bath or shower water within 48 hours (Dealey 1994a).

Trevelyan (1996) found that cleansing wounds with swabs could traumatize granulating or epithelializing tissues and suggested that another method of cleansing should be used.

Chlorhexidine and wound cleansing

Chlorhexidine solutions have the characteristics of an ideal antiseptic. They have a low toxicity to living tissues and are effective against a wide range of Gram-negative and Gram-positive organisms (Morrison 1989). Sebben (1983) also noted that chlorhexidine combined good antimicrobial action with minimal effects on healing wounds. Brennan et al. (1985) found chlorhexidine to be as innocuous as normal saline.

Chlorhexidine is said to be deactivated in the presence of pus to a lesser extent than povidone-iodine (Sheikh 1986). In fact Vistnes and Pardoe (1976) claimed that chlorhexidine has a wide range of bactericidal activity and retains its antiseptic effect even in the presence of blood and pus and was the chosen regimen used successfully in one of the UK's largest outbreaks of epidemic methicillin-resistant *Staphylococcus aureus* (Beedle 1993). However, the solution can harbour *Pseudomonas* and Gram-negative organisms, at certain concentrations (as when used in floor cleansing buckets). This problem is avoided by use of prepared sachets.

Chlorhexidine was first synthesized in 1950 and the low toxicity, high antimicrobial activity and strong affinity for binding to skin and mucous membranes led to its development for wound care and dental use (Denton 1991). Soluble chlorhexidine digluconate cannot be isolated as a solid and is manufactured as a 20 per cent aqueous solution (chlorhexidine gluconate). The solubility of chlorhexidine salts in alcohol is higher than in water. However, chlorhexidine gluconate solution should not be added directly to neat alcohol because precipitation may occur (Denton 1991). Chlorhexidine is rendered inactive by certain organic materials such as alginates. Therefore, the use of chlorhexidine when alginates are used as haemostatic agents (as in dental work), may be an unnecessary waste of the product.

Alcohol-based chlorhexidine solutions are particularly suitable for final-stage skin preparation of the operation site. However, the area should be kept wet for at least two minutes to achieve maximal effect (Denton 1991). The immediate bactericidal action of chlorhexidine surpasses that of other antiseptics, including povidone-iodine, and the residual effect also prevents the immediate regrowth of bacteria (Denton 1991).

There is a potential for bacterial resistance to antiseptics (Leelaporn et al. 1994). However, this fear is negated in skin cleansing prior to surgery because:

- skin cleansing is essential to prevent clinical infection post-operatively;
- the solution will be used only once on the pre-operative tissues and resistance would probably rely on repeated applications.

Chlorhexidine is highly effective in prevention of wound sepsis (Colombo et al. 1987) and workers in France found irrigation of chlorhexidine to be effective for controlling existing wound infection.

Collier et al. (1978) found bathing patients in baths containing aqueous solutions of chlorhexidine gluconate at concentrations ranging from 0.01 per cent to 0.05 per cent was a valuable adjunct to the local infection control protocols.

Given that the idea of chlorhexidine being toxic to wounds is correct there may be a concern that this process may damage healthy granulation. However, the slight damage that may occur could promote inflammation within the wound and thereby 'kick start' the healing process. However, as chlorhexidine is only applied to sloughy or contaminated wounds where granulation is not present, healing is unlikely to be affected or traumatized by the procedure. Treatment would discontinue once granulation is apparent.

Chlorhexidine has only a small possibility of absorption through the tissues (Denton 1991). A study into use of chlorhexidine and blood levels showed no detectable blood levels in any of the volunteers (Denton 1991). Denton also writes that 'chlorhexidine has been in use for over 30 years and, in this time, the occurrence of sensitivities remains very low'. Denton also cites many studies reviewing the use of chlorhexidine and wound healing and found that it did not delay healing and actually reduced wound inflammation.

The antimicrobial activity of chlorhexidine is pH-dependent with the optimum range of 5.5–7, corresponding with the pH of the body. However, bacterial activity of chlorhexidine is altered by the type of encountered bacteria. Antimicrobial activity of chlorhexidine will rise, along with the pH, when *Staphylococcus aureus* is encountered but will reduce in the presence of *Pseudomonas aeruginosa*. This has implications for treating *Staphylococcus aureus* with chlorhexidine but not when *Pseudomonas aeruginosa* is the colonizing bacteria (Denton 1991).

McLure and Gordon (1992) write 'Studies evaluating antiseptics are often poorly designed and executed so that valid conclusions concerning efficacy are difficult to substantiate'. The future for bacteria and the lessons for mankind are clear. Unless further work is completed on the destruction of bacteria, then organisms will continue to mutate through natural selection and antiseptics and disinfectant use will be as limited as antibiotics are now. Experience suggests that whatever mechanisms are produced to combat infection, the bacteria will continue to mutate and develop resistance (Hampton 1997d).

Therefore, in wound cleansing, the conclusion is: only clean those wounds that have debris to be removed. Clean with warmed saline or warmed tap water. Use either irrigation with warmed saline or short periods of soaking in a bath or bucket. Use a clean procedure for chronic wounds but continue asepsis for acute wounds for 48 hours post-operatively.

Gloves

It is now accepted practice to wear gloves for all procedures involving body fluids, particularly when undertaking wound care (Gould 1997). However, superficial or clean wounds can be cleansed quite safely with ungloved, well-washed hands (Cruse and Foord 1980). An enormous amount of money is spent unnecessarily on purchasing sterile gloves for use in chronic wounds that are contaminated with bacteria and are likely to be recontaminated only with the patient's own commensals; this will not be altered by the use of sterile gloves.

However, gloves should be worn in wound care to protect other patients from cross-infection. This does not negate the need for excellence in hand washing as minor cuts in the gloves will allow the entry of bacteria. Sterile gloves should always be considered when handling an acute wound or patients who are immunocompromized.

Prevention of cross-infection

There is some evidence that nurses' uniforms become contaminated with bacteria during clinical procedures (Hambreaus 1973) and that plastic aprons will offer a high degree of protection. However, the aprons should never be reused.

At the time of dressing wounds:

• the bedside fan should be turned off as it can distribute bacteria over a wide area;
• beds should not be made prior to or during dressing changes as shaken sheets can distribute bacteria;
• the floor should not be swept when a dressing is being changed.

Bacterial resistance to antiseptics and disinfection

There is an awareness of resistance to antibiotic occurring as MRSA emerges. However, little has been thought about the emerging bacterial resistance to antiseptics. The next section will review the potential for bacteria to develop immunity to antiseptics.

Bacteria may become resistant either by chromosomal mutation and selection or by plasmid transfer (Kelly and Chivers 1996). Mutation is generally a chance genetic change in a cell that alters the protein synthesis and if the new protein protects the cell against an antibiotic, the bacteria can be considered resistant. Multidrug export genes, residing on plasmids within the cell, are responsible for resistance in bacteria. The resistant markers on the plasmids are genetically linked and *Staphylococcus aureus* is coded by at least one of three separate multidrug determinants (Leelaporn et al. 1994).

Littlejohn et al. (1992) wrote 'multiresistant strains of *Staphylococcus aureus* frequently encode resistance to antiseptics and disinfectants and resistance to a broad range of antiseptics may be of particular importance to an organisms potential to survive in the hospital environment'. Plasmids that have a broad range may disseminate genetic information through bacteria of different species.

Reduced susceptibility to some disinfectants is predominantly encoded by the same multiresistant plasmids that confer resistance to certain antibiotics (Irizarry et al. 1996). Stickler and Chawla (1987) found a significant correlation between resistance to antiseptics and multiplicity of antibiotic resistance. This was supported by Irizarry et al. (1996) who found that 80 per cent of MRSA strains collected for research were resistant to more than one antibiotic and reduced susceptibility to antiseptics were predominantly encoded by the same multiresistant plasmids. Irizarry also stated that minimal inhibitory concentrations for a wide range of antiseptics and disinfectants are greater for MRSA than for penicillin sensitive *Staphylococcus aureus*.

The Leelaporn et al. study characterized the occurrence, distribution and phenotype of quartenary ammonium compound (qac) genes in clinical isolates of coagulase-negative staphylococci (CNS). This confirmed that resistance was particularly found in two multidrug export genes (qacA and qacC) and that 40 per cent of resistant CNS isolates contained both qacA and qacC.

The results revealed that most of the resistant CNS strains had resistance to high concentrations of antiseptics/disinfectants, particularly if the plasmid contained both qacA and qacC genes. During the study, plasmids were specifically encoded with the qacA gene and it was found that subsequent elimination of plasmid-encoded qac gene also eliminated the qacA gene. The results of the study emphasized the importance of bacterial resistance to disinfectants and antiseptics and supported evidence that *Staphylococcus aureus* and CNS strains share a 'common pool of resistance determinants'.

Leelaporn et al. (1994) reported that multidrug resistance is a worldwide concern and is of growing importance in foreign body implantation such as prosthetic surgery, intravenous catheters and dialysis catheters and also in immunocompromized patients. Certainly there is worldwide evidence, and concern, that there is multidrug resistance of *Staphylococcus aureus* to antiseptics and disinfectants and this resistance has also been found in other coagulase-negative organisms. Leelaporn et al. (1994) claim the resistance is 'mediated by active export of the toxic compounds from the cell by means of the proton motive force'. Littlejohn et al. (1992) supports this view but also claims that some resistant determinants require ATP to energize transport.

Leelaporn et al. suggest that the broad substrate specificity of the resistant determinants is a possible explanation for the organisms survival in the hospital environment. Littlejohn et al. (1992) underlined this view by stating: 'Resistance to a broad range of antiseptics may be of particular significance to an organisms potential to survive in the hospital environment'. This belief is also supported by evidence that Australian strains are displaying resistance to >20 antimicrobial compounds including antiseptics (Gillespie et al. 1986, cited by Marples and Cooke 1988). There is, however, little evidence that bacteria can develop iodine resistance (Prince et al. 1983).

Cookson et al. (1991) questioned the results of bacterial resistance to antiseptics as high-level concentration still had some efficacy and researched evidence of resistance came from use of low-level concentrations. This finding was not reflected in Leelaporn et al.'s work where it was found that strains that contained both qacA and qacC genes were resistant to higher concentrations of antiseptic than strains that contained qacA alone. QacC had low-level resistance to the antimicrobial compounds discussed above.

If this work is accurate, then 40 per cent of the resistant isolates (containing both qacA and qacC) will be resistant to high-level concentrates; of those containing qacA alone, some will be resistant to high levels; those containing qacC (10 per cent) will be resistant to low-levels. The figure for high-level concentrate resistance will, therefore, be greater than the figure for low-level resistance.

Hedin and Hambraeus (1993) established that long-term use of chlorhexidine largely prevented colonization of resistant organisms although it is noted that their definition of long term covered a two-week period and actual long-term use may well show an increase in resistance.

McLure and Gordon (1992) found that all antiseptic potency dropped in time and with dilution. Leaper (1987) had already reported that antiseptics are deactivated in the presence of pus. Therefore, as potency drops, there is increased potential for resistance to develop.

QacA genes are found on large plasmids, whilst qacC are generally found on small plasmids (Leelaporn et al. 1994). Duckworth et al. (1988) found that smaller plasmids are associated with chloramphenicol resistance, whilst large plasmids have a wider resistance and show an interrelationship between other large plasmids. Littlejohn et al.'s study (1992) identified four determinants encoding antiseptics (qacQ, qacB, qacC and qacD).

Coagulase-negative staphylococci (CNS) have emerged as major nosocomial pathogens with blood-stream infection rates of 1.9/1000 admissions and accounting for 25 per cent of bacteraemias. Mortality can be as high as 14 per cent of those patients with CNS bloodstream infection (Perdreau-Remmington et al. 1995).

In addition to the large circular chromosomes, most bacterial cells contain DNA molecules called plasmids. These plasmids can be transferred between cells in sexual conjugation, transferring new characteristics on the recipient cell (Lehninger 1975). Some plasmids have been known to cross species, thereby transferring resistance.

Plasmid transfer is the more common type in development of resistance as the resistance is transferred from donor bacteria to recipients by one of three methods.

1 Conjugation: cell-to-cell contact when DNA is transferred via cytoplasmic bridge called a sex pilus.

2 Transformation: the bacteria take up naked DNA and incorporate it into their genome.
3 Transduction: transfer of genes by bacteriophages (virus) (Kelly and Chivers 1996). There is evidence that transduction can occur between species.

Due to the increased resistance of antibiotics, antiseptics and disinfectants are increasingly being seen as an important factor in the prevention of infection (Cooper 1996b). However, there are problems that arise from this:

• antiseptics are toxic to wound tissue (Leaper et al.1987);
• frequent use of antiseptics may increase potential of resistance (Johnson 1987);
• antiseptics are inactivated by pus or wound exudate (Leaper et al.1987);
• routine cleaning does not kill bacteria and may increase potential of resistance (Walsh and Ford 1992).

Disinfectant and antiseptic action on bacteria is either bactericidal or bacteriostatic through inhibiting bacterial plasma membranes, causing leakage of cellular constituents and coagulation of cytoplasmic proteins (Cooper 1996a), or by preventing reproduction of the cells but not destroying them. The bactericidal method works well on *Staphylococcus aureus* as Gram-positive bacteria possess one cell wall whereas Gram-negative cells have two outer walls and limit the affect of the agent (Cooper 1996a).

Use of dressings in infected and colonized wounds

There is a belief that occlusive dressings (such as hydrocolloids) provide a moist warm condition that is an ideal environment for bacteria to breed. This is not supported by research. Handfield-Jones et al. (1988), Gilchrist (1990) and Hutchinson (1990) all confirm that bacteria do not proliferate under hydrocolloids and sometimes actually decrease in the hypoxic environment. However, this is in the case of colonized wounds. Selection of an occlusive dressing for a clinically infected wound would be pointless. If a wound is clinically infected, with cellulitis, increased production of exudate and malodour, the dressing selection should be based on removing excess exudate and bacteria as quickly as possible.

Some modern dressings are considered to possess infection control properties by acting as a physical barrier to dispersal of wound pathogens and through immobilization of bacteria within the dressing matrix (Bowler et al. 1999). A hydrofibre and two alginate dressings were shown to be effective in their ability to absorb and retain organisms (Bowler et al. 1999). Dispersion therapy would also be an ideal dressing as it removes exudate and locks exudate, and potentially bacteria, in the central layer of the dressing.

The action of the cells in prevention of infection

Leucocytes

Leucocytes are white blood corpuscles of two types: granulocytes, which have large granules within the cytoplasm and agranulocytes, which lack granules in the cytoplasm. These form several different subtypes of leucocyte, each with its own specific function: neutrophils, macrophages, basophils, lymphocytes and eosinophils. Leucocytes are the primary effector cells against infection and tissue damage. They require oxygen to perform their function and any decrease in blood oxygen can affect their performance and increase the risk of clinical infection.

Neutrophils

Neutrophils make up approximately 60 per cent of all white blood cells. They are found in blood and bone marrow and have a life of 12–20 hours. They are a very efficient bactericidal agent and are essential in prevention of infection throughout the body and in tissue injuries. Neutrophils crawl out of the blood vessels and into the tissues but are unable to swim in water. Therefore, they become static in oedematous tissues (Majno and Joris 1996) and are ineffective against bacteria in oedematous legs. The granules of the neutrophils contain three antibacterial proteins: lactoferrin, lysosyme and cobalophilin. When these granules are released into the wound bed, the bactericidal action destroys the remaining bacteria (Majno and Joris, 1996). The neutrophils have high levels of glycogen reserves that they use for energy for phagocytosis when oxygen is deplete. Nevertheless, Rabkin and Hunt (1988) found that leucocytes cannot work effectively in oxygen concentrations lower than 30 mmHg, which is common in injured tissues.

As the neutrophil kills the bacteria, a burst of energy is required and this frees enzymes, prostaglandins, proteins and bactericidal oxygen-derived free radicals. This enriches the exudate with a mixture that is capable of destroying dead tissue and sometimes destroys even living tissue, making it harmful to the wound (Majno and Joris 1996).

Macrophages

Macrophages are monocytes which are produced in the bone marrow and then circle the body for six days until they 'mature' into macrophages and settle in the tissues (see Figure 1.5). Macrophages are thought to live for months in the static state and are activated by chemotaxins released by tissue injury. When they rush to the injured site they stimulate:

- phagocytosis;
- initiation of the immune response;
- angiogenesis;
- fibrosis;
- clotting;
- secretion of proteins;
- recognition and ingestion of all foreign antigens.

(Majno and Joris 1996)

Macrophages process antigens and present them to T cells (lymphocytes), thereby activating the immune system. They also release many mediators that are involved in activating wound healing, stimulating growth factors and fibroblast activity. Therefore, macrophages are one of the most important elements in wound healing and tend to be reduced or missing in chronic wounds. This could account for the slow healing of old wounds.

Mast cells

Mast cells and basophils are filled with large granules that will release histamine and other mediators related to wound healing.

They are, therefore, almost as important to wound healing as macrophages and, like macrophages, are a part of the initial inflammatory process. Once that process becomes slowed through wound ageing, the activity of the mast cells cease and the mediators are no longer released to stimulate wound healing. The mediator from these cells is histamine, which is usually the first to be released in inflammation along with serotonin from platelets. The histamine, derived from the mast cells, can dilate small arteries and contract large arteries and is, therefore, valuable in introducing the essential blood constituents into the wound bed.

Mast cells multiply in response to a T-cell lymphokine now named interleukin. The mast cells can cause localized skin flushing in response to sensitized stimuli such as dressings.

Factors affecting wound infection

Diabetes

Diabetic patients are more susceptible to clinical infections as the inflammatory response of the diabetic can be altered by their disorder. Capillary basement membrane thickening may interfere with leucocyte migration to the wounded tissue and chemotaxis is impaired in patients with diabetes. Hyperglycaemia also impairs leucocyte function by impairing the transport of ascorbic acid into cells, impairing the ability of polymorphonuclear leucocytes to ingest bacteria (Laing 1998). These factors will increase the infection risk of the diabetic patient.

The deficient blood supply in the diabetic foot causes a chronic deterioration of newly formed tissues and a large release of free oxygen radicals (Im 1995a), which also causes damage to newly formed tissues. The tissue injury, combined with poor oxygen delivery, will lower resistance to infection. Therefore, the diabetic patient is at higher risk of clinical infection.

Perioperative normothermia and wound infection

Kruz et al. (1996) claim that mild pre-operative hypothermia, common during major surgery, can promote surgical-wound infection by triggering thermoregulatory vasoconstriction, which decreases subcutaneous oxygen tension. Reduced levels of oxygen in tissue repair will impair oxidative killing by neutrophils and will decrease the strength of the wound by reducing deposition of collagen (Kruz et al. 1996).

Kruz et al. studied wound infection following surgery through a randomized controlled trial with 20 patients randomly assigned to either routine care or additional warming. The results showed that patients in the control group had average temperatures of 34.7 ± 0.6°C with 19 per cent developing infections post-operatively. The experimental group had average temperatures of 36.6 ± 0.5°C with only six per cent developing wound infections. Hospital stay was prolonged by 2.6 days for the patients in the control group. This led to the conclusion that hypothermia may delay healing and predispose surgical patients to wound infections.

Conclusion

Very few exuding, malodorous wounds will be clinically infected and antibiotics should only be given if there are clinical signs of infection confirmed by swab results. If this rule is not complied with, bacteria will continue to mutate and antibiotic and antiseptic resistance will increase. This will become a problem in the near future with wounds increasingly becoming infected and thereby reflecting on poor healing rates.

Activity

1 List five symptoms that would suggest clinical infection in a wound.
2 Identify a patient with a wound with surrounding erythema. Does the patient have a pyrexia, pain or increased exudate? Does the swab result confirm infection?
3 Write a 500-word reflection on what has been learned from this exercise. Place the work in the professional profile.

CHAPTER 5

Assessment, management and treatment of leg and foot ulceration

Leg ulcers are very common with one per cent of the UK population suffering chronic leg ulceration (Callum et al. 1985). Roe et al. (1994) found that leg ulcer care by nurses often falls short of what is ideal. Nevertheless, the management of leg ulcers is a major challenge to general practitioners and nurses who bear the burden of caring for a difficult problem. There is also a wide variation in treatment of ulcers with a poor knowledge base in some nurses (Bell 1994). Emmott (1992) found that nurses were unable to identify the factors that delay healing and had difficulty in applying the physiology of wound healing to practice. Bell (1994) found that nurses, working in a Dublin outpatient department did not recognize poor blood supply or immobility as significant factors in delay or enhancement of healing of leg ulceration. These studies identify the importance of education in the prevention, treatment and management of wounds. Kane (1990) reviewed sources of nurse knowledge in leg ulcers and found that most knowledge was obtained from nursing colleagues, with nursing journals and company representatives ranked second and third. Very few nurses actually obtained knowledge from study days.

Ruckley (1998) claims that up to 70 per cent of ulcers can be healed in 3–6 months using compression therapy and, therefore, failure to assess with a Doppler and failure to employ appropriate use of compression bandaging is unacceptable practice. Nevertheless, as many as 80 per cent of people with leg ulcers, in the community, will not have been assessed using Doppler ultrasound. Superior assessment leads to appropriate selection of evidence-based treatment and this can lead to cost-effective treatment, particularly when symptoms are identified and corrected. Appropriate treatment enables the ulcer to heal, almost in spite of the type of dressing used (Backhouse et al. 1987).

Therefore, a clinical history and careful physical examination is the first step toward healing the ulcer and the dressing is almost of little importance and should be the last consideration.

Graduated compression therapy

Graduated compression therapy is rapidly becoming the treatment of choice in venous leg ulcers as it is cost-effective and offers faster healing rates. Compression bandaging of many types are now available on prescription and should be made available to all patients with assessed and diagnosed venous leg ulceration. However, inappropriate and incorrectly applied bandages can cause increase in size of an ulcer and, if used on ischaemic limbs, may lead to amputation (Callum 1987). Therefore, education in assessment of ulcers and bandaging techniques is extremely important and skilled holistic assessment is essential. Education of the patient is also important as Nudds (1987) found that patients who were given detailed information were more committed to compression therapy and had faster healing rates than those who were not given information. It is a requirement of any practitioner applying compression therapy, to be aware of research-based evidence and good practice and to have a clear understanding of how approved techniques can achieve the objectives of treatment. The RCN (2000) clinical practice guidelines in the management of patients with venous leg ulcers recommend that all assessment and clinical investigations should be undertaken by a health care professionals trained in leg ulcer management.

Compression therapy is becoming known as the main treatment option for venous ulceration (Stemmer et al. 1980; Blair et al. 1988; Charles 1991) as research and experience in applying bandages demonstrates the effectiveness of short-stretch, multilayer and long-stretch bandages. These methods of bandaging increase venous return, allowing the lower extremity tissues to recover from the affects of venous hypertension and offers faster healing rates (Stemmer et al. 1980; Charles 1991). Cherry (1990) reported an estimated cost for treatment of £300 to £600 million per year in 1990 and this is possibly a conservative figure as a comparative cost today. However, inadequate knowledge of assessment and poor skill in bandage application can lead to tissue necrosis. The damage depends on the following :

- bandages incorrectly applied with high bandage elasticity;
- whether the bandage is overstretched when applied;
- how many times the bandage has been washed;
- how long the bandage has been in place;
- whether the bandager is skilled in Doppler assessment.

(Eagles 1999)

Callum et al. (1985) observed 'several cases in which injudicious use of compression in a limb with occult arterial disease had apparently led to severe skin necrosis and, in a few instances, to amputation' (Figure 3.1, page 86). This statement emphasizes the urgent need for nurses to obtain knowledge and to become skilled in the application of compression bandages. Compression therapy should not be undertaken by any professional unless they have been taught those required skills, are competent and have accompanying knowledge.

Although full compression is the optimum choice for treating venous ulceration, reduced compression is better than no compression for patients who cannot tolerate the tightness required for providing the necessary sub-bandage pressures (Arthur 2000).

The principle aetiology of ulcers is chronic venous insufficiency afflicting 70 per cent of people with ulcers. Some ulceration (8–10 per cent) is arterial and there are also those people with mixed aetiology, neoplasms or vasculitic ulceration associated with rheumatoid arthritis.

Arteries

The arterial walls are thick and strong and are made up from three layers:

- intima: a thin inner membrane covered by flat endothelial cells;
- media: a thick strong coat made of muscle fibre mixed with sheets of strong elastic tissue;
- aventitia: a thick outer coat of connective tissue.

The artery divides, becoming smaller and thinner until the aventitia disappears and the artery becomes an arteriole and part of the microcirculation. A capillary is approximately 0.8 cm long and just wide enough for a red corpuscle to pass through. Nourishment and oxygen cannot pass through arteries but can pass through the thinner walls of the capillaries. The blood takes a few seconds to pass through the capillary and, during that time, there is a quick exchange of gasses and dissolved substances, supplying the tissues with the required oxygen and nutrients and ridding the tissues of matter resulting from cellular metabolism. Arterial ulceration occurs when there is an interruption of this process of exchange due to atherosclerosis and poor delivery of blood to the tissues.

Doppler ultrasound is used by nurses to exclude arterial disease prior to applying compression bandaging and is not used to diagnose venous disease. The sounds of the arteries can be heard through a Doppler probe; these sounds identify the elasticity of the arterial walls and can lead to assisted diagnosis of atherosclerosis. The walls of the arteries are elastic and 'rebound' with each beat of the heart. The first stage is expansion, second stage is recoil and the third stage is a reactive rebound. This can be heard as three distinct or 'triphasic' sounds. As the artery ages, some of the elasticity is lost and the third reactive sound is lost, leaving only two (biphasic) sounds. Once athrosclerotic plaques are laid over the arterial walls, the arteries lose the elasticity completely leaving only one (monophasic) sound. The inelasticity of this last condition forces blood to enter and leave the artery under great pressure and the sound that can be heard is a distinctive 'whoosh', a little like a dog bark. If this sound is identified, even when elevated blood pressure readings are found, the patient requires specialist assessment and vascular surgical referral is essential.

Pathology of arterial ulcers

Arterial ulcers can be divided into two groups: (1) macro-vascular disease and (2) micro-vascular disease.

Macro-vascular disease

Local and temporary deficiency of blood to the tissues is called ischaemia. If blood supply is stopped to the arm, pain does not occur for two or three minutes. However, if the arm were exercised, the pain would begin in seconds. This reaction is similar to the reaction that occurs in intermittent claudication. Exercise demands increased metabolism and, when the arteries are unable to deliver enough blood to cope with the demand, ischaemia and pain ensue. Arterial insufficiency increases and may result in rest pain (an ominous sign), which is most commonly experienced at night when the sufferer is in bed. Signs of arterial insufficiency are:

- pain at night;
- pain on walking, patient has to stop after a few minutes and pain is relieved by rest;
- the foot is cold;
- numbness;
- skin pallor;
- leg is hairless;
- shiny, smooth thin, tautly stretched skin;
- trophic skin changes;
- pinching the nail bed shows sluggishness of refilling time – longer than two seconds;
- lifting the leg higher than the heart produces a cadaveric pallor and on lowering the leg shows a delay in returning to normal colour with a possible final dependent dark red discolouration (rubor). The time of refilling, from pallor to some colour is 10–15 seconds for normal; 15–25 seconds for abnormal; 25–40 seconds for severe ischaemia; greater than 40 seconds for very severe (Bryant 1992);
- foot can be dark red in colour (rubor);
- absence or decrease in foot pulses;
- a sudden darkening in colour to a navy or black/blue, suggestive of arterial thrombosis.

Warmth is important to the patient with vascular disease as this causes a vasodilation and increased delivery of blood to the starving tissues. However, heat can aggravate ischaemic pain due to the increased demands of metabolism and, as the arteries are undoubtedly sclerosed, there will be only minimal or possibly no vasodilation response to warming.

Arteriosclerosis is the most common disease of the arteries and literally means hardening of the arteries. There is a loss of elasticity and a thickening in the arterial walls which reduces the size of the lumen and prevents or reduces the flow of blood within either the macrocirculation (large arteries) or the microcirculation (arterioles).

The patient with atherosclerosis will possibly have a dark coloured foot when in the dependent position. This is caused by the delay of delivery of blood and the haemoglobin becomes deoxygenated causing the discolouration of the tissues. Many patients can tolerate up to 70 per cent occlusion of the artery (Bryant 1992). In atherosclerosis, monocytes adhere to the lining of the arterial wall, encouraging macrophages to release growth factors, stimulating growth and migration of vascular smooth muscle cells. Platelets then adhere, resulting in a plaque that narrows or blocks the lumen of the artery (Bryant 1992). In diabetes, this process is accelerated.

Many non-healing ulcers on the feet and leg are vascular in origin (8–10 per cent) and, without Doppler assessment may be misdiagnosed. Arterial ulcers are complex and the most difficult type of wound to heal due to the lack of arterial perfusion to the tissues.

Cigarette smoking lowers skin temperature, causes vasoconstriction, promotes atherosclerosis, decreases prostaglandin production and reduces production of fibrinogen (Siana et al. 1992). Patients who are diabetic and smoke are severely jeopardizing arterial perfusion (Bryant 1992).

The main arteries for the leg begin as the femoral artery in the thigh. This becomes the popliteal artery at the knee and, below the knee it separates to become the anterior tibial artery, peroneal artery and posterior tibial artery. The anterior tibial artery runs down over the middorsum of the foot as the dorsalis pedis and the posterior tibial artery runs behind through the grove behind the medial malleolus at approximately 3 o'clock. It is the anterior tibial artery, the dorsalis pedis and the posterior tibial artery sounds that are investigated with Doppler assessment.

Gangrene

Gangrene is a result of continued ischaemia, which occurs sooner with high pressures but can also occur with very low pressures applied over sufficient time (Laing 1998). Gangrene can be dry, with tissues that mummify and demarcate naturally, or wet with malodorous and probably infected tissues. Dry gangrene is best kept dry with either dry dressings (or no dressing) as healing at this point is not an option and moist dressings will promote rehydration of the hard necrotic tissue promoting infection. Wet gangrene will be treated with a dressing to remove the anaerobes that are causing the malodour. Occasionally oxygen is a treatment option for anaerobic infection.

The patient with gangrene requires an urgent vascular consultant assessment for angioplasty, femoral popliteal bypass or amputation. Angioplasty is a positive and simple solution, if it is successful, and preferable to amputation.

When deciding which, among several therapeutic options to prescribe, the clinician should weigh the cost of each therapy against its potential for improving the patient's functional status and quality of life (Reiber et al. 1998).

A vascular ulcer, due to macro-vascular circulatory disease, is likely to have caved sides (punched out) to the wound and likely to be deep. The bed of the wound may be very pale and bloodless, indicating the ischaemic process that occurs within the tissues. The ulcers will appear anywhere on the leg or foot and will probably be multiple. There are often tendons exposed and the wounds can be wet but are more likely to be dry with very low exudate. Usually, arterial ulcers are painful particularly when the leg is elevated, due to the ischaemia. However, complaints of increased pain at night will normally be leg pain rather than ulcer pain. Often the wound bed is very pale – almost white in appearance – due to the poor blood delivery and may contain yellow/ grey nonviable tissue.

Treatment options for arterial ulcers are limited. However, referral to a vascular consultant is the highest priority. Wound treatment involves keeping the wound moist and encouraging the blood supply and this can be done in various ways:

- larvae therapy;
- negative pressure therapy;
- warmth.

Although all of these methods increase blood supply to the wound, they all have the ability to increase pain and, therefore, care should be taken to reassess quickly following application. It would be wise to refer to a vascular consultant prior to these treatments. When these dressings are not an option, then the wound should be kept moist with hydrogels or hydrocolloids. Anecdotally, arterial ulcers appear to respond to potassium permanganate soaks.

Microcirculatory disease

Vasculitic ulceration

Rheumatoid arthritis is a chronic systemic disease with inflammatory changes occurring in the connective tissues. This includes the connective tissues within the walls of the blood vessels, which become chronically inflamed leading to vasculitis. It is known that 6–8 per cent of inpatients with rheumatoid arthritis have active leg ulcers (Wilkinson and Kirk 1965). Although vasculitis is most often found in patients with rheumatoid arthritis, it can also be associated with diabetes, scleroderma, bowel disease and polyarteritis.

Vasculitis affects the arteries, veins and capillaries when the small arterioles become inflamed and the lumen of the arterioles become smaller due to the oedema caused by the inflammation process. Small clots may form within the larger vessels resulting in local tissue necrosis. When small vessels are involved, localized bleeding may occur, producing small dark spots. This is due to an autoimmune failure or localized infection of the capillaries and often found in people with rheumatoid arthritis. Ulcers, caused by vasculitis, are often small and multiple with a darkened centre and erythema surrounding the peri-wound area (in the acute stage) with caved edges and symmetrical lines (Figure 5.1). They are acutely painful, often have a yellow necrotic base to the wound, are very difficult to treat and normal wound care does not support healing in the acute stage of these ulcers.

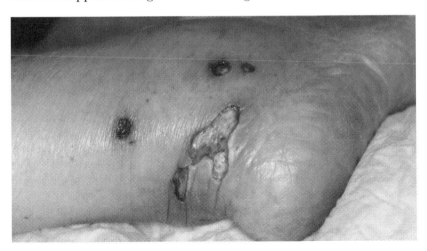

Figure 5.1 Vasculitis.

Generally, vasculitis is related to either rheumatoid arthritis or the conditions described above. However, the patient in Figure 5.2 had none of these conditions and yet he presented with a non-healing ulcer. He was a young man of 48 with no obvious venous disease and with a normal ABPI of 1.0, but his wounds were refusing to heal. There was no evidence of clinical infection but the wounds continued to deteriorate. The wounds were round in shape, extremely painful with dark blue margins, all indicative of vascular disease and in particular, pyoderma gangraenosum. A short course of steroid therapy was given: 40 mgs Prednisolone for eight days and 5 mgs for five days. The wounds suddenly began to heal, shrinking in size by one half in the first week of treatment. This was only one case study, but it offers a rationale for investigating non-healing ulcers for vasulitic changes.

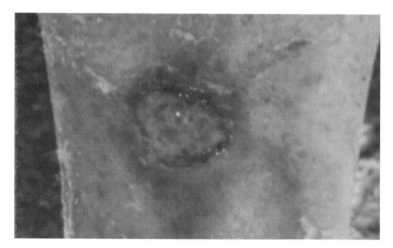

Figure 5.2 Round ulcer with dark blue margins – indicative of vasculitis – possibly pyoderma (see Plate 27).

Common treatment for vasculitis is corticosteroids, administered possibly through pulse therapy, to reduce the inflammation in the arterioles. The reduction of inflammation reduces oedema within the vessels and allows blood to return to the tissues. Iloprost may be of some value, but that is unproven at present. Analgesia is of utmost importance and probably needs to be morphine based to control the pain, with Entinox possibly required at dressing change. Patients find some relief in moist dressings such as hydrocolloids or hydrogels whereas dry dressings, such as alginates or iodine cadexomers, are likely to increase pain because of the hydrophilic/osmotic pressure caused to the wound. The patient in Figure 5.1 had extreme pain and became debilitated through lack of sleep and difficulty of eating during painful episodes. Topical analgesia still has not been licensed for wound care although there are those professionals who claim success with EMLA cream (see Chapter 3). There may be some value in maggot therapy as the action of the maggots in the wound may encourage blood flow.

Pyoderma gangraenosum

Pyoderma gangraenosum (PG) is a rare, destructive, inflammatory ulcer and is probably fundamentally an autoimmunological problem, particularly as it is often found in patients with rheumatoid arthritis or inflammatory bowel disease. Brunstring et al. (cited by Samuel and Williams 1996) noted the first reports of PG in relation to bowel disease, although PG is not necessarily connected to the disease. It may also be associated with haematological malignancies such as acute myeloid leukaemia and chronic myeloid leukaemia (Samuel and Williams 1996). PG is difficult to diagnose and can be misclassified as chronic wounds of prevailing aetiology. It should be suspected in patients with wounds that do not respond to standard therapy, especially if the patient suffers with a PG associated disease (Lorentzen and Gottrup 1998) and particularly if a dark blue/mauve band is present on the wound margins.

The patient can present with a fever and a rapidly enlarging ulcer with an area of surrounding erythema. The clinical appearance is unique. It generally has smooth symmetrical outlines with a border of blue directly around the margins of the wound. The wound bed can often contain slough and necrotic tissue that remains hydrated. The wounds can appear anywhere on the body but are most commonly found on the proximal part of the calf.

Dressings can only support symptoms of PG but will not promote healing. The wounds are nearly always very painful and treatment relies on reducing the pain and administering steroid therapy. Corticosteroids will reduce the inflammation and associated oedema, and, until that is achieved, dressings (hydrogels, hydrocolloids) should be used to moisten the nerve endings and reduce pain. Dry dressings may well increase the pain in an already painful wound through a hydrophilic 'pull'.

There has been some work looking at the use of immunopressives such as cyclosporin, which has shown some promising results (Samuel and Williams 1996).

Veins

The superficial and deep veins of the leg are linked together by the perforator veins with the deep veins under high pressure and the superficial veins under lower pressure. Blood is returned to the heart through intrathoracic pressure (breathing), compression of the calf muscle and through a system of non-return valves within the veins (Figure 5.3). The sounds of intrathoracic pressure can be heard by placing a Doppler probe over a vein within the arm. As inspiration and expiration occurs, the blood can be heard rushing through the vein and then pausing in time to the breathing pattern.

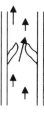 In normal physiology, muscles contract, forcing blood toward the heart. The valves in the walls of the veins, open to allow the passage of blood. When the muscle is relaxed, the valves close.

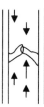 The calf muscle relaxes and the pressure is released from the artery. Blood tries to obey gravity but the valves are competent and prevent the back-flow of blood.

Figure 5.3 Normal physiology of the veins.

Normal physiology

Normal physiology of venous return requires the calf muscle to compress the deep veins during exercise. The action of the muscles in the foot and calf is to contract and this causes a rise in pressure in both superficial and deep veins. When the muscle relaxes, the pressure ceases and the blood is held from returning to the feet by competent valves found within the lumen of the veins. When the muscle is contracted, the pressure in the deep vein system rises higher than in the superficial system.

Dale and Gibson (1997) found that the most effective way to return blood to the heart was through exercise and recommends that patients are encourage to walk as much as possible. Gardener and Fox (1983) discovered a venous pump mechanism in the sole of the foot that returns blood upward with no assistance from muscular action as weight bearing simultaneously on the heel and the metatarsal heads of the foot empties the deep plantar veins upward toward the calf. Ertl (1991) discusses the 'foot pump' and its importance in venous return, and claims that it operates independently of any muscular action and ankle movements have no effect on the response but 'on weight-bearing, emptying of the plantar venous complex is dramatic'.

The plantar arch is the arch in the sole of the foot formed by the anastamosing branches of the plantar arteries. The plantar venous plexus comprises the lateral plantar veins, saphenous vein, posterior tibial vein and the superficial dorsal veins. The plantar plexus fills when the foot is dependent and empties immediately when weight is placed on the arch of the foot. Blood is collected in the plexus veins from the deep spaces of the foot and from the superficial veins. It is then transported into the deep venous system and this outflow from the plexus is independent of calf muscle contraction (White et al. 1996). Foot impulse technology uses the foot pump mechanism to stimulate venous return by an increase of 250 per cent. This increases the healing rate of venous ulcers, increases blood flow in ischaemic limbs and reduces the potential of deep vein thrombosis (Hutcheson 1999).

Negative intrathoracic pressure

The negative intrathoracic pressure, previously described, will cause a 'suction' effect to occur within the veins, drawing blood toward the heart. Exercise will lead to increased air intake and higher intrathoracic pressure, which, combined with the calf venous pump, gives effective venous return.

Venous insufficiency

When the calf muscle relaxes, in a person with venous insufficiency, the superficial system tries to refill but, due to the increased pressure in the vein and the damaged valves (Figure 5.4), it is unable to refill fully. This leads to venous hypertension and a potential for venous ulceration. Damage to the vein often follows a history of deep vein thrombosis (Hopkins 1987) or because of occupational requirements (such as hairdressers who stand in one position for many hours) resulting in venous stasis. Two generations ago, women remained on bedrest for up to two weeks following childbirth and many experienced a condition referred to as 'white leg'. They were unaware that they had developed deep vein thrombosis and many of these mothers are now presenting in later life with venous leg ulceration. When the calf muscle fails to effectively return the blood to the heart there is a reflux or pooling of blood in the lower extremities resulting in venous hypertension (Ertl 1993). Normal pressure in the venous system is 30 mmHg. However, when pressures within the deep or perforating veins are insufficient, the systolic pressures in the superficial veins can be considerably higher at 60–80 mmHg (Mekkes 1998). The increased pressure within the deep veins creates a back-pressure and morphological changes in the capillaries, such as stretching the walls and causing permeability with resultant capillary leakage.

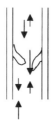 Incompetent valves allow back-flow of blood into the lower extremities causing venous stasis and venous hypertension. This prevents exchange of gases and nutrients. Blood is unable to effectively return to the heart and the tissues become oedematous.

Figure 5.4 Incompetent valves permit return of blood.

Deep vein thrombosis

As deep vein thrombosis (DVT) can be related to venous ulceration later in life, it is worth reviewing this condition at this point. Three elements are required to cause a DVT:

1 venous stasis (follows travelling distances when seating compresses the back of the leg or through long periods of standing) and disturbance of the coagulating system;
2 non-functioning valves within the superficial veins (valvular dysfunction occurs following previous episodes of deep vein thrombosis or due to age or occupation, e.g. long periods of standing);
3 viscous blood (occurs during dehydration, when unwell, in smokers or in women on the pill). Blood viscocity relies on the haemocrit (the percentage of the blood volume which is composed of red blood cells) and to a much lesser extent on the concentration of plasma proteins and white cells (Bliss 1998). Dehydration (such as occurs during air flight) will increase the percentage of red blood cells in the blood. To counteract this problem, it is advisable to drink increased amounts of water when travelling by air.

When these three conditions (known as Virchow's triad) are present, there is an increased potential for thrombosis to occur. Approximately 40 per cent of venous leg ulcers are caused by a previous DVT (Lindholm 2002).

Fibrin cuff theory

Fibrinogen is one molecule that leaks into the interstitial fluid where these small molecules unite (polymerize) to form fibrin (Robinson 1988). There is a theory that the insoluble fibrin is deposited around capillaries where it forms a 'cuff' and effectively prevents the diffusion of nutrients and oxygen to the tissues and reduces removal of metabolic wastes (Robinson 1988). This will lead to atrophy of the skin and a potential for ulceration (Morison 1993). This remains largely an unproven theory and is seriously questioned by Mekkes (1998).

White cell trapping theory

There is another, perhaps stronger, theory of 'white cell trapping' (Coleridge-Smith et al. 1988) where the capillary loops are blocked by trapped white blood cells. 'This blocks further circulation, producing ischaemia which aggravates trophic changes already occurring in the skin. The trapped white cells become activated, releasing toxic metabolites which alter capillary permeability and precipitate the leakage of fibrin and other large molecules' (Ertl 1991).

Free radical theory

Leucocytes are found in healthy subject's legs when venous insufficiency is present. It is thought that the leucocytes become trapped, possibly brought about by hypoxia (Angle and Bergan 1997). The leucocytes are responsible for releasing free radicals, which then injure the surrounding tissues. The adherence of the white cells to the vein walls then further reduces delivery of nutrients and oxygen to the area. This also remains a largely unproven theory. Hayes (1996) claims that the possibility of free radical formation is combined with proteolytic enzyme release to cause ulceration.

Large molecule trapping theory

Another hypothesis, put forward by Falanga and Eaglestein (1993) looked at peri-capillary leakage of macromolecules such as alpha-macroglobulin and fibrinogen. They suggested that leakage of these large molecules would trap and bind growth factors, preventing them from repairing pre-damaged tissues.

However, it is likely that leg ulcers are the result of many contributing multifactorial and sequential processes and that no one theory is entirely responsible.

Pathology of venous ulceration

Pressures caused within the veins when muscles contract, along with hypertension caused by incompetent veins and capillary dilation, creates a localized venous hypertension. The lumen of the veins are then stretched, leaving 'gaps' in the cells of the veins and fluid begins to leak into the tissues causing oedema. Normal physiological response to leakage of fluid into the interstitial spaces would be drainage via the lymphatic system, thereby relieving the congestion. In venous hypertension, this system becomes overcharged and blocks (Mekkes 1998), consequentially leading to excess fluid, debris, lipids and proteins forming within the interstitial spaces. The capillary dilatation continues to allow leakage of plasma contents including red blood cells, which causes pigmentation, leaving a brown stain (haemosiderin) on the skin (Figure 5.5). Haemosiderin is a classic precursor to venous ulceration and should alert the practitioner to potential of ulceration in otherwise healthy patients.

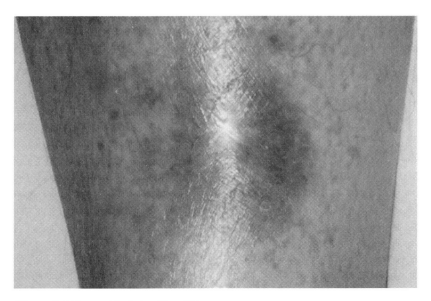

Figure 5.5 Haemosiderin (see Plate 28).

Lack of nutrients and oxygen exchange causes an overall deterioration of the tissues and continued deposit of waste products in the tissues (particularly fatty deposits) all results in lipodermatosclerosis (Robinson 1988). However, the physical appearance of lipodermatosclerosis (the skin feels 'woody' to the touch combined with fat necrosis and, possibly, upside down champagne-bottle shaped legs), does not exclude arterial involvement in ulceration and the potential for mixed aetiology is high. Cornwall et al. (1986) recommends that every patient with an ulcer, particularly older patients, should be given Doppler assessment prior to applying compression therapy (see later in this chapter).

Atrophy blanche and ankle flare

Atrophy blanche is small avascular areas of scarring that can be found around ulcers or in areas of haemosiderin and in the gaiter area. The physical appearance is a white or grey area of tissue. The pathological process seems to involve thrombosis and the obliteration of capillaries in the middle and deep dermis (Vowden 1998). Ankle flare, which is tiny dilation of 'spider naevus' vessels on the medial aspect of the foot, is often a precursor to venous ulceration. Atrophy blanche can be considered an extreme form of lipodermatosclerosis and is a state where spontaneous ulceration can occur (Mekkes 1998).

Exudate in venous ulceration

Exudate production in ulcers is largely due to hydrostatic pressures within the lower extremities. This hydrostatic pressure can cause the loss of protein-rich fluid, which can lower serum albumin. Compression therapy reduces hydrostatic pressures and will reduce the loss of protein within the fluid. Another reason for excessive exudate is bacterial contamination as bacteria will cause vasopermeability.

Assessment

The selection of treatment and final healing of an ulcer is dependent on the skilful and knowledgeable decisions made by the practitioner. Knowledge of how medical problems can cause, or interrelate with, venous ulceration can only complement the physical assessment. Therefore, assessment of the patient begins with sitting with the patient and taking a history.

Holistic assessment

The practitioner should discover:

- the patient's history:
  has any member of the family had leg ulceration?
  does he or she smoke?
  nutritional status?
- the patient's medical history. Has the patient any record of:
  rheumatoid arthritis?
  previous DVT?
  heart disease?
  diabetes?
  steroid therapy?
  chemotherapy?

All these conditions will effect wound healing.

The practitioner should also gain the history in the patient's own words. Patients will generally identify one or two symptoms as the primary problem such as pain, smell or the ulcer is weeping, requiring large dressings and a lot of attention. They rarely identify the ulcer itself as their actual problem.

The length of time that the wound has been present will effect healing times. A wound of 50 years is unlikely to heal in 3–6 months. Whereas, a wound of two days could be expected to heal rapidly as inflammation and growth factors are present to stimulate healing.

The speed of ulcer development can be an indication of its aetiology. An arterial ulcer is likely to be rapid in development, whereas venous ulceration is slow in progression and possibly develops in size over months or even years. However, a venous ulcer can develop following a knock, such as with a shopping trolley. The patient often wrongly identifies the source of the knock as the reason for the ulcer. It is difficult to understand that the ulcer was waiting to happen and only required a small knock to open the wound.

The history of the ulcer is important, such as: what initiated it, has it enlarged recently, has the malodour increased, and what dressings have been used in the past? This often reminds the patient of problems they have experienced with particular dressings such as allergies or sensitivities to dressings.

Pain

The time at which the patient experiences pain can be informative. Venous ulcers are often more painful when the leg is dependent. This is due to the pooling of blood in the lower extremities. Arterial ulcers are likely to increase in pain when the legs are elevated due to the fact that blood is not efficiently being delivered to the extremities and elevation plus gravity will further reduce the delivery of blood. Patients with arterial insufficiency often complain that they must sit out of bed at night for relief of pain.

If the patient experiences pain when walking it would alert the practitioner to the possibility of intermittent claudication. Pain experienced in bed at night causing the patient to get up usually (although not always) indicates arterial involvement. The patient typically gets out of bed at 2 am and sits in a chair for the rest of the night.

If the patient complains of continuous pain it is important to discover whether is the continuous pain in the ulcer or in the leg. Patients will often complain that their ulcer is painful but further questioning reveals that the pain is not in the ulcer but in the ankle or in the lower tissues. If this fact is not identified, it may effect decisions

on dressings as wet dressings (hydrogels and hydrocolloids) are soothing to a painful wound and dry dressings (alginates, hydrofibres) can
increase pain. However, if the pain is not actually in the wound itself,
then a wet dressing is not necessarily required.

If an accurate holistic assessment is completed, the practitioner
should have already made a decision about the ulcer pathology prior
to physical assessment. This decision must be confirmed or denied
by Doppler assessment.

Physical assessment

The practitioner should always be able to view the removed dressing.
There is often an informative discolouration or malodour in the
dressing that is not apparent in the wound and the selection of
wound dressing relies on how much exudate is lost in the dressing or
which malodorous bacteria may be colonizing the wound.

What colour is the wound?

This will help decide on the stage of healing and will affect treatment. A
red or pink wound with red lumps in the base would suggest a healing
wound that requires protection and support. A green wound would
indicate a *Pseudomonas* colonization and this could lead to enlargement
of the wound (Madsen et al. 1996). A brown or red discharge would
suggest possible haemolytic streptococci or *Staphylococcus aureus*.

What size is the ulcer?

A large ulcer will require different treatment to a smaller ulcer
and will heal slowly in comparison. A small ulcer may require a simple
support dressing whereas a large ulcer would require a dressing to
absorb the quantities of exudate that may be lost from the wound.

Where is it sited?

Arterial ulcers are usually multiple, with caved sides and can be
anywhere on the leg or foot. Venous ulceration usually occurs within
the gaiter area and the wounds are generally shallow sided, they
progressively enlarge and are unlikely to be multiple. Matorell ulceration generally occurs on the shin and is shallow with a necrotic
base (Cameron 1996). Matorell ulcers are generally secondary to
hypertension.

Causes of intractable or non-healing ulcers

There are some ulcers that resist all efforts to heal them and the most knowledgeable practitioner appears to be unable to assist. There may be several occult causes of this intractability and it is not helpful for the practitioner to feel frustrated at their inability to heal the wound. Finding the cause of the poor healing is often extremely difficult and beyond the limits of the nurse.

The cause may be pyoderma gangraenosum, the exceedingly painful cryofibrinogenaemic cutaneous ulcer (Falanga 2001), cancer, peripheral vascular disease or many other delaying factors. Many of these require medical intervention and that is not always easily obtained and often takes many months to organize.

The results of physical examination of the leg

Oedema, discoloured tissues, ankle flare, lipodermatosclerosis all can indicate venous insufficiency. Pale cold toes, slow refilling time when the nail is pinched, dark blue toes, white and hairless legs, can all indicate there may be arterial involvement. A 'fixed' ankle joint will prevent natural movement of the leg and, therefore, the calf venous pump will not be quite as active and venous return may be poor although Ertl (1991) believed the ankle joint has little effect on the calf pump.

Once the physical assessment is completed, the practitioner should be certain of the diagnosis and have an idea of the treatment required. This decision must be followed by making a Doppler assessment. The assessment results can be easily documented using an assessment form. The form can be introduced by the practitioner or a ready-prepared form obtained from some companies.

Laser-Doppler velocimetry

Laser-Doppler velocimetry (LDV) is useful in measurement of relative tissue blood flow. Lucarotti et al. (1988) found a change in both the variability of the LDV waveform and its absolute level when measured in the supine and dependent limb, in patients with venous reflux. These changes correlated with simultaneous photoplethysmographic assessment of venous reflux and were more pronounced in patients with leg ulcers. The changes were also reduced by compression bandaging.

Photoplethysmography

King and Brereton (1998) describe photoplethysmography as 'developed to investigate venous haemodynamics of the lower limb using a special sensor and is the term given to recording changes in limb size due to tissue fluid or pooled blood within the veins. A light-emitting diode is placed above the medial malleolus to measure the speed at which the capillary bed becomes filled with blood following calf muscle exercise'. Doppler ultrasound is used regularly by nurses to identify arterial disease. Likewise, photoplethysmography can and should be used by nurses to identify the presence of venous insufficiency.

Doppler assessment

The hand-held Doppler ultrasound probe usually contains two piezoelectric crystals, one of which acts as a transmitter of the ultrasonic wave whilst the other receives the reflected signals (Wheston 1996). The probes are obtained in differing strengths with 5 mmHz, 8 mmHz and 10 mmHz. The mmHz required depends on whether there is oedema present.

Ankle brachial pressure index (ABPI)

1   Patient rests with legs elevated for 20 minutes, preferably with the feet in line with the heart. This is an important way to equalize the blood pressure in the legs and arms and to get a true reading for the ABPI.
2   Sphygmomanometer cuff is placed around the leg just above the malleoli. Too far up the leg and the cuff will not occlude the artery enough to get a true reading. The cuff must be a standard adult size for limb circumference up to 32 cm. Larger legs should have the larger cuff.
3   A sterile dressing and/or cling film may be used to protect the cuff from open wounds.
4   Select an 8 MHz probe (for a normal non-oedematous leg) and attach to the Doppler.
5   Palpate the foot arteries in at least two places. Preferably the dorsalis pedis on the dorsum of the foot, and the posteria tibial artery just behind the medial malleolus.

6   Apply ultrasound gel to the skin and the Doppler probe is placed, in the gel, at a 45° angle over the previously identified artery.

7   The cuff is inflated until the sound has gone.

8   Slowly deflate the cuff. The point at which the sound can be heard is the systolic pressure.

9   Using the cuff and Doppler probe, record the highest systolic pressure from at least two pulses in the ankle and/or foot.

10   Using the Doppler probe, record the highest systolic pressure from the brachial artery.

11   Place A (ankle) over B (brachial) = 1.0 or ABPI >1.

12   ABPI > 1 is normal. If the patient has an ulcer, consider referral to the vascular consultant for vein stripping.

13   ABPI < 0.8 shows arterial involvement. Compression should not be applied and the patient should be referred to a vascular consultant for advice on potential light compression or angioplasty.

14   ABPI > 0.6 patient should be urgently referred to a vascular consultant.

15   ABPI > 1.3 practitioner should be aware of atherosclerosis. Atherosclerosis hardens the walls of the artery, preventing total occlusion of the lumen. Therefore, arterial sounds can still be heard even though the artery lumen is a fraction of normal diameter size. The sounds from these arteries are often monophasic with a dull sound.

The sounds of the artery should be:

- Clear with a triple beat or triphasic sound.
- As the patient ages, the sounds may reduce to double beats or a biphasic sound.
- With atherosclerosis the artery loses its elasticity and gives one solid sound and the dull 'woof-woof' monophasic sound informs the assessor that there is atherosclerosis present. Particular care should be taken if elevated blood pressure readings are found.
- A clear and continuous 'whoosh' sound, which sounds a like wind through trees, is a vein. The artery is often hidden behind the vein and by tilting the angle of the probe, the artery can often be found. The sound of the vein can alter when the patient breathes. This is due to intrathoracic negative pressure causing a suction effect in the vein.

Warning

- Patients with monophasic dull sounds should not be compressed without advice from a vascular surgeon. It is possible that the patient with mixed aetiology can receive compression therapy. However, this should **never** be undertaken without express orders from a vascular consultant.
- Patients with ankle circumference of less than 18 cms should not be compressed without the use of wool padding to enlarge the circumference of the entire leg.
- Diabetic patients should not be compressed without the opinion of the diabetic consultant and/or vascular consultant as tissue perfusion may be low and compression bandaging can reduce the perfusion by 44.2 ± 13.1 per cent (Mayrovitz et al. 1997). In future, the microcirculation may be judged through application of an oximeter.
- Medial calcinosis can result in unusually highly elevated blood pressure in patients with diabetes with possible ABPI ratio of greater than two or even more. This indicates there are atheromatous plaques within the vessels and these plaques are preventing occlusion of the artery although the actual arterial lumen is quite small. This means the sounds can still be heard long after a normal vessel would have experienced occlusion. Therefore, patients with ABPI greater than 1.3 should not be compressed without the agreement of the vascular consultant. Therefore, elevated blood pressure and a dull monophasic sound should alert the practitioner to possible narrowed lumen, particularly in diabetic patients.
- Care should be taken with rheumatoid patients as their ABPI may be normal but microcirculation can be poor and tissue perfusion may be low. Compression bandaging can reduce the perfusion by 44.2 ± 13.1 per cent (Mayrovitz et al. 1997).
- Patients should always be questioned about intermittent claudication as they may have normal ABPI when at rest but abnormal during exercise.

Plate 1
Formation of an
endothelial plug by
platelets (page 6).

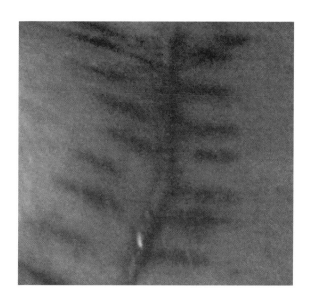

Plate 2 This wound
will heal through
secondary intention
(page 7).

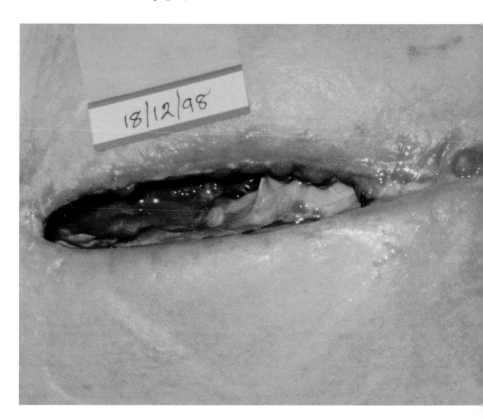

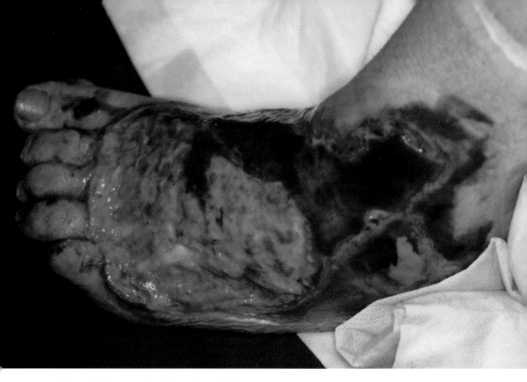

Plate 3 Extravasation injury (page 31).

Plate 4 Contact dermatitis is frequently mistaken as a clinical infection (page 33).

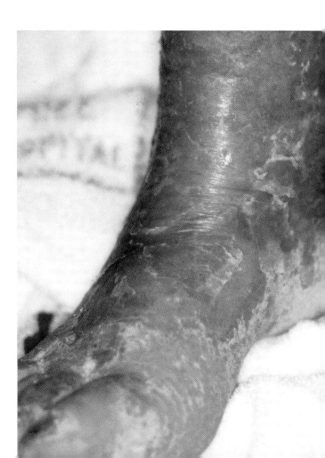

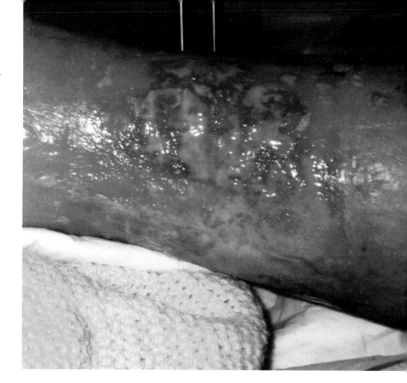

Plate 5 The demarcation line of erythema is less defined in clinical infection (page 33).

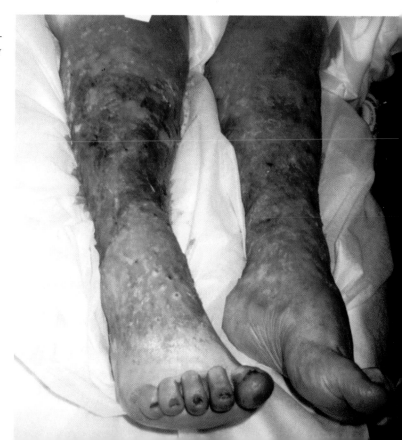

Plate 6 This patient has multiple sensitivities, possibly partially due to her own exudate (page 35).

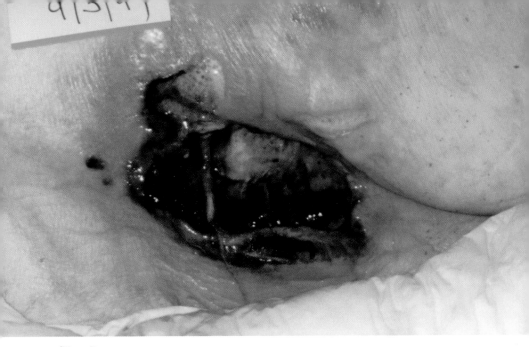

Plate 7
Black wound
(page 52).

Plate 8
Yellow wound.

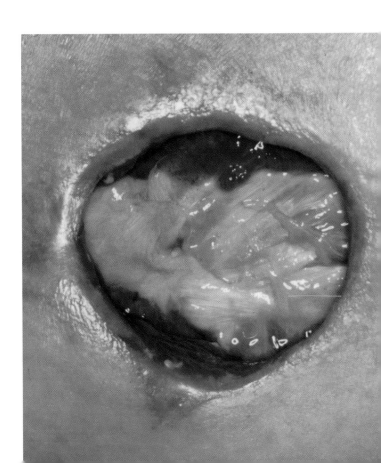

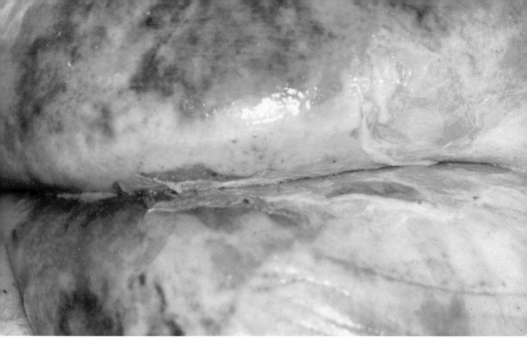

Plate 9 (above) The areas of devitalized tissue and blistering can clearly be seen (page 53).

Plate 10 (below) A green wound, indicating *Pseudomonals* colonization (page 54).

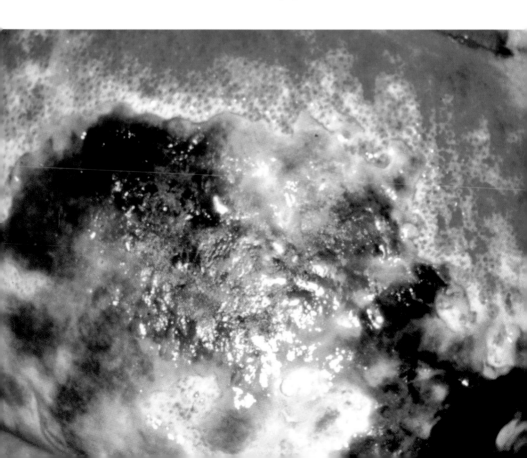

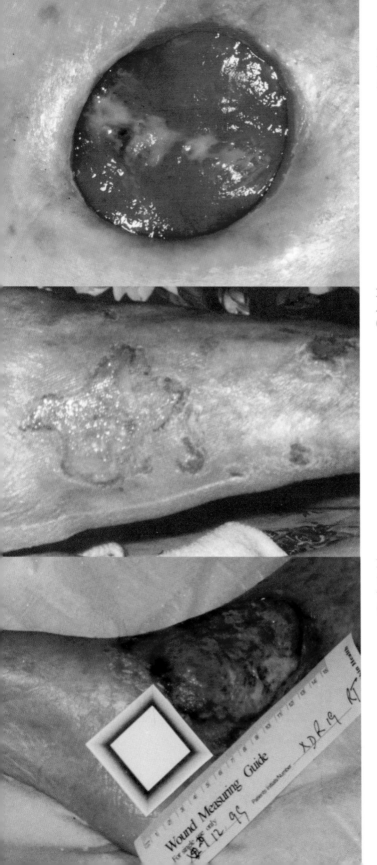

Plate 11 A red wound, showing signs of granulation. (page 54)

Plate 12 An epithelializing wound (page 56).

Plate 13 Computer tool for measuring wound dimensions (page 59).

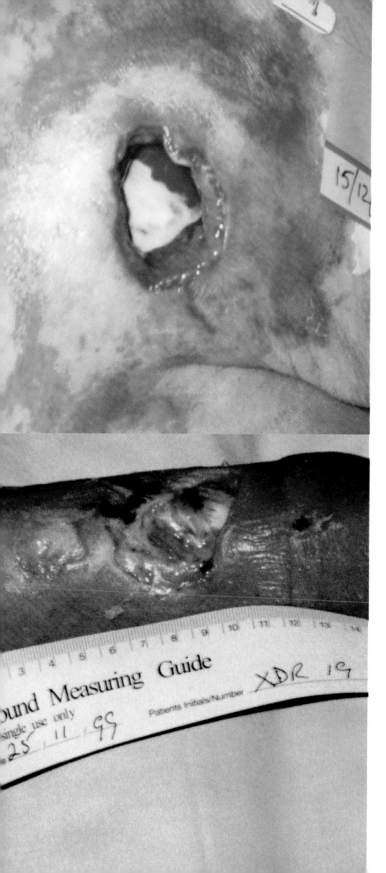

Plate 14 Tissue maceration (page 67).

Plate 15 Tendons exposed as a result of poor bandaging techniques in mixed aetiology leg ulcers (page 86).

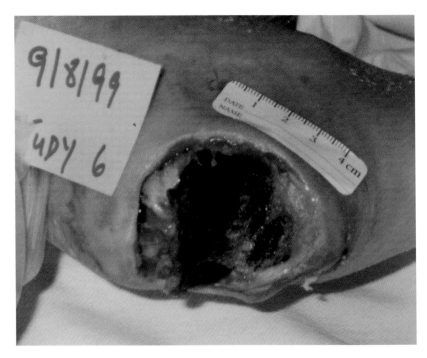

Plate 16 (Above)
Hard eschar requires
debridement (page 87).

Plate 17 (Below) Sharp
debridement (page 87).

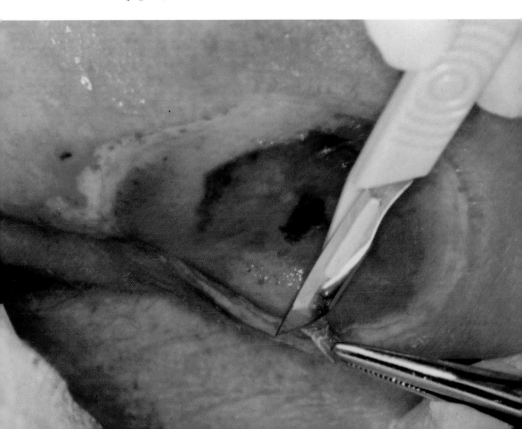

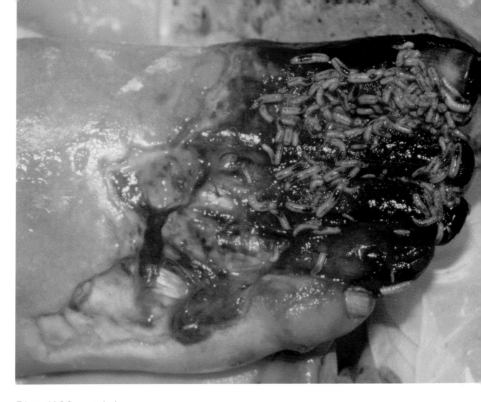

Plate 18 Maggots being used to debride gangrenous tissue (page 93).

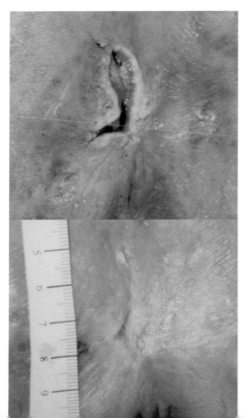

Plate 19 Wound prior to mud pack application (page 113).

Plate 20 Healed wound after five weeks following regular mud applications (page 113).

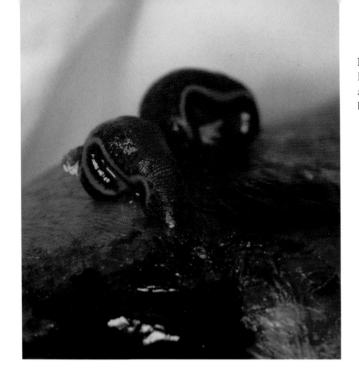

Plate 21
Elderly lady with
a haematoma treated
by leeches (page 119).

Plate 22 Initial
application of
leeches (page 120).

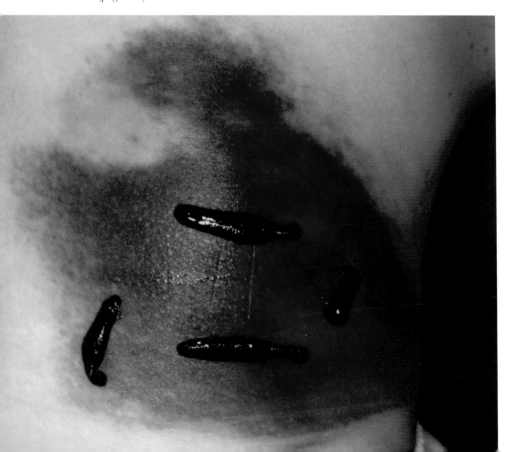

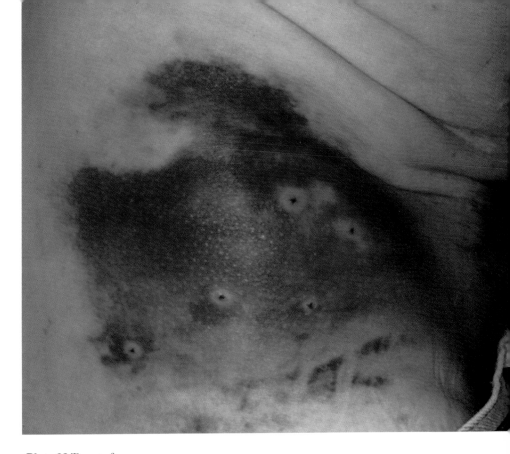

Plate 23 Twenty-four
hours post leech
application (page 121).

Plate 24 A clear
demarcation line created
by an inappropriate
dressing (page 124).

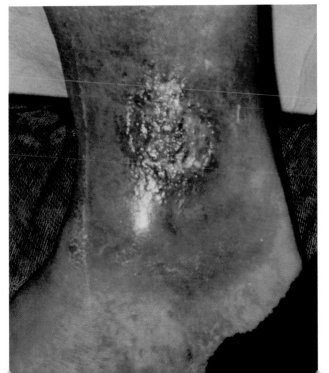

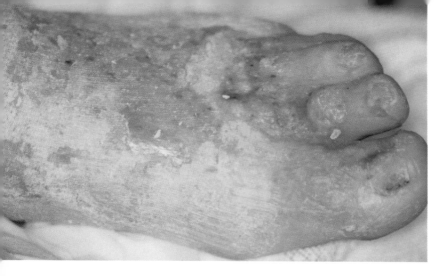

Plate 25 This gentleman had not had his feet in water for three years because the nurse believed the ulcer should not be wet (page 147).

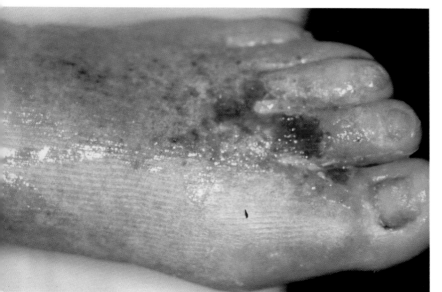

Plate 26 The same gentleman after soaking the foot for five minutes a day for three days (page 147).

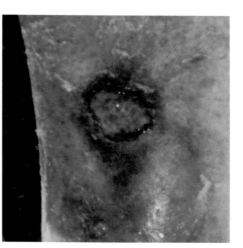

Plate 27 Round ulcer with dark blue margins – indicative of vasculitis – possibly pyoderma (page 168).

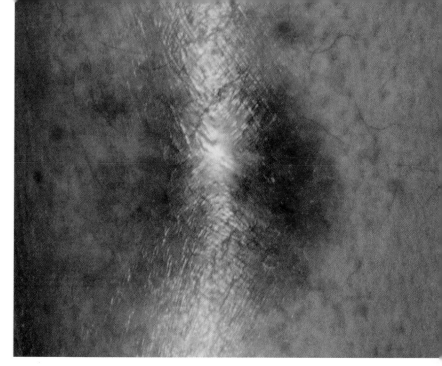

Plate 28 Haemosiderin
(page 175).

Plate 29 (Below) This
wound had healed in 10
days following skin
grafting (page 200).

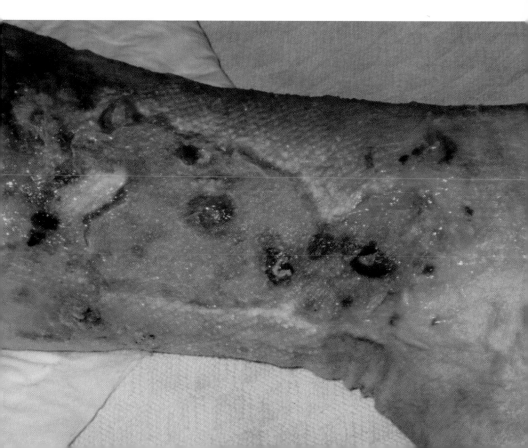

Plate 30 A donor site can be painful and difficult to heal (page 230).

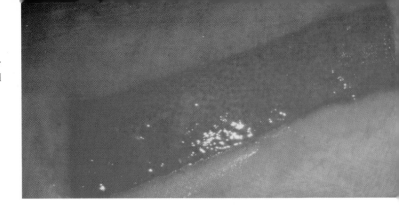

Plate 31 Necrotic toe (page 233).

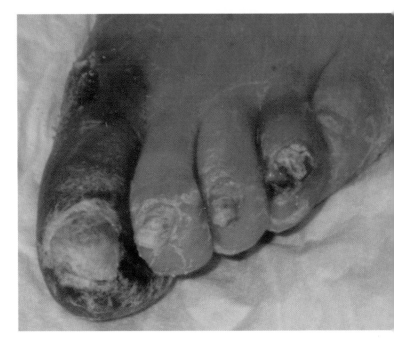

Plate 32 Basal cell carcinoma (page 242).

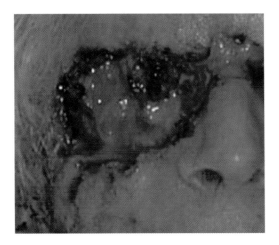

Plate 33
Pressure ulcer
with evidence of
undermining
(page 258).

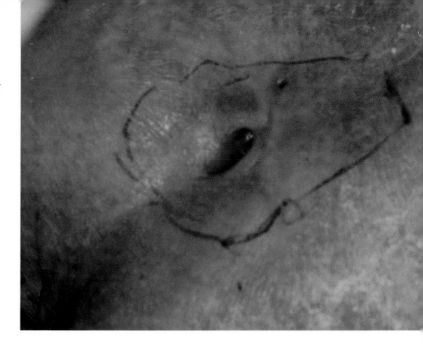

Plate 34
Pressure ulcers
are often difficult
to classify until
fully debrided
(page 277).

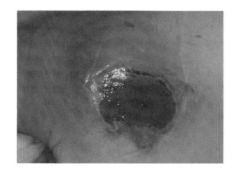

Plate 35
Stage 5
pressure ulcer
(page 278).

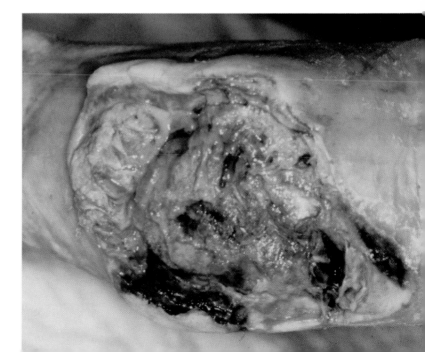

Plate 36 Small area of ulceration (page 345).

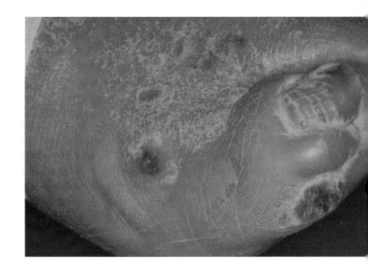

Plate 37 Macerated sacrum (page 346).

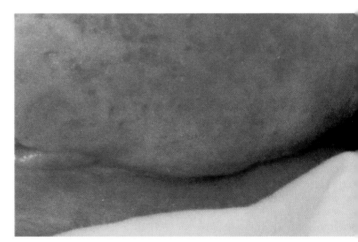

Plate 38 Neuropathic ulcer (page 348).

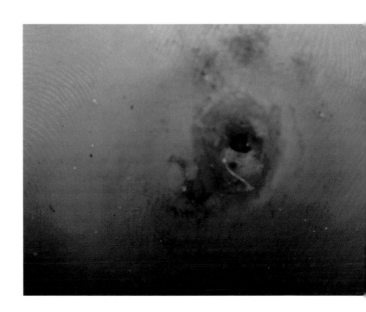

Patients who are to be given anti-embolism stockings should always be assessed prior to application. Any indication of potential arterial disease should lead to Doppler assessment. Failure to do so can lead to tissue damage, potential ulceration and even amputation. Callum (1987) found 38 cases of damage caused through inappropriately used antiembolism stockings. Damage, caused by antiembolism stockings, can be to the heel or over the foot (Figure 5.6).

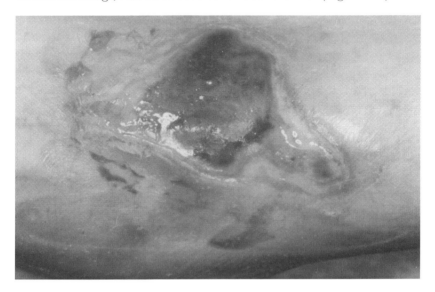

Figure 5.6 Injury caused by anti-embolism stockings across the astralagus on the foot dorsum.

Doppler assessment is the most important assessment in identifying arterial disease and should be the minimum investigation prior to applying compression. However, it should be complementary to a professional and experienced holistic patient assessment. It is important to remember that patients with diabetes, rheumatoid arthritis or any disease leading to calcified arteries may have abnormally high ABPI even in the presence of arterial disease.

Compression therapy

There are a many different types and makes of bandages and many differing techniques in compression therapy. Long-stretch, short-stretch and multilayer bandages, all applied by different methods, all requiring distinct skills and all with various cost implications, causing possible difficulty of choice for the practitioner. All of these methods will achieve graduated compression when applied correctly and randomized controlled trials undertaken by Scriven et al. (1998) and Duby et al. (1993) found no significant differences in healing rates between short-stretch and multilayered bandages.

Graduated compression

Graduated compression is achieved through the natural shape of the leg (Moffatt 1992a) which is generally narrower at the ankle and wider at the knee. The pressure produced by the bandage is calculated by using Laplace's law (Moffatt 1992a), which has implications for irregularly shaped lower limbs and skill of bandage application. Laplace's law

$$P = T \times N \times Constant$$
$$C \times W$$

1 P = sub-bandage pressure. This is pressure exerted by applying a bandage under tension to a curved surface (Nelson 1996). The bandage tension is provided by the choice of bandage and by the skill of the nurse applying the bandage.
2 N = number of layers. Two layers of bandages provide twice as much pressure as one layer and, therefore, the application of bandages should ensure a 50 per cent overlap on each turn of the bandage to ensure there are only two layers of bandage applied. Overlap greater than 50 per cent would increase sub-bandage pressure.
3 C = limb circumference. Compression, correctly applied with a 50 per cent overlap, should achieve graduated pressure of 40 mmHg at the ankle and 17 mmHg at the knee. However, the shape of the limb can affect the sub-bandage pressure. Laplace's law dictates higher pressure on a small compressed limb than a large compressed limb. Therefore, pressure will be greater on a thin ankle than on a thick calf. Venous ulceration often leads to 'champagne-bottle' shaped legs and, therefore, part of the skill of bandaging is ensuring the leg is correctly shaped by the use of orthopaedic wool giving graduated compression along the length of the leg.
4 W = width of bandage. The average size of a bandage is 10 cm, which is probably the safest (Keachie 1992). However, thinner legs tolerate 8 cm well and larger legs will take 12 cm comfortably.

The four-layer system can be purchased as a package with the size of bandage pre-selected.

Sub-bandage pressure should be 40 mmHg at the ankle and 17 mmHg at the calf, giving graduated compression. This pressure can be achieved by bandaging at the same strength compression from toe to knee (Laplace's law), practice and through the understanding of the process. Companies that produce bandages may often loan machines to measure sub-bandage pressure so practitioners can practise achieving correct pressures. Experience in the technique is essential and not easily achieved. Stockport et al. (1997) assessed bandaging skills of doctors and nurses with half being experienced and half being inexperienced at compression bandaging. The results showed that inexperienced practitioners were more likely to apply dangerously high levels of sub-pressure with single-layer bandages and recommended that only experienced practitioners should be allowed to bandage using single-layer. However, there is not a transition period between 'inexperienced' and 'experienced'. If the 'inexperienced' practitioner is not allowed to bandage, 'experience' is not achievable. Therefore, education and practice is infinitely important if optimum healing rates are to be achieved with compression therapy. Training has been shown to improve bandaging skills (Nelson 1995) and it is therefore important to ensure increased education in bandaging techniques for hospital and community nurses, and for continual assessment in bandaging to be promoted as part of practice.

Here are some tips:

- Always start bandaging with the bandage roll upward. If the bandager tries to roll the bandage with it pointing down, they will have difficulty in maintaining the 70–90 per cent compression.
- The patient should be on a bed or couch to enable the bandager to apply the bandage easily. However, if this is not possible, seat the patient comfortably in a chair with the legs elevated on a stool. It is easier if the bandager has an apron and a protective cover for the lap. The patient's foot can then be placed on the lap whilst the bandager sits on the stool.
- The patient will often complain that the bandage is too tight because they are not used to the supportive nature of the

bandage. A full explanation of what to expect, prior to applying the bandages will reduce the anxiety about the bandages.

- When bandage is left over at the top of the leg, do not continue applying around the leg at full stretch as this can cause a tourniquet effect and negate the benefits of compression. Either apply with no stretch, or double the bandage back on itself and secure with tape.
- Doubling the bandage layers increases sub-bandage pressures and is inadvisable unless it is part of the recommended bandaging technique.

Short-stretch bandages

There is sometimes confusion over what constitutes a short-stretch bandage, particularly as other bandages can be given a class 2 classification (Elastocrepe) and the misnomer is further supported by studies referring to Elastocrepe as 'short-stretch' (Gould et al. 1998). However, Elastocrepe does not maintain compression (Gould et al. 1998) and is, therefore, not suitable for use in compression therapy. In this section, short-stretch bandages will refer only to the cotton bandages (Comprilan, Rosidal K and Actico). The bandages are made of cotton, and the extensibility comes from the weave of the 100 per cent cotton fibres. Because they are cotton, they are unlikely to cause skin sensitivity. The stretch of the material is retained even after 12–20 washes and this makes it a very cost-effective bandaging system.

Short-stretch bandages are applied at 90 per cent compression from the toe to just below the poplitial crease and this provides the graduated compression required. The firmness of the bandage application forms a rigid 'tube'. The calf muscle rebounds against the sides of the 'tube' and compresses the superficial veins, which reduces hypertension and effectively aids venous return (Simpson 1997). It is thought that the action of short-stretch bandages requires mobility in the patient as venous return relies on the 'rebound' action of muscle contraction. However, the bandage is applied tightly and this compression will offer some venous return. It has been successful in healing ulcers in paraplegic patients. There is also an issue that some immobile patients are on bedrest and this may well be the factor that heals the ulcer rather than any external treatment such as dressings or bandages.

The bandager should be able to run their hand up the completed bandage without the edges of the bandage rolling back, whilst at the same time, a finger can be placed under the bandage around the ankle. This informs the bandager that compression is correct.

Short-stretch bandages offer lower resting pressures and are safer when used in ulcers of mixed aetiology. However, a bandage should never be applied when ABPI<0.8 without assessment and agreement of a vascular consultant. Short-stretch bandages are easily applied with little training. Long-stretch and multilayered bandages require more training. The patient or carer can often manage to apply short-stretch bandages with education and support from the professionals. This provides an opening for patient independence. Long-stretch and multilayer bandaging can also be taught to some carers.

Short-stretch bandages are not as hot or as bulky to wear as the multilayer system. They are made of cotton and, as there is no rubber content, they are less likely to cause sensitivity. Multilayer and long-stretch bandages have rubber content.

Short-stretch bandages can be washed as many as 13–20 times and are therefore cost-effective. Some long-stretch can be washed (Tensopress and Setopress). Multilayer bandage are cut from the leg and, therefore, are not reusable.

Short-stretch bandages have proven efficacy (Charles 1991) but there is no evidence to show that it performs differently to any other compression bandage (Fletcher and Callum 1997).

Short-stretch bandages are safer in ulcers of mixed aetiology as there is little residual compression when the leg is at rest (Dale and Gibson 1997) whereas long-stretch and multilayer bandages have higher resting pressures. Short-stretch bandages do not require removal at night whereas, some long-stretch bandages have high resting pressures and removal at night is recommended.

Shoes usually fit over the short-stretch bandages and they are available on the drug tariff.

New types of short-stretch bandages are cohesive (Actico) and do not require tapes to hold them *in situ*. The bandage will hold in place for a week without moving or falling down. However, these are removed through cutting and it is not possible to wash them.

Short-stretch bandages are an excellent alternative treatment to multilayer and long-stretch bandages and can achieve high healing rates when applied correctly. However, it is imperative that education in both assessment of venous ulcers and application of bandages is offered so that practitioners can continue to offer high quality, research-based treatment for patients with venous leg ulcers (Hampton 1997e).

Short-stretch method of application

1   Measure the ankle. The ankle should be above 18 cm to safely
    apply compression. An ankle less than 18 cm could still be given
    compression providing the leg was padded with orthopaedic wool
    to give a full and graduated shape with the ankle measuring
    greater than 18 cm. The dimensions are important because
    Laplace's law dictates that the thinner the diameter, the higher
    the pressures need to be. To achieve 40 mmHg of pressure at the
    ankle it needs to be larger than 18 cm. Protect bony prominences
    with orthopaedic wool – toe to knee. The orthopaedic wool can
    either be bandaged toe to knee or strips can be cut over the bony
    prominences (Figure 5.7).

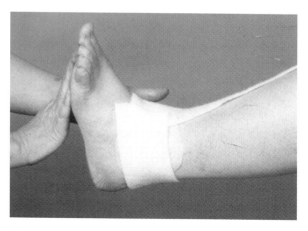

Figure 5.7 Orthopaedic wool padding.

2   Foam pads or shaped chiropody felt may be required below the
    malleolus as this will ensure that pressure is equally applied in the
    required area. Extra orthopaedic wool may be necessary to
    reshape misshapen legs.
3   Keep foot flexed at 90° angle when bandaging. Ask the patient to
    point the 'toes toward the nose'. This ensures a correct fit of the
    bandage around the heel. If it is not applied in this manner there
    is the potential for the bandage to loosen.
4   Remove the clips from the bandage and throw away. These clips
    are largely used in Europe where short-stretch bandages are used
    as multilayered bandages. They must never be used to secure

single or double layered bandages as the clip teeth can cause trauma to the tissues.

Technique

- Start with two complete turns around the foot at 50 per cent extension (the double layer increases compression) (Figure 5.8).

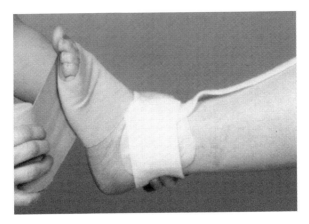

Figure 5.8 Two turns over the toes.

- Take the bandage around the heel with 50 per cent bandage above the heel and 50 per cent below (Figure 5.9).

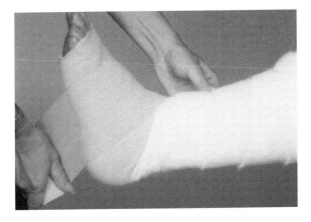

Figure 5.9 Taking the bandage around the heel and over the foot in a figure of eight.

- The next turn is a figure of eight around the base of the foot; this is at 70–90 per cent extension. Ensure that all the foot is covered with bandage.
- The next turn is above the heel at 70–90 per cent extension.
- Each turn of the bandage is 50 per cent above the previous spiral ensuring that only two layers of bandage are in contact with the leg. Each turn is 70–90 per cent extension of the bandage.
- The bandage is best applied in a spiral, not a figure of eight.
- The bandage should finish at the popliteal crease (or two fingers below the knee).
- Change the bandages as required and this is preferably weekly.
- Do not wrap excess bandage at the top as this will increase the sub-bandage pressure. However, the bandage must not be cut as this interferes with the weave of the bandage. With experience the bandager can often finish without excess bandage. If necessary, the bandage can be turned back on itself and loosely secured.
- A second bandage may be required for a large leg to ensure that the tension is correct. If a second bandage is required, it should be applied in the opposite direction to the first bandage.
- Apply tape to secure the bandage (Figure 5.10).

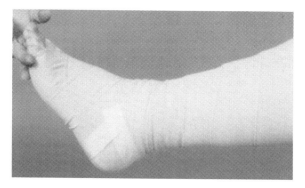

Figure 5.10 Apply tape to secure the bandage.

- Check the comfort of the patient.

Modified Pütter technique

- Place two turns of the bandage over the malleoli;
- take the bandage to the toes and cover the heel and ankle in a figure of eight;

- spiral the bandage from the malleoli to mid-calf;
- take the bandage up round the back of the calf to just below the knee;
- spiral back down the calf at low tension;
- apply a second bandage, beginning again at the malleoli but reversing the direction of the of application;
- take the bandage to the toes and then spiral up the leg;
- secure well with tapes;
- place tapes around the toes and around the heel in a V shape to prevent shoes from dislodging the bandage.

A study by Ertl (1992) suggested that short-stretch bandaging is the safest method for those patients with an arterial component to the ulcer.

Multilayer bandages

The Charing Cross method of bandaging has been shown to have healing rates of 69 per cent in 12 weeks (Moffatt et al. 1992) and has the advantage of maintaining the required degree of compression. The action of the bandage is the opposite of short-stretch. Whereas the non-elastic immovable bandage forces the energy back into the leg, the elastic bandage absorbs the energy from the calf muscle and then 'springs back' into the original position, thereby encouraging venous return. All bandages are applied at mid-stretch so that compression is achieved by elasticity and overlap rather than by the tension applied by the bandager (Simpson 1997). Application requires skill and training.

The multilayers form a supportive 'tube', which maintains shape and stays *in situ* whereas short-stretch bandages may slip down, particularly after the first 24 hours when oedema is reduced by the compression. Multilayer bandaging applies a therapeutic level of compression by using a combination of weaker bandages, which prevent excessive pressure being applied to the limb (Moffat 1997). They do not require the patient to be ambulant, whereas short-stretch may require the patient to be ambulant to achieve the 'massage' effect of the bandage. There is a proven efficacy for multilayer bandages (Nelson 1997), although patients may find it difficult to wear shoes. Multilayer bandages are available on the drug tariff.

The requirements for Charing Cross multilayer bandage are:

- orthopaedic wool (may require more than one if the leg is thin) – used to provide padding for protection and to absorb exudate;
- a light cotton crepe bandage – offers some elasticity and support;
- light compression bandage (Litepress);
- cohesive bandage (Coplus);
- a knitted viscose dressing (Tricotex) is generally used as a standard dressing with the multilayer bandage.

An alternative system of multilayer bandaging was found to have similar healing rates as the Charing Cross bandage system (Wilkinson et al. 1997). This was a useful alternative prior to multilayer bandages (i.e. Profore) being placed on the drug tariff:

- a light-weight elasticised tubular bandage (Tubifast) applied over the dressing;
- lint, applied around the leg in strips;
- high compression bandage (Setopress);
- lightweight tubular bandage (Tubifast).

The method of application of this multilayer bandaging is as follows:

1 Measure the ankle. The ankle should be above 18 cm to be suitable for compression. Ankles under 18 cm will require extra padding to bring the leg into a suitable shape for compression.
2 Ankle measurement of greater than 25 cm may require double bandage compression.
3 Keep foot flexed at 90° during bandaging. This ensures a correct fit of the bandage around the heel. If it is not applied in this manner there is the potential for the bandage to loosen.
4 Apply orthopaedic wool in a spiral from toe to knee. This may require more than one orthopaedic wool bandage if the ankle is small or the leg misshapen. Pad misshapen legs until graduation of shape (smaller at ankle), is achieved.
5 Apply the 10 cm crepe bandage from toe to knee in a spiral with a 50 per cent overlap at each turn of the bandage.
6 Apply 10 cm elastic, conformable compression bandage in a figure of eight from toe to knee. This method used to be called the 'fish tail' method of bandaging and requires some skill. The stretch applied to this bandage should be approximately 50 per cent.

7 Ensure a 50 per cent overlap to prevent over-compression through too many layers as doubling the bandage will increase the sub-bandage pressures and may cause tissue damage or discomfort for the patient.
8 Apply the cohesive bandage layer. This bandage is a useful addition to bandaging as it clings to itself and will support the lower bandages, keeping them *in situ* until removal.
9 Change the bandages when required, preferably weekly.

Long-stretch bandages

Long-stretch bandages have true extensibility and stretch a 'long way'. It is this extensibility that encourages venous return. They are applied at 50 per cent stretch, which requires a skilled and experienced bandager as long-stretch has an extensibility greater than 100 per cent of the original length (Charles 1999) and there is a potential for the bandage to be applied too tightly. As the calf muscle contracts and pushes the bandages outwards, the elastic component recoils and compresses the muscle. This 'massages' the veins and encourages venous return. There are some long-stretch bandages that have a high resting pressure and require removal at night (blue line bandage) and the bandager should be aware of the company literature prior to applying the bandages, particularly when a patient is infirm and unable to reapply bandages themselves.

As the bandages are applied as one or two layers, shoes usually fit over the bandage. Not all long-stretch bandages can be washed, however, Tensopress and Setopress are washable (Ertl 1992). Tensopress and Setopress are also available through the drug tariff (Ertl 1992).

Applying long-stretch bandages requires practice and skill to achieve the correct tension as they can possibly be over-extended causing excess pressure. Some long-stretch bandages require removal at night and reapplication each day (Ertl 1992).

Long-stretch bandage are applied as follows:

1 Measure the ankle. The ankle should be greater than 18 cm to be suitable for compression. Ankles less than 18 cm will require extra padding to bring the leg into a suitable shape for compression.
2 Keep the foot flexed at 90° during bandaging. This ensures a correct fit of the bandage around the heel. If it is not applied in this manner there is the potential for the bandage to loosen.

3 Apply orthopaedic wool in a spiral from toe to knee. More than one wool bandage may be required if the ankle is small or the leg misshapen. Pad misshapen legs until graduation of shape, smaller at ankle, is achieved.
4 Apply the long-stretch bandage from toe to knee using a figure of eight around the foot. Keep the bandage extended by 50 per cent during application.
5 Ensure a 50 per cent overlap at each spiral. Either a figure of eight or spiral method can be used.
6 Finish below the popliteal crease (or two fingers below the knee).
7 The bandage can then be covered with a layer of stockinette to keep it in place.
8 Change the bandages when required, preferably weekly.

There is a satisfaction in bandaging long-stretch bandages correctly. They look, and generally feel, very comfortable. The outcome of using these bandages is similar to that of short-stretch and multilayered bandages and ulcers will heal in 3–6 months. However, it requires a skilled practitioner to apply them and education of the bandager is an important element in the healing process.

Modified compression

A modified treatment for leg ulcers is used by the wound healing clinic in Cardiff (Melhuish et al. 1998). The leg is measured for Tubigrip. Three lengths are cut, a short, medium and long length. The three lengths are applied to legs assessed for venous disease and comply with the idea that double layers increase sub-bandage pressures. The three lengths, applied with the first length from the toes, ending at the malleoli. The second length toe to mid-calf and the final length extending from toe to just below the knee. This will give graduated compression according to Laplace's law and make application easier for individual patients, giving them independence.

Compression hosiery

Graduated compression hosiery is useful in the management of lymphoedema, venous ulceration, prevention of venous ulceration and prevention of deep vein thrombosis. Graduated compression hosiery works in a similar way to compression bandages with the shape and elasticity of the stocking providing graduated compression.

The dangers of compression hosiery are also similar to those of compression bandaging as poorly fitted stockings can cause pressure necrosis and application to an arterial limb can reduce blood flow, increase the potential of pressure necrosis and may even lead to amputation of the limb.

Too long a stocking can cause the stocking to roll down, creating a tourniquet effect. This may reduce blood flow to and/or from the feet and may increase the potential for deep vein thrombosis. The material may increase potential for contact dermatitis.

Compression hosiery is difficult for elderly patients to apply, particularly when there is a limited degree of mobility and hand dexterity. Therefore, it may require the time of a carer or nurse to put on and take off the stockings every day. A polythene bag placed over the foot before the stocking is put on, assists with application. The bag can be pulled off the foot once the stocking is applied. Producers of the hosiery may offer a nylon stockinette, free of charge, to aid application. Talcum powder applied to the legs and feet aid application. However, the talcum can be clogging and drying for the skin and is probably not generally advisable. Medi-Valet is a device that aids application. The stocking is placed over a metal frame, the frame supports the application of the stocking and is removable once the stocking is in place on the leg. However, this still requires a little strength and dexterity and may not suit all patients.

Two types of compression hosiery may be considered for the patient who requires independence. The Jobes stocking has a zip at the back which allows the stocking to be applied easily and then the zip is done up once the stocking is in place. Activa stockings are provided with a special applicator that makes applying the stockings simple for the patient.

There are three classes of compression hosiery:

1 Class 1: applies 14–17 mmHg of pressure and is used for 'tired legs', varicose veins and mild oedema.
2 Class 2: applies 18–24 mmHg of pressure and is used for severe varicose veins, prevention of ulcers, reduction of severe oedema and reduction in risk of ulcer recurrence.

3 Class 3: applies 25–35 mmHg of pressure and is used for lymphoedema, ulceration, very severe varicose veins, post phlebitis or cellulitis.

Accurate measurement of the limb is vital and should always be completed by a nurse or technician experienced in measuring and applying stockings. If the legs are measured at the end of a day, the measurement will be entirely different to the same leg measured at the beginning of the day. The optimum time for measuring would be the beginning of the day or if the patient has been on bedrest throughout the day.

Prior to fitting the patient should be assessed using a hand-held Doppler. An ankle brachial pressure of <0.8 should exclude the patient from wearing compression hosiery. An experienced practitioner, to ensure correct fit of the stockings should measure the limb. Skin should be checked daily as should heels for signs of erythema caused by pressure. The patient's compliance should be assessed as, without commitment to treatment, the ulcer will not heal.

Intermittent compression theory

Intermittent compression therapy is another way of encouraging venous return that can either be the main method of compression or can complement compression bandaging. The machine has a small compressor to which one or two tubes can be connected. The tubes will be connected from the proximal end to one or two boots. The boots come in a range of sizes and lengths and can be worn as one or as a pair. The use of one boot will see the air expanding the boot for a short period of time and then releasing the air. As a pair, the boots alternate in expanding with air and 'squeeze' the legs, causing reduction in venous hypertension and encouraging the patient to relax whilst the therapy is on. The patient can use the boot in the morning for an hour and in the evening for two hours and the boot can also be applied over compression bandaging (NHS Centre for Reviews and Dissemination 1997).

Bedrest

Bedrest with bed elevation is known to be an excellent way of achieving venous return (Mekkes 1998). The elevation level of the bed equates to the level of pressure applied by compression bandages but the bed must be clearly above heart level to achieve venous return.

However, for patients with congestive cardiac failure, elevating the bed to such a degree can embarrass the heart when leg oedema floods the venous system with a clear danger of complete heart failure. There is also the danger of reducing mobility in patients, leading to permanent immobility. For example, one patient walked into hospital for leg ulceration treatment. The treatment was leg elevation with the legs higher than the heart. Treatment was successful but three months later, she had to be wheeled out in a wheelchair to a nursing home, minus her leg ulcer but with a greatly reduced quality of life.

Treating venous ulcers

Activate the calf venous pump by introducing exercise. Walking at a steady pace is recommended. For immobile patients, leg exercises may be introduced and referral to a physiotherapist is helpful. However, the simple fact is that standing and transferring from bed to chair will activate the foot pump. Therefore, immobile patients who are able to transfer, could be asked to stand every hour.

To aid venous return when resting, the leg should always be elevated higher than the heart. However, elderly patients will find this particularly difficult when sitting in a chair. Nevertheless, it is recommended that the legs are not kept dependent for any longer than a few moments.

The patient and the ulcer should be assessed and, if the ulcer is venous in origin, a dressing should be selected according to holistic and physical findings. It is wise to care for the whole leg by washing in a bucket of water and applying ointment such as 50 per cent, oil or creams. Care must be taken with applying creams as they can contain preservatives (such as parabens) and these can act as allergens. Oils such as Oilatum or olive oil, can be added to the bath water or soaking bucket.

Measure the wound and record size, colour and describe malodour. Photographs are a useful assessment tool and can provide a detailed history of wound changes.

Zinc paste or ointment bandages are useful additions to any bandaging regime as it cares for the entire leg and also aids healing in the wound (Allen 1988). However, care should be taken as zinc bandages contain preservatives and paste bandages are the most common cause for identified sensitivities in leg ulcers (Dale 1984). Zinc may influence wound healing by reducing free radical activity, improving cell mitosis, strengthening collagen cross-bonding and inhibiting bacterial growth (Dickerson 1993). Zinc paste bandages may donate sufficient zinc to increase the levels of zinc at the site and accelerate wound healing. Appropriate compression therapy should then be applied.

At each dressing change, the wound status must be reassessed, remeasured and any changes recorded. The wound status may have changed since the last assessment and the dressing may need to be reviewed. However, the dressing type should not be changed without a rationale but if the wound is obviously static, it would not be good practice to continue using the same dressing for weeks. In this case, consider a dressing that may 'kick start' the wound (see Chapter 3).

The patient must be reassessed every six months using Doppler assessment.

Pinch grafting as an alternative to full skin graft

Pinch grafting is a simple procedure that can be performed at the bedside by a nurse trained in the technique. The donor site is injected with lignocaine 0.5–1 per cent or the site can be covered with EMLA cream or Ametop Gel and an occlusive dressing (Greenwood et al. 1997b) one hour prior to harvesting. Small pinches of skin can be harvested by the use of a scalpel and forceps (Figure 5.11). The harvested skin should be thinly cut; too deep and the graft will not take and the donor site would have an increased potential for clinical infection. Pinch grafting is a skill that could be learned and practised by district nurses, particularly as Öien et al. (2001) found that pinch grafting in the community was 3.3–5.9 times cheaper than in hospital.

Prior to harvesting, the donor sites should be identified as clean (not highly contaminated with bacteria or clinically infected). The donor site should be cleansed prior to harvesting, using the local protocol for skin cleansing (chlorhexidine is popular for this purpose). Once harvesting is complete, the donor site and the grafted site can be covered with Mepital and an absorbent secondary dressing and left for 5–7 days. The outer, secondary dressing can be changed in this time if required. Pinch grafting requires only small patches of skin which can be taken from various sites, whereas, skin grafting requires a large piece of tissue removed from one site. Mekkes (1998) found pinch grafting to be superior to skin grafting in regards to graft take, the speed of healing process, the quality of the healed skin and the functional and cosmetic appearance of the donor site.

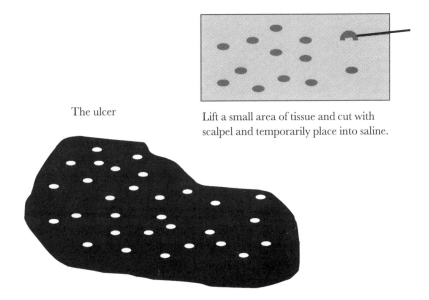

The ulcer

Lift a small area of tissue and cut with
scalpel and temporarily place into saline.

Pinch grafting provided areas of epithelial tissue that will migrate
outward to the wound margins. Wounds heal faster with this method.

Figure 5.11 Method of pinch grafting.

Skin graft

Skin grafting is a surgical procedure requiring possible theatre time
although it can be accomplished at the bedside. Graft edges can be
sutured into place and/or negative pressure can be applied to the
grafted wound. If it is policy to use paraffin gauze over the graft, it is
important that several layers are used to prevent adherence. Donor
sites are often the more difficult of the two wounds to manage. Skin
grafting may lead to a wound that heals faster (Figure 5.12),
although it should be noted that this can lead to difficulty with healing two wounds if the graft does not take.

Surgery for correcting venous insufficiency and arterial incompetence

Referral to a vascular surgeon may lead to removal of the veins,
injection or ligation. As venous insufficiency occurs due to incompetent valves, removal of the veins containing these valves, may correct
venous hypertension. Injection and ligation will have the same effect.

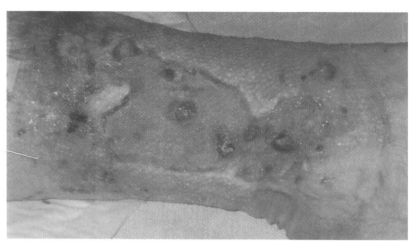

Figure 5.12 This wound had healed in 10 days following skin grafting (see Plate 29).

Arterial ulcers will particularly benefit from vascular surgery with a femoral popliteal by-pass or angioplasty restoring the potential for blood delivery to the tissues. Both systems can offer dramatic results of healing as blood is successfully restored to the tissues. However, these methods are not always successful and are often not possible due to poor medical status of the patient.

Quality of life for the venous leg ulcer patient

The patient must live with the treatment once it is applied and often this is difficult. When alone at night, a firm bandage can feel very tight indeed. Or, a dressing that increases in odour or discharge can seem far worse when visiting friends. These patients may be unhappy with their dressings and have difficulty with compliance. Dale and Gibson (1997) write 'A patient who has suffered a leg ulcer for many years may have developed low self-esteem as a result'. Such a patient may have lost the motivation to persevere with treatment and given up any hope of the ulcer healing, a belief that becomes a self-fulfilling prophecy as the patient ignores treatment advice and the ulcer does not heal. For these patients, in compression therapy, dietary advice and exercise are of prime importance and, combined with a compromise, may lead to increased compliance. Full concordance will hopefully come when the patient sees improvement in the ulcer healing rate.

There are also patients who are reluctant for the ulcer to heal (Poulton 1991). Perhaps because their ulcer is their life and their point of reference or their link with the outside world through the district nurse visits. Improving their contact with outside, through dinner clubs, home visits from voluntary organizations, and arranging for the patient to visit the clinic instead of home visits, will help to decrease their loneliness and need for contact.

House (1996) identified several factors that may affect compliance:

1 complexity of the treatment procedure;
2 degree of change to individual lifestyle required;
3 length of treatment;
4 whether the treatment is seen as potentially life-saving;
5 level of patient's knowledge, individual health and spiritual beliefs;
6 level of physical independence;
7 motivation;
8 failure to understand medical jargon;
9 difficulty with recalling information;
10 social isolation.

The practitioner assessing the patient should be aware of all these factors and be prepared to address the issues. Charles (1995) looked at quality of life and found that two main themes emerged: the effect on patient's working lives and human interaction. Charles found that these two themes frequently overlapped as, when a person is unable to go to work, the opportunity of making social contact is either lost or greatly reduced. Charles writes 'Work satisfies a variety of psychological needs such as achieving a sense of personal identity, being a part of a group and feeling a sense of self-worth. When a person's network of social relationships is deficient, loneliness is a likely result'.

Walshe (1995) found that pain was the most overwhelming feature of leg ulceration that prevented people from going out. Very little work has been completed in reducing pain in leg ulceration and analgesics often leave the patient feeling nauseous or lethargic, which are often not acceptable and, therefore, do not increase quality of life.

The basis of any compression treatment must be the professional's empathy and understanding of the patient's social and medical problems. Keeling et al. (1997) found that patient's perception was, generally they received little social support. The professional will need to build up trust, between themselves and the patients and carers, and education must be the cornerstone of that trust.

The effect of clinical governance

Clinical governance is a new concept, introduced by the Labour Government (1999–2000) to ensure that practices, throughout the health service, are based on clinical evidence; that no task or practice is undertaken in isolation, without excellent rationale for why it is done. The concept will lead the health service into a new era when the senior nurse or consultant cannot demand a junior to undertake a procedure without being able to give evidence of why that procedure is required. This is particularly strong in the area of leg ulcer treatments. There is a dearth of evidence to show that patients with venous ulcers must receive Doppler assessment and, if suitable, must be given the option of compression bandages. With Clinical Governance, those areas not complying with this standard will be sought out and brought into line. Therefore, it is imperative that all nurses and general practitioners are aware of the treatment options for leg ulceration, follow the standards set by the leaders in the field and complete audit in treatment and healing rates of leg ulcers.

Malignant ulceration

A non-healing wound, particularly one with rolled edges or one with a cauliflower appearance should be biopsied to rule out malignancy. It is wise to question malignancy in wounds that have been present for some years, particularly if not responding to modern therapy such as compression.

Lymphoedema

Lymphoedema is a chronic swelling of the limbs due to a failure of the lymph drainage system to remove the protein rich interstitial fluid. Lymph has two primary functions, achievement of tissue homeostasis and support of the immunological system. It comprises of a system of vessels, similar to the venous system, which drains fluid from the interstitial spaces, returning it to the blood stream.

Approximately 90 per cent of the tissue fluid returns via the venous system, the other 10 per cent returns via the lymph system (Jeffs 1993).There are four main components to lymphoedema: excess protein in the tissues, oedema, chronic inflammation and excess fibrosis (Mortimer and Regnard 1986). Identified by a positive Stermmer's sign where the skin at the base of the toes cannot be pinched. The skin will be pitted and fibrous and the limb will be grossly swollen and distorted and exaggerated skin folds occur. The skin is compromised by the oedema in the tissues and easily breaks into ulceration. Treatment is reduction of the oedema through compression therapy, leg elevation, exercise and wound care.

Theories of causation of venous ulceration are still being debated with the white cell and fibrin cuff theories remaining largely conjecture and unproven. However, an increase in the rates of leg ulcer healing is occurring and this success can only be attributed to the increased knowledge and experience found in interested and committed clinical professionals.

Prevention of recurrence

The focus of good management and treatment of leg ulceration is on compression therapy with the issue of prevention of recurrence largely ignored. Use of compression stockings should be encouraged for the prevention of recurrence (Effective Health Care 1999). However, there are many different manufactures' compression stockings available on the drug tariff and selection may be difficult. If possible, the patient or carer must accept responsibility for the prevention of ulcers in the healed leg.

The following points offer support for the prevention of recurrence. Prescribe appropriate and measured compression stockings. The patient must either be able to apply the stockings independently or have a friend or carer who can be trained to apply them. Aids for application can be obtained from several manufacturers:

- Actiglide: a simple idea providing easy application of stockings;
- vinyl gloves to aid grip and reduce damage to the stockings from fingernails;
- a plastic bag can be placed over the foot, the stocking slips over the top and the bag can be withdrawn once the stocking is in place.

Gentle application of compression stockings should be carried out before rising in the morning or, once the leg is dependent, the oedema will return.

Provision of exceptional skin care is vital to the maintenance of tissue viability. Application of creams, ointments or oils will help to keep skin supple. However, care should be taken to ensure the patient is not sensitive to whichever product is being used. Most creams contain preservatives and it is these that generally cause sensitivities. Ointments, such as 50/50 (50 per cent paraffin, 50 per cent petroleum jelly) rarely contain substances that cause sensitivities. Oils may be a problem in cases of hypersensitivity, particularly if the patient is allergic to nuts; it is probably safer to use emollients in the bath water rather than olive oil or arachis oil.

The patient should be warned to protect the leg against trauma. Wheelchair footrests must be retracted when mobilizing. Coffee table corners can be dangerous. Supermarket trolleys cause untold and unresearched damage to legs and many leg ulcer victims claim the first trauma and initiation of the ulcer was from a supermarket trolley.

The patient should be advised to elevate the legs when resting although mobilization will increase venous return and advice should include a plan of mobility for the individual patient.

> Numerous articles have been published under the title 'The final cause of venous ulceration'. Theories reflected methodology, trends and new discoveries of those days. Vascular anomalies, clotting disorders, fibrin cuffs, iron deposition with formation of free radicals, leucocyte and thrombocyte accumulation, diffusion barriers for cytokines, increased expression of endothelial adhesion molecules and other immunological phenomena were considered to be the final cause of leg ulceration.
>
> (Mekkes 1998)

It is likely that some, or many, of these are present in venous ulceration. The jury remains out but scientists continue the struggle to identify the 'final' cause.

Foot ulceration in patients with diabetes mellitus

Hyperglycaemia is the common characteristic in the two types of diabetes:

* Type 1. The pancreatic islands of Langerhans's cells fails to produce insulin.
* Type 2. There is an insulin resistance and impaired insulin secretion, combined with environmental and genetic factors (Reiber et al. 1998).

At any one time there are more patients occupying hospital beds with diabetic foot complications than by all other patients with complications of diabetes, and 50 per cent of all non-traumatic amputations are performed on diabetic patients (Barnett 1992). Foot ulcers remain one of the most costly aspects of treatment of diabetes and 15 per cent of all patients with diabetes will experience foot ulceration (Effective Health Care 1999).

Patients with diabetes mellitus are more likely to develop atherosclerosis, but in six patients with circulatory insufficiency, it is generally the smaller tibial, peroneal arteries (Bryant 1992) and the microcirculation that are occluded. Often the main arteries are not particularly occluded and Doppler readings can be >0.8. Nevertheless, the patient is not suitable for compression as the micro-circulation is not delivering necessary blood to the tissues. Therefore, extreme care must be taken when making a decision to treat an ulcer with a venous component in a diabetic patient in case there is mixed aetiology, even when Doppler readings are normal.

There are four main factors leading to necrosis of the tissues:

1 Ischaemia with impairment of effective circulation is the single most important factor responsible for delayed healing in diabetic foot ulcers (Macfarlane and Jeffcoate 1999). However, ischaemia can result in macro-vascular or micro-vascular disease. Doppler readings or palpation of pedal pulses can only assess for macro-vascular disease and does not identify abnormal capillary function. Peripheral vascular disease is one of the most important factors (a 46 per cent causal factor) associated with amputations and linked to 62 per cent of non-healing ulcers (Reiber et al. 1998).
2 Sensory neuropathy or damage to the sensory nerves in legs and feet can lead to loss of sensation and potential injury, which goes unnoticed and may result in necrosis.
3 Autonomic neuropathy may result in loss of blood flow to the feet and loss of sweating.
4 In motor neuropathy, the wasting of muscles in the feet causes defor-mities and pressure from shoes can lead to necrosis.

Diabetic neuropathy

Neuropathy is the commonest complication of diabetes, and usually arises within five years of the onset of the disease (Barnett 1992). Patients with diabetic foot ulceration on the plantar, medial and lateral surfaces of the foot will almost all have clinically significant peripheral neuropathy. These patients generally have adequate blood supply and develop foot ulceration because of high pressures, possibly through tight-fitting shoes, and direct and unnoticed injury from treading on a nail or pin. Some patients however can develop ulceration through repetitive moderate stress (Brand 1978). Pathogenesis of neuropathy is generally ascribed to abnormalities of the sorbitol pathways. However, defects in the myosnositol, glutathionine and related pathways may also be important (Bessman and Sapico 1992).

Diabetic ulceration, more often found over bony prominences on the foot, is often caused by ill-fitting shoes or because neuropathy has not alerted the patient to tissue injury. Neuropathy can lead to a Charcot joint, which is a result of neuropathy, osteoporosis and sometimes trauma. The main characteristic of the Charcot joint is a flattening of the medial longitudinal arch, often with a 'rocker bottom' shape to the foot. Build up of callosities offers abnormal pressure loading on the tissues and can often lead to ulceration. A wound over a Charcot joint can be very difficult to treat as it is, necessarily, a weight-bearing joint and osteoporosis, hyperostosis, osteolysis, pathological fracture, spontaneous dislocation of the joint and generalized joint or bone damage can occur.

Charcot foot occurs in more than one per cent of all patients with diabetes and develops unilaterally in 80 per cent of patients but can present bilaterally in 20 per cent. It is a chronic, painless degenerative process affecting the weight-bearing joints of the foot, involving the midtarsal joint in 60 per cent of patients (Laing 1998). It is thought to be due to repeated minor trauma in the neuropathic foot caused by the inability to feel the trauma because of diabetic neuropathy.

Charcot joint is generally not seen in the ischaemic foot but has been noted following revascularization (Laing 1998), leading to a belief that increased blood flow from autonomic neuropathy may bear some responsibility for the Charcot joint (Laing 1998). The Charcot joint develops through three stages:

1 Acute inflammation associated with hyperaemia and erythema. The bone softens and fragments and fracture dislocations occur.
2 Bony coalescence occurs with a reduction in swelling in the foot with periosteal new bone formation.
3 Bony consolidation and healing occurs (Laing 1998).

This process can last up to three years, although it can be much more rapid.

A well-designed back-slab fibreglass boot can be an excellent way of relieving pressure during mobilization. Because of the poor blood supply, due to diabetes, negative pressure therapy is helpful, as is dispersion therapy dressing. Fifty per cent of patients with neuropathic joints, require amputation within five years (Barnett 1992). Ischaemic ulceration and gangrene are common in patients with diabetes.

Tyrell (1995) is concerned with the effect that fashion shoes may have when worn by people with diabetes. Tyrell writes 'During the stance phase (the time during walking when the body passes over the top of it) the increase in foot length and width leads to impaction of the forefoot in the forepart of the shoe'. Due to diabetic neuropathy, the walker may not be aware of the damage that is occurring within the shoe. Therefore, advice on footwear should be given to those with diabetic neuropathy, suggesting adequate width, length and girth with enough room for extension of the forefoot without impaction (Tyrell 1995).

Other factors that increase the load on the diabetic foot are: insulin deficiency, which is associated with depressed collagen formation with fewer granulocytes and fibroblasts; non-enzymatic glycosylation of collagen leading to a thickening of the dermis; and loss of elastic fibres, which makes the tissues thicker, less flexible and resistant to digestion by collagenase (Laing 1998). Keratin also becomes glycosated and leads to and contributes to the overall thickening of the skin (Laing 1998).

These factors increase joint stiffness, reduce mobility and increase the risk of ulceration.

Autonomic neuropathy

Autonomic neuropathy can result in a loss of sweating and can cause dryness of the skin and cracking (Knowles 1996). Diabetic patients also suffer from yellowing toenails and fungal infections. Therefore, skin care is a necessary part of the general care given to the patient and education in keeping the feet clean and dry and the skin moistened is imperative. Surgical spirits can be useful in prevention of fungal infections when sprayed between the toes. However, a patient with diabetes should always be referred to a chiropodist who will be the prime advisor on care of the feet. Peri-wound areas can always be protected from maceration (prior to applying dressings), with a liquid, non-sting barrier film such as Cavilon or SuperSkin.

Blood sugar is an important element in formation and non-healing status of diabetic ulceration. Without maintenance of acceptable blood sugar levels, wound healing will definitely be compromised. Blood sugars (glucose) can react chemically with fats and proteins within the blood and destroy the proteins' ability to function (glycation reactions). When the level of sugar remains high it increases the potential for protein destruction to occur and the continued interference with the protein function will eventually lead to destruction of cellular function and the well-recognized tissue injuries that are related to diabetes.

Diabetes and the potential for clinical infection

Patients with diabetes are at higher risk of acquiring infection and Steed (1998) states 'A vigorous search for infection is important in patients with diabetes'. Impairment of leucocyte function, reduced cellular immune responses, prolonged persistence of abscesses and delayed wound healing all predispose the diabetic patient to infection. Acute infections in patients who have not recently received prescribed antibiotics are often caused by a single organism, whereas infections treated previously with antibiotic therapy are often polymicrobial. Once an infection is established, it can sometimes spread with frightening rapidity, leading to involvement of the whole foot and septicaemia in a short period of time (Laing 1998).

Despite the fact that they have diminished sensation, many patients with diabetes develop pain in their foot when infection is present. Patients with diabetes have multiple microorganisms within their wounds and 25 per cent of patients will have anaerobic bacteria present, which may not show on swab cultures. Systemic antibiotics are regarded as part of standard treatment for invasive infections in diabetic foot ulcers (Effective Health Care 1999). However, Jeffcoate (1999) is concerned that as antibiotics encourage resistant organisms, there is a risk that any infection of bone with methicillin-resistant *Staphylococcus aureus* (MRSA) may be difficult to eradicate and may threaten the whole limb. Jeffcoate recommends that antibiotics are only given appropriately and are avoided when ulcers are clinically clean and clinically uninfected. Edmonds (1999), on the other hand, recommends that early use of antibiotics should not be ruled out and that diabetic patients should be examined at every visit for clinical signs of infection, swabs taken if indicated and antibiotics prescribed for a positive swab.

The foot ulcers in diabetic patients can track and cause deep-seated problems with the potential of osteomylitis. Pressure ulcers on the diabetic foot will occur at the point of maximal pressure on the plantar of the foot and next to the bone. This will form an underlying ulcer, which will track outward forming a smaller sized wound on the surface of the foot. There is often a hard 'scab' on the base of the foot, which, when debrided, will release the abscess and reveal the larger hole underneath. It is important that an ulcer, suspected of tracking, should be X-rayed to eliminate osteomylitis and the wound explored to establish the depth of the diabetic ulcer is vital as the necrotic and hard tissue may cover a pocket of pus beneath it.

Debridement is an important component of treatment; it permits full examination of the wound bed and identifies tracking. However, a professional, skilled in the diabetic foot, must undertake debridement as the consequences of poorly debrided tissue in the diabetic patient can lead to amputation.

Vasculopathy is associated with diabetes and can be macro-vascular or micro-vascular in origin and is more commonly found in type 1 diabetes. Macro-vascular disease is easily identified through Doppler assessment. Micro-vascular disease is less easily identified and, because of the problems of identification and the possibility of poorly perfused tissues, compression should only be applied following vascular assessment and authorisation of a vascular consultant. Arterial calcification can be found in 94 per cent of patients who have had diabetes for 35 years (Laing 1998).

The newest form of treatment for diabetic ulceration is tissue engineering (see Chapter 3) and there has been considerable success using this method.

The diabetic ulcer is a significant healthcare problem and inadequate or improper therapy may lead to amputation. Therefore, careful monitoring, patient education and education for the professionals caring for diabetic foot ulcers is imperative.

Aspirin in treatment of leg ulcers

There has been interest recently in the use of aspirin in healing venous ulcers. Layton et al. (1994) undertook research in this area. They used a double-blind, randomized placebo-controlled method using 20 subjects. Ten patients were supplied with 300 mg of enteric coated aspirin and compared to standard therapy in the other 10 patients. Of the patients taking aspirin, 38 per cent healed completely and 2 per cent improved compared with 0 per cent healing and 26 per cent improving on the standard therapy, providing evidence that aspirin is a useful adjunct in treatment of chronic ulcers. If future studies demonstrate similar results, this will form a strong argument for patients with venous ulcers receiving aspirin therapy.

Conclusion

Leg ulcer treatment has progressed enormously since the early 1990s and compression has been largely responsible for the increase in healing rates. The most important elements of the treatment is the involvement of the patient and the education of those caring for the ulcers. Without knowledge of how leg ulcers occur, whether arterial or venous in origin, there will be a lack of understanding of how they heal. High wound healing education is required for the medical teams who are responsible for caring for patients with leg ulcers.

Activity

1 Learn the concepts of compression bandaging.
2 Practise applying short-stretch compression bandaging; identify the point at which confidence in the technique is gained. Ask an experienced bandager to assess you in practise.
3 Practice applying multilayer compression bandaging; identify the point at which confidence in the technique is gained. Ask an experienced bandager to assess you in practice.
4 Enlist the assistance of a nurse experienced in Doppler technique. Learn how to use the Doppler and become familiar with the three different sounds of arteries.

CHAPTER 6

Nutrition and wound healing

KATHARINE MARTYN

In this chapter, nutrition and the basis of the healthy diet is reviewed; specific nutrients and their effects on wound healing are identified and the implications of malnutrition are discussed. The final section reviews how diet may be used as a form of therapy by modulating the immune response and influencing inflammation.

The relationship between nutrition and wound healing is complex. Evidence suggests that malnutrition will influence the wound healing process but despite this the majority of wounds heal (Carlson 1999). This may contribute to the low profile of nutritional support that is evident in care settings. It is thought, however, that good nutrition is essential for ultimate wound strength and that the critical period is in the early phases.

Observations based on populations and the incidence of disease have led to a greater understanding of the impact of nutrition on health and also to the development of nutritional guidelines. These are based on the reference nutritional intake (RNI) for nutrients (MAFF 1995). A reference nutritional intake is the amount of a nutrient that is required by 97.5 per cent of the population to prevent signs of deficiency occurring. In calculating this figure, it is assumed that the population is normally distributed. Individuals may require a nutrient intake that is greater or less than that recommended and it is important in health care that each individual's nutritional needs are assessed to ensure adequate intake.

The Health Education Authority (HEA) has taken the dietary recommendations and devised 'The Balance of Good Health' documentation, which acts as a guide to the types of food that need to be eaten to achieve a healthy, balanced diet (HEA 1994).

As health professionals it is important that nurses understand the healthy diet and how dietary requirements may change due to ill health. Whilst all diets should contain a balance of nutrients, the amount of differing nutrients, for someone who is ill, may differ to that in their healthy state due to altered physiological need. Understanding the basics of nutrition will enable the nurse to make informed decisions as to the foods that she will advise her patient to eat.

Food is without doubt the most economical source of nutrients and a balanced diet will contain all the nutrients required by an individual. The nutrient content of food can be divided into the macronutrients: fat, carbohydrate and protein and the micronutrients: vitamins and minerals.

Macronutrients

Protein, fat and carbohydrates each contain carbon, hydrogen and protein. They are each a potential source of energy although the preferred energy source for body tissues is glucose predominantly derived from carbohydrate.

Fat

Dietary fat, whilst more energy dense, is not used for an immediate energy source but will provide a source of stored energy in the fat cells, adipocytes. Fats are composed of fatty acids attached to a glycerol backbone. It is these fatty acids that determine to which group a fat or oil belongs. Saturated fatty acids have each carbon atom attached to hydrogen; mono-unsaturated fatty acids have a double bond between two carbon atoms, which are not then attached to hydrogen. Polyunsaturated fatty acids have more than one double bond. Of these, the polyunsaturated must be part of the dietary intake. They consist of the essential fatty acids, N6, linolenic and N3, linoleic fatty acids (Table 6.1). Once ingested dietary fatty acids undergo elongation and desaturation, which lead to a range of products that play important roles in cell membrane structures and cellular function. Some of these products are the cytokines, prostaglandins and leukotrienes, which are important within the inflammatory response.

Table 6.1 Fatty acids

Saturated fatty acid
Found in coconut oil, palm oil, dairy products and meat.

Mono-unsaturated fatty acid with one double bond
Found in olive oil, rape seed oil, peanut oil, cows milk and beef

---

Polyunsaturated fatty acid N-6 PUFA Linoleic acid
Found in corn oil, soybean oil, sunflower oil, poultry and meat.

Polyunsaturated fatty acid N-3 PUFA Linolenic acid
Found in flaxseed oil, cod liver oil and oily fish such as herring.

Fats are also a source of fat-soluble vitamins A, D, E and K although the majority of vitamin D, in adults, is derived from the action of sunlight on the skin.

Carbohydrates

Carbohydrates are the main source of energy and include single or multiple units of glucose, starch, non-starch polysaccharide (NSP) and cellulose. NSP and cellulose will largely enter the colon unchanged and provide a substrate for bacterial fermentation, producing short chain fatty acids (SCFA), which are an important energy source for colonocytes and may play a role in energy balance in times of stress or acute illness.

Protein

Proteins provide a source of amino acids of which 20 are important. Of these, nine are essential as they cannot be synthesized within the body. Others such as arginine and glutamine are semi essential and play an important role during periods of stress and tissue trauma (see section on nutrition therapy). Amino acids are important for cellular growth, repair, communication and cellular products such as hormones and enzymes. Unlike energy, derived from fats and carbohydrates, there is no store of amino acids. Instead there is a continuous turnover of amino acids derived from the diet and normal cell degradation.

Micronutrients

Vitamins are organic substances whilst minerals are inorganic and are derived from the environment from which the food is produced. Both vitamins and minerals act at a cellular level and will be required in differing amounts reflecting cellular function and health status. The bioavailability of vitamins and minerals can be influenced by other foods within the diet and the aging process. The main vitamins and minerals are listed later in this chapter.

Nutrients and wound healing

Several nutrients have been directly linked to wound healing and deficiency states may impair wound strength and delay the healing process

Protein

Following tissue damage there is a predictable physiological response as the immune system is activated and healing begins. This response requires amino acids and to meet that demand a catabolic response, the breakdown of body tissues, ensues. As a consequence a negative nitrogen balance occurs. The extent and duration of this response will reflect the extent and nature of the tissue damage.

The amino acids are required for the formation of antibodies and leucocytes, which are needed to prevent infection. They are also a vital component of fibroplasia, required for wound contraction, collagen synthesis and in the formation of granulation tissue.

The healthy adult needs 0.8 g protein daily per kilogram body weight. In the presence of tissue damage this can increase further to 1.2–1.5 g/kg/day for partial thickness wounds and 1.5–2 g/kg/day for full thickness or extensive wounds with exudate. Increasing the dietary intake any greater than this will not influence the negative nitrogen balance, which tends to be present even when nutritional needs are met, and can be detrimental by increasing the workload of the liver.

Carbohydrates and fat

Both carbohydrates and fat provide a source of energy and in health are consumed to excess leading to stores within the body. During periods of ill health the energy requirement can increase whilst the appetite is suppressed. This leads to a breakdown of energy stores. The utilization of glycogen from the liver provides a supply of glucose. When this is exhausted the body catabolizes protein and to a lesser extent, stored fats to produce the glucose required. In addition the metabolism of fat results in the production of pro-inflammatory substances such as prostaglandins and cytokines, which mediate the inflammatory responses. This depression of appetite and mobilization of stores is considered to be the mechanism by which optimum nutrients are supplied to the immune system without the need of the energy dependent processes of eating, digestion and absorption.

Wound healing is a catabolic, energy dependent process. Carbohydrate not only provides energy but glucose fuels fibroplastic migration, phagocytic activity and cellular proliferation (Murray-Kiy 1997).

Maintaining a balance between energy demand and energy supply is essential during periods of ill health (see section on Management and interventions later in this chapter). Individuals who are underweight, or have a negative energy balance, prior to becoming ill are more prone to complications. It has been estimated that as many as 40 per cent of patients admitted to hospital are malnourished on admission and for many their condition will worsen (McWhirter and Pennington 1994).

Vitamins, minerals and trace elements

Vitamins (see Table 6.2) and minerals play important roles in cell metabolism, often acting as co-factors. During wound healing, cell activity increases and it is likely that the demand for micronutrients will also increase, although precise requirements are generally unknown. Some vitamins and minerals have been shown to play a specific role in wound healing.

Vitamin C

Vitamin C is a water soluble antioxidant. Its main function is as a co-substrate in oxygen requiring hydroxylation reactions. As such it is essential in the hydroxylation of proline and lysine in the production of pro-collagen. During acute illness, stress, injury and increased metabolic rate vitamin C use and excretion increases. Smokers may have a vitamin C requirement that is twice that of a non-smoker.

Table 6.2 Vitamins and their sources

Vitamins	Source
A Retinol B-Carotene	Liver, meat and meat products. Milk and milk products. All vegetables especially carrots, red and orange fruits.
D Calciferol	Fatty fish (herring, sardines) margarine. Low fat spreads, evaporated milk. Breakfast cereal.
E	Vegetable oils, margarine, whole grain cereals, eggs, dark green vegetables, nuts.
K	Green leafy vegetables, dairy produce, vegetable oils, cereals and meat.
Thiamin	All cereals especially bread, breakfast cereal and potatoes.
Riboflavin	Milk and milk products. Fortified breakfast cereals.
Niacin	Meat and meat products, bread, fortified breakfast cereals.
B6	Many differing foods. Potatoes and breakfast cereals are a high souce.
B12	Meat and liver products, milk products.
Folic acid	Green leafy vegetables, fortified breakfast cereal, milk and milk products.
C	Citrus fruit and jucies, green vegetables and other fruit.

Healthy adults require 60 mg/day, some people recommend an intake of between 100 mg and 200 mg for those with chronic wounds, although cell saturation with vitamin C has been noted at 100 mg/day.

Vitamin A

Vitamin A is important for cellular differentiation and proliferation. It enhances the inflammatory response probably by increasing the influx of macrophages. This in turn results in the increased release of growth factors in the wound (Thornton et al. 1997). The RNI for vitamin A is 600 µg /day for adults.

Zinc

Zinc is critical to healing because it is a component of many enzyme systems such as carbonic anhydrase, the immune system and a co-factor in collagen formation. Zinc deficiency can occur as a result of diarrhoea, renal failure, diuretic use, laxatives, enteral and parenteral nutrition. These conditions or situations are often present in patients with wounds and as such zinc deficiency needs to be considered. Hypoalbuminaemia may also account for lower serum zinc concentrations, as zinc is transported bound to albumin. The RNI for zinc is 7–9 mg/day.

Iron

Iron is important in the transportation of oxygen and as a factor in collagen hydroxylation. In most cases the iron intake matches that of loss but there is evidence of iron deficiency in children, the elderly and menstruating women. Iron is widely found in animal and vegetable sources. It has greater bioavailabilty from animal sources but its total absorption is limited from both. In many cases the level of deficiency is insufficient to effect wound healing. The RNI for iron is 8.7–14.8 mg/day.

Other nutrients may play a specific role in wound healing, for example arginine (see section on nutrition therapy, page 221).

Assessing the nutritional status of patients with wounds

The aim, during wound healing, is to ensure adequate nutrition to:

1 Provide adequate calories and protein for metabolism and to reduce loss of body tissues.
2 Prevent malnutrition occurring or minimize the impact of disease on nutritional status.
3 Provide an optimum environment for wound healing.
4 Return patient to their former nourished status.

Assessment is the first stage in ensuring that adequate nutrition is provided for the patient (MEREC 1998). All nursing frameworks cover areas that can identify altered nutritional status or nutritional intake. Alternatively nutritional screening, using risk scores, will effectively identify those patients most at risk. All members of the multidisciplinary team can use them.

There are several factors that can indicate malnutrition or the potential for malnutrition in the patient with wounds. These should be explored and documented during the assessment process.

Weight

Weight should be recorded on admission and discharge from hospital and at regular times in the community. It is a useful indicator of energy intake and when coupled with the height can be used to predict the body mass index (BMI). The BMI is a measure of body composition and can indicate the relative fatness of an individual.

Sudden unplanned weight loss of more than 10 per cent in three months could be significant. Weight loss during the period of ill health is not uncommon but excessive and continued loss indicates a negative energy balance and increases the risk of complications. Weight loss may also be associated with lethargy and tiredness, which may make it difficult for the patient to mobilize; this in turn may influence venous return. Excessive weight loss can also lead to depression, which may influence compliance to treatment.

Excess weight may also indicate poor nutrition, and can be detrimental to wound healing due to reduced mobility and increased body mass. Abdominal wounds may be at risk of dehiscence due to the excessive fatty tissue. Wipke-Tevis and Stotts (1998) demonstrated that many patients with leg ulcers are obese. Although it is unclear whether obesity precedes the development of leg ulcers or develops as a result of decreased activity once the ulcer had appeared.

Skin, hair and nails

Observations of the skin, hair and nails can give information about micronutrient and macronutrient deficiency. The presence of pressure sores may indicate poor nutrition prior to ill-health (Banks 1998).

Monitoring patients with wounds, recognizing delays in wound healing, secondary infections or excess exudate can also indicate reduced nutritional status or the potential for a worsening condition. Individuals with excessive exudate loss are more at risk of protein depletion.

Mouth and dental care

Patients with ill-fitting dentures or poor dental condition may have difficulty eating a wide range of foods. The more limited the diet the more likely the individual will suffer from deficiency in nutrients. Sores in the mouth, angular stomatitis can also indicate nutrient deficiency.

Mobility and dexterity

Alterations in mobility and dexterity can reduce access to shops and food purchase. It can also limit cooking activities and subsequently reduce dietary intake. Many ready-prepared meals are packaged in such ways that make them difficult to open. Elderly patients with hip fractures are often malnourished prior to coming into care and this may influence recovery (Unosson et al. 1995).

Social factors

The home situation including access to cooking and food storage facilities can reduce food purchase and regular hot meals. In addition old age, living alone and bereavement are all risk factors for malnutrition. Dietary recall can outline the normal diet an individual has and suggest potential deficiencies in macronutrients or micronutrients.

Cognitive function

Confusional states, short-term memory loss and dementia can make food intake irregular. This can be made worse in hospital or care situations that have rigid and inflexible mealtimes. Poor nutrition is also associated with lethargy and depression, which may make it difficult for individuals to comply with new medications and treatment regimens.

Illnesses and medication

Certain conditions predispose an individual to malnutrition these include patients with cancer, gastro-intestinal disease such as Crohns disease or ulcerative colitis, metabolic disorders such as diabetes, and trauma. Patients with chronic leg ulcers show diminished levels of vitamin A, vitamin E, carotenes and zinc (Rojas and Phillips1999).

Patients undergoing surgery or who were admitted with cerebral vascular accidents (CVA) can be without food for considerable periods of time.

Patients on multiple medications are also at risk of malnutrition. Drugs can alter taste, absorption and metabolism of nutrients others such as steroids and chemotherapy can depress the immune response.

Biochemical assessment

Several biochemical measurements can be of use in determining nutritional status. They are objective but can also be influenced by stress, infection and other concurrent disease states.

Serum albumin is a common indicator of the patient's total protein status. However, it is not very sensitive as it can be influenced by sepsis, nephrotic syndrome, liver disease, burns and altered fluid status, all of which lower serum albumin levels. It has a half-life of 21 days and large amounts are stored in the body. A patient may already be malnourished before serum albumin levels drop significantly:

> 3.5 g/dl   reflects adequate stores

< 3 g/dl   hypoalbuminaemic tissue oedema

<2.5 g/dl   deficiency of stores.

Serum transferin is a more accurate indicator of protein stores and is more sensitive than serum albumin. Levels can be lowered in liver diseases, burns and cortisone therapy whilst being elevated in iron deficient anaemia. It has a short half-life and smaller body stores

> 200 mg/dl   normal

< 100 mg/dl   depleted stores.

Insulin like growth factor (IGF) or somatomedins are low molecular weight peptides produced by the liver. In particular IGF-1 has a short half-life of a few hours and is unaffected by the acute phase response. It may be a more accurate and sensitive reflection of nutritional status independent of concurrent disease activity.

Management and interventions

- Ensure nutritional care is planned. Where nutritional teams involving the multidisciplinary team are evident, nutritional care has been shown to improve.
- Complete a regular assessment or screen for risk of malnutrition.
- Ensure there are clear protocols for referral to dieticians and provision of nutritional support.
- Ensure support is available during mealtimes in order that individuals can access and eat their food. In the hospital, reducing other activities such as wound dressings, ward rounds or investigations during mealtimes can help.
- Whilst in the community providing support over the mealtime can improve nutritional intake.
- Prepare the individual to have a meal, offer hand washes prior to meals. Ensure dentures fit and that teeth are cared for, ensure correct eating utensils, plate guards, non-slip mats or beakers are available.
- Offer drinks with food. Ensure food is of the correct consistency and temperature.
- Monitor and record dietary intake. If energy intake is poor offer supplements, such as Build up or Complan, consider fortifying food. Add butter or cream to soup, have whole milk, whilst adding skimmed milk powder can make foods more energy dense. Offer snacks between meals such as milky drinks or sandwiches. If a complete feed is required, take advice from the dieticians and ensure all feed is given.
- If additional protein is required, consider fortifying food.
- Encourage intake of fruit and vegetables. However if appetite is poor this may decrease total energy intake and you may need to consider supplements of vitamins and minerals such as zinc, iron and vitamin C. This is particularly important for the frail elderly with small appetites.

Nutrition as therapy

Nutrition and the immune response

Studies increasingly demonstrate how nutrients are interacting with cellular functions. This has led to a resurgence of interest into what is known as immuno nutrition where the addition of specific nutrients modulates immune responses.

Fatty acids

Fatty acids are found in cellular membranes and their relative amounts reflect the dietary intake of fat. The essential fatty acids derived from the N3 and N6 polyunsaturates are precursors of pro-inflammatory substances. Fatty acids have also been shown to influence the function of cells of the immune system (Miles and Calder 1998). Manipulating the intake of PUFA through addition or deletion of dietary sources such as fish, seeds and oils may influence the immune response, although consumption is likely to be in excess of that normally considered.

Anabolic support

Studies have demonstrated how the clinical use of anabolic agents such as recombinant growth hormone or Oxandrolone has improved wound healing and promoted weight gain (Demling and De Santi 1999). Ziegler et al. (1988) demonstrated how the use of recombinant growth hormone in patients with burns reduced protein catabolism and enhanced wound healing. Oxandrolone has been used to combat the weight loss in patients with thermal wounds and AIDS.

Arginine

The semi-essential amino acid, arginine, enhances wound healing and the lymphocyte immune response. Supplementation with arginine has been shown to increase both collagen deposition in small test wounds and the lymphocyte response to mitogens (Barbul et al. 1990).

Conclusion

Studies will continue to illuminate the relationship between diets and wound healing, providing evidence for the relationship between nutrients and cell activity. Currently although the evidence for a direct effect of diet on wound healing is limited there is a growing body of evidence to suggest that good nutrition will not only enhance the immune response but also ensure optimum healing of wounds through a range of mechanisms. Secondary effects of good nutritional care including an improved sense of well-being, and increased energy levels will also impact on the compliance to treatment and subsequent recovery. It is therefore essential to consider nutritional care as part of the managed wound care that will lead to increased and improved wound healing in patients.

CHAPTER 7

Surgical wounds

The successful culmination of any operation is a healed wound. Failure of a wound to heal leads to increased hospitalization times, increased costs and a decrease in patient quality of life. There is also an increased risk of post-operative complications, with deep vein thrombosis, chest infections and nosocomial infections being three of the many potential problems resulting from reduced mobility.

During the past century remarkable advances have been made in surgery, associated with the lowest recorded rates of infection or sepsis (Leaper 1995). Surgical wounds are brought in direct apposition during suturing and are exposed only briefly to potential contaminants (Briggs 1997). Cruse and Foord (1980) found that risk of post-operative infections doubled for every hour the patient remains on the operating table. Eight to ten hours following surgery, the wound will be filled with blood clot. Within 24–48 hours, the epithelium will be united during the acute inflammatory stage of wound healing. Therefore, surgical wounds united and healed by first intention are not normally a problem of healing. However, dehiscence may occur when the inflammatory stage is extended and healing delayed.

Dehiscence is the term used when separation of a surgical wound occurs and usually arises between the sixth and eighth post-operative day (Figure 7.1). The degree of separation may be from partial to complete separation with joints or viscera exposed. Most wounds separating in the early stages of healing are due to poor suturing technique or poor suturing material (Perkins 1992). Late wound dehiscence is probably due to infection or formation of haematoma. The presence of a foreign body (e.g. silk suture) reduces the number of bacteria required to cause a wound infection by 10 000[26].

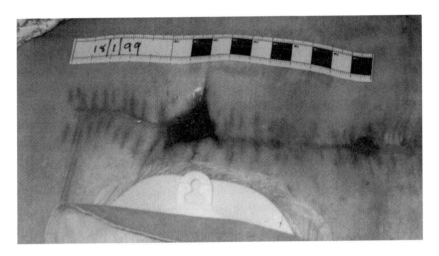

Figure 7.1 Dehisced wound.

Other responsible factors are:

- obesity;
- formation of haematoma;
- medication that interferes with the healing process (steroid therapy, chemotherapy);
- poor nutrition;
- anaemia;
- diabetes;
- age;
- malignant disease.

Surgical wound infections are generally primary in origin (Lockett 1983) and most infected and dehisced wounds will heal by secondary intention (see Chapter 1).

Pre-operative preparation

Given that a wound dressing remains *in situ* for 48 hours post-operatively, and given that the surgical line is sealed within 24–48 hours post-surgery, then most clinical infections in surgical wounds are potentially primary and obtained intra-operatively. Therefore, consideration must be given to prevention of infection prior to theatre. Cruse and Foord (1980) showed reduction of wound infection rates from 2.3 per cent if the patient did not shower, 2.1 per cent if showered using soap to 1.3 per cent if hexachlorophene was used during showering. Garibaldi et al. (1988) demonstrated a similar result. Cruse and Foord also showed a reduction from 2 per cent clinical infection to 1.6 per cent when a 3-minute chlorhexidine preparation was used immediately pre-operative. In order to prevent post-operative infection, Leaper (1995) states:

> Adequate surgical scrub, appropriate suture materials and antibiotic prophy-laxis, perioperative correction of dehydration and poor nutrition are examples of effective therapy which can be conformed to by all surgeons. Other factors, such as the use of wound guards, drains and surgical dressings are less easy to estimate for effectiveness or be sure that they could be changed or left out of surgical ritual.

Bowel preparation in elective colorectal surgery has often been stressed by following a survey Duthie et al. (1990) into current practice of bowel preparation and chemoprophylaxis amongst surgeons in Wales and the south-west of England. They identified one surgeon who used no pre-operative bowel preparation. One hundred consecutive colorectal cases were studied from one surgeon and this identified a seven per cent incidence of wound infection and one anastomosis leaked. None of these patients had mechanical bowel preparation but all had antibiotic chemoprophylaxis. Mechanical bowel preparation is usual in the UK but these results demonstrate that its importance as a factor in wound infection and anastomotic dehiscence may be overstated (Duthie et al. 1990).

Pre-operative shaving

Shaving has been found to be the most significant factor in post-surgical wound infection. The skin is more likely to support bacterial growth than hair (Meers et al. 1990). Shaving with a razor produces an infection rate of 2.5 per cent, dropping to 1.4 per cent if an electric razor was used and dropping further still to 0.9 per cent if hair was left. Bacteria are the most abundant life form on earth and the skin is an ideal environment to support the microscopic colonies. Bacteria cause very little problems to the skin, which provides protection for the body. However, once the skin surface is injured through shaving, the bacteria are allowed to enter and to infect the lower tissues. When the surgeon introduces a cut over the infected area, the bacteria are spread deeper and over a larger area, leading to post-operative clinical infection.

Wound closure

Healing by primary intention is when the edges of the wound are brought into approximation by the use of sutures, clips, adhesives, skin tapes or wound closure zips and the best cosmetic result is obtained by good apposition of the skin edges and deep layers (Leaper 1992). Approximation of the tissues will allow the healing process (see Chapter 1) to continue in the enclosed space of the two wound edges and the closed suture line will prevent post-operative entrance of microbes.

Healing by secondary intention is when the wound is left unsutured and granulation tissue formation with contraction and epithelialization leads to final wound closure.

Delayed primary closure is closure of new or reopened wounds that is delayed for a few days but is sutured prior to emergence of granulation tissue.

Skin closure

Sutures are chosen for their strength, absorptive properties and handling characteristics (Leaper 1992) and are designed to either degrade over a period of time (Maxon and PDS) or to retain the strength and require removal (Nylon and Prolene). The cosmetic appearance following removal is largely due to the skill of the applier. If the sutures are too tight, the site of the suture can become inflamed, even infected and this can also have an affect on the cosmetic appearance of the wound, leaving scar tissue over the suture site.

Staples are metallic, easy and quick to apply, inexpensive and do not penetrate deeper than the dermis and are useful in wounds of low tension (Galvani 1997). Stapling devices have been developed mainly for bowel surgery, particularly for anterior resection (Leaper 1992). Skin tapes are easily applied, inexpensive and used largely in minor wound treatment, particularly in accident and emergency departments. Skin adhesives are easily applied but expensive. The adhesive may act as a barrier against healing (Galvani 1997). Wound closure zips are two rows of polyamide teeth on flexible ribbons held on to the skin with adhesive strips (Galvani 1997).

It has become increasingly obvious that monofil sutures cause fewer post-operative infections compared with braided sutures (Gottrup 1999). The duration of time between trauma and closure is crucial. If the injury occurred more than six hours previously, the principle is not to close the wound although safe closure is possible after this time in clean wounds, particularly face wounds (Gottrup 1999).

Warmth in healing and reduction of infection

Wounds are hypoxic, due to the vascular response to injury and vasoconstriction resulting from injury, and are also affected by any drop of temperature in the wound bed. Hypovolaemia, hypothermia, anxiety and pain all increase the potential of vasoconstriction (Hopf 1999). All surgical patients are at risk of hypothermia. Many patients spend time, pre-surgery, dressed in a paper gown with a single blanket over them and are given sedatives pre-operatively leading to a lack of awareness of feeling cold. They may then be wheeled through cold corridors to theatre where their temperature is further compromized by the use of anaesthetics. Hypothermia and resultant vasoconstriction will effect delivery of oxygen to the surgical incision site.

An exciting research project was conducted in pre-operative, intra-operative and post-operative warming of patients and the relationship to pressure sore formation and post-operative clinical infections. The patients are warmed with a Bair-hugger blanket and all intravenous fluids are warmed during administration (Scott et al. 1999a). The results proved to be quite startling with 58.7 per cent reduction in pressure sore formation and a reduction in post-operative clinical infection with the rate of infection being three times higher in the hypothermic group than in the normothermic group (Mortensen et al. 1996).

Surgical wounds will heal rapidly if blood perfusion is maximized, thus delivering oxygen, nutrients and cells of the immune system to the site of injury and providing minimal opportunity for microorganisms to colonize and proliferate (Bowler et al. 2001). Bowler used wounds in the anus to demonstrate this statement as the wounds – despite being susceptible to gross microbial contamination – are very well perfused and rarely become infected. Intra-abdominal infections normally reflect the microflora of the resected organ (Bowler et al. 2001). Minimizing the incidence of post-operative wound infection relies on adequate asepsis and antisepsis and preservation of the local host defences (Bowler et al. 2001).

Langer's lines

Langer's lines are the natural skin creases and surgical incisions along these lines are not conducive to healing and are best avoided. However, there may be occasions when it would be unavoidable.

Dehiscence

The aim of the surgeon should be to achieve a post-operative strength similar to that pre-dating the procedure; it should be pain free and aesthetically pleasing (Foster 1994).

Abdominal wounds that are healing normally develop a ridge that can be seen 5–7 days post-operatively. Wounds at risk of dehiscing do not form a ridge (Perkins 1992). Other signs of potential wound dehiscence are:

- sudden discharge of fluid from the wound;
- obvious weakness in the suture line that can be easily noted;
- cellulitis at one end or all along the suture line;
- patient feels that something is 'giving way'.

Treatment of a dehisced wound would be either a return to theatre for resuturing, possibly deep tension sutures, or the wound will be healed by secondary intention. When pus is noted within the wound, resuturing would not benefit the wound healing process.

Skin grafting

Cells recognize each other by recognition of chemical messengers and recognition of the surface of other cells. If the recognition is not there, the unrecognized cell will be rejected and destroyed by the host's efficient immune system. However, if a skin graft is taken from the person who is to be grafted, then few problems will be found with 'take up' of the graft. Swabs should be taken prior to grafting as certain bacteria (e.g. haemolytic *Streptococcus* Group G) are particularly damaging to the uptake of grafts.

Donor sites

Skin grafts can be a useful means to healing ulcers quickly. However, the donor site can be a difficult and intractable wound to heal (Figure 7.2). Donor sites are superficial wounds and, as such, expose raw nerve endings leading to considerable pain. The hair follicles remain intact and, therefore, epithelial tissue will migrate out from the follicles making healing fairly rapid (8–16 days) depending on the wound condition. Should the wound become infected, the pain will be increased, exudate will be copious and healing will be slowed. There are many surgeons who use the traditional dressing paraffin gauze on skin grafts and donor sites and this dressing can become firmly stuck to the wound if several layers are not applied. If firmly adhered to the wound, paraffin gauze can be removed by application of a hydrogel to the surface of the dressing followed by gentle massage into the dressing. This generally lifts and frees the paraffin dressing.

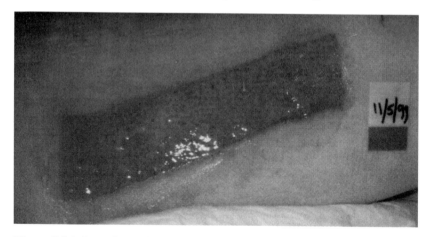

Figure 7.2 A donor site can be painful and difficult to heal (see Plate 30).

Although classified as an epithelializing wound, the raw and exposed dermis of the donor site produces more fluid than any other superficial wound (Fowler and Dempsey 1998). As an acute wound, the donor site is particularly susceptible to infection and treatment would ideally provide protection against invasion of organisms; that is, leave dressings *in situ* as long as possible.

Hydrocolloids offer an ideal wound healing environment and are excellent for donor sites, providing the wound is not producing excessive exudate. The dressing will also be easily and painlessly removed. Alginates will reduce blood loss (see Chapter 3) and, when combined with a vapour permeable film dressing, will also provide an ideal wound healing environment.

The primary concern of theatre staff is to prevent infection entering the wound, particularly as there may be a 4.53 per cent incidence of infection in surgical wounds (Yalcin et al. 1995). Treatment of infected surgical wounds is fairly straightforward with removal of sutures to allow drainage (Cutting 1998) and systemic antibiotics may be required.

Pilonidal sinus disease

Symptoms of pilonidal disease can cause discomfort, pain, loss of earnings and excessive hospitalization. A survey completed in 1985 showed that 7000 patients were admitted that year for pilonidal sinus treatment for an average stay of five days (Berry 1992). It is thought that pilonidal disease originates within the natal cleft in a hair follicle, which becomes distended with keratin (Berry 1992). The follicle develops inflammation and is occluded by the resultant oedema. The occluded follicle ruptures, creating a pilonidal abscess.

Treatments include:

- incision, drainage and curettage;
- wide excision – popular method that allows the wound to heal by secondary intention;
- excision and primary closure;
- laying open the sinus – this allows pus to escape freely and healing is through secondary intention;
- antibiotics – not always successful in practice (Berry 1992);
- conservative treatment for chronic sufferers with minor symptoms is shaving the affected area daily and twice daily baths or showers.

Dressings for post-operative pilonidal sinus wounds were (traditionally) Proflavin soaked gauze packs. However, removal of these packs, post-surgically, is very distressing and extremely painful. Use of modern dressings such as alginates, hydrofibres and gels are less painful on removal and offer an excellent wound healing environment. An excellent dressing for this purpose is Aquacel although an alginate may be preferred if bleeding is a possibility (it has been noted at Eastbourne Hospital that use of some dressings increase the number of post-surgical bleeds from pilonidal sinus excisions). However, that has yet to be audited or researched.

Fistulae and sinus wounds

The greatest challenge in wound healing comes from the treatment and management of fistulae. High fluid loss with resultant electrolyte and serum protein loss can cause major problems in healing the wounds and the loss of bodily fluids from the fistulae can macerate peri-wound areas and increase the size of the surface wound.

Treatment is individual to the patient and the wound. However, there are many wound management bags obtainable today that can cope with large amounts of drainage and these are possibly an excellent way of providing the optimum wound-healing environment when exudate and faecal contamination may be responsible for damaging the fragile surface of the wound bed. However, if a wound dressing is required, there are several options such as Allevyn (a hydrophilic foam cavity dressing), Aquacel, Cavicare and Tenderwet.

Aquacel, alginates, etc. will soak up fluid from within the sinus. Care must be taken to ensure that these do not act as a 'plug' in a sinus wound. Cavicare is a foam that is prepared by mixing two catalysts together and can create a foam that will fit the wound. This can be removed daily, washed, soaked in chlorhexidine, rinsed in saline and placed back into the wound. It is an excellent way of judging wound healing as less mixture is required as the wound heals. However, care should be taken that the dressing is removed regularly as it could act as a 'plug', thereby preventing drainage. There is also the possibility that, placed in a narrow channel, the dressing could become fixed and cause trauma on removal.

Tenderwet is a dressing that contains a gel that is soaked in Hartmann's solution. The gel has an affinity for protein and will release Hartmann's into the wound in exchange for exudate. This has the effect of cleansing the wound and increases healing rates. However, this dressing must be changed twice daily and is unlikely to fit into a narrow channel.

Amputation

Amputation is generally the result of poor vascularization of tissues and this can hold a poor prognosis for healing. Added to this is the problem of trying to anastomose two tissue edges that do not belong together. This always adds to healing difficulties. Also, a majority of amputations are among the population who smoke or those with diabetes.

Ischaemic toes and feet are difficult to treat; however, mummified necrotic toes can be safely left to dry and demarcate naturally (Figure 7.3). When the surgeons make a decision on the extent of the amputation, they will consider the vascular status of the leg and will cut at the point they can expect to find a reasonable blood supply so that the wound will heal.

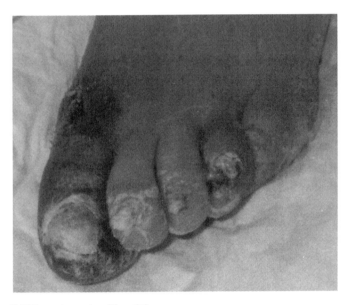

Figure 7.3 Necrotic toe (see Plate 31).

Wound care immediately post-operatively should be protective and should keep the wound warm and occluded. However, wound dehiscence following amputation should be viewed seriously because of the poor blood supply and the risk of associated osteomylitis. Negative pressure therapy (vacuum) would increase healing rates within the wound as it promotes blood supply to the area, and is likely to reduce the potential of osteomylitis as it draws bacteria away from the site. If negative pressure therapy is not an option, absorptive dressings that keep the wound moist would aid healing (Aquacel, hydrocolloid paste, alginates, Tenderwet dressings, warm-up dressings, etc.).

Pain is frequently a post-operative complication of amputation with phantom limb pain commonly felt within the first few days; this is often non-responsive to analgesia. Many nurses believe that complete pain relief after surgery is not possible and is not, therefore, part of their nursing aim (Saxey 1986). Liaison with the pain control specialist nurse is important as transcutaneous nerve stimulation (TNS) may help along with administration of carbamazepine and strong analgesia.

Briggs (1996) found that leaving a vapour permeable film *in situ* until suture removal considerably lowered the amount of pain patients experienced against those whose wounds were exposed on day three. Briggs believed this raised an argument against exposing wounds until suture removal.

Degloving injuries

The commonest cause is the limb being trapped between the road and a moving vehicle tyre. Avulsion of the skin and subcutaneous tissues by a twisting mechanism ruptures the musculocutaneous and fasciotaneous perforating vessels, devascularizing the outer tissues (Whiteside and Moorhead 1999).

External fixator pin sites

External fixator pin sites are often used in orthopaedic surgery and are used to stabilize fractures that have either soft tissue loss or have failed to heal. The pins may have to remain in position for several weeks and attention to the pins is required to maintain their integrity. As the pin site creates a loss of the protective skin surface, the site has a high potential for infection and this has a potential to lead to osteomyelitis. The motion around a pin can result in the formation of a membrane, which lies between the tissues and the pin with direct access to the outside environment (Wallis 1991). The Sheffield Limb Reconstruction Service recommends (Sims 1996):

- massaging the pin-site twice daily as it prevents pulling of the skin, particularly during physiotherapy;
- daily cleaning of the site with sodium chloride;
- that the patients are encouraged to shower and to dry the sites well;
- use of unsterile cotton buds to remove the crusts to facilitate drainage;

- that gauze dressings are only applied to discharging pin sites;
- that ointments and paraffin gauze are not used for pin sites.

Care of central lines

Central line use is becoming increasingly common and most nurses, at some point, will be faced with the care of a central line. Central lines allow microorganisms easy access to the bloodstream and the most pressing problem arising from this is prevention of infection. There is a possibility that infection rates can reach as high as 42 per cent through central lines (Conly et al. 1989). Contamination can enter the bloodstream through the site of the line, catheter hubs, connections and the solution itself. Care should be taken when introducing drugs or solutions to the line and a reduction in the frequency of use of the ports would decrease any potential risk.

Dressings are fairly simplistic and are often selected for user preference. Gauze and tapes are commonly used (Perry 1994) and are simple to apply and cost-effective. Adhesive, vapour permeable film can be used and this allows visual inspection of the site (Perry 1994). Arglaes, an adhesive film dressing containing silver, has the potential of reducing bacterial contamination of the site and this may decrease the risk of clinical infection.

Cleansing protocols for central line sites are likely to be individual to each hospital or community area. Nevertheless, the sites should be cleaned away from the exit site taking care not to drag on the line (Perry 1994).

Blisters

Blistering, particularly following orthopaedic operations, is a common problem with no documented research and little recorded in the literature (Wright 1994). The actual cause appears unknown although it is thought to be related to the dressings used following surgery (Williams 1994). If dressings are applied by being stretched across the wound, it creates a pulling action on the skin. As the patient moves or flexes the joint, the dressing pulls tighter on the fragile tissues and may lead to blistering. There is also a possibility that the application and subsequent removal of film dressings, sometimes used during surgery, may cause stress on the tissues and lead to blistering. Williams (1994) and Wright (1994) found an incidence of 35 per cent of patients developing blisters following total hip replacement and Wright found that this was particularly related to the application of Mepore dressings, with 85 per cent of patients from the Mepore group developing blisters.

Prevention of blistering post-operatively could be addressed in the following way:

- consensus in use of wound dressings would be required with each surgeon following a recognized policy;
- adhesive dressings should never be stretched prior to being applied;
- a barrier film (Cavilon or Opsite spray) could be applied to the skin prior to using adhesive tape;
- discontinue use of adhesive tape – review alternative tape;
- standardization of wound care is required with a clear protocol for nurses to follow.

Stoma skin care

The very nature of the stoma function is likely to cause skin problems in the peri-stoma area. The following may be causes of skin damage:

- faecal leakage;
- strong adhesive that pulls on the skin during removal;
- inappropriate skin cleansing;
- hypersensitivity to materials used in the stoma appliance;
- fungal infections generated by the warm, moist peri-stoma skin;
- excretion of drugs;
- radiotherapy;
- bacterial contamination;
- poorly advised diet.

Hypersensitive reactions are easily identified in comparison with infections as the reaction of contact will leave a very clear demarcation line the shape of the dressing. Erythema from infection will have an uneven line often extending beyond the dressing outer edge.

Solutions to peri-stoma skin irritation

No-sting barrier films such as Cavilon or SuperSkin place a clear, painless barrier over the traumatized skin. They create a strong base for adherence of the appliance and prevent further trauma on removal of the appliance. Also, no-sting barrier creams help the adherence of the stoma appliance. Another barrier cream (Comfeel) contains aluminium paste, which helps to dry the damaged skin. Unlike Cavilon, this cream must be allowed to dry prior to application of appliance. Stomahesive will protect against stoma discharge on the skin as will a stomahesive flange.

Nutrition and surgery

Nutritional assessment prior to surgery is a vital part of post-operative wound management. Sub-clinical nutritional deficiencies may not be uncommon and will be significant if wound healing is impaired (Telfer and Moy 1993). Prior to elective surgery, there is an opportunity to provide the optimum nutritional status for the patient and this can be achieved through improved diet, nasogastric feeding, central feeding and not allowing starvation periods to exceed allotted times (e.g. six hours).

Surgical pain

It is likely that nurses do not imagine patients' wound pain correctly and are disinclined to administer sufficient analgesics to relieve pain completely (Ketovuori 1987). Hayward (1975) showed that post-operative pain could be reduced by giving good information pre-operatively. The Royal College of Surgeons (1990) found that 75 per cent of patients experienced moderate to severe pain post-operatively. Pain can have a negative effect on wound healing as pain causes stress, which promotes physiological reactions such as vasoconstriction and leads to poor delivery of nutrients and oxygen at the wound bed. Work by Briggs showed that covering a surgical wound with a film dressing reduces pain and, therefore, analgesic requirements.

Patient controlled analgesia (PCA) is the easiest and most successful way of controlling pain. The result of this is reduced anxiety for the patient and an added benefit is that patients receiving PCA were discharged earlier than those not receiving PCA (Clark et al. 1989).

An easy assessment for patient pain is to use a pain analogue scale with patients being asked to place their pain on a scale of 1–5 or 1–10 with 1 as no pain and 5 or 10 as the worst pain ever suffered. Most people find the scale system is easy to use and can fairly accurately place their pain level on the scale.

Wound care

Smith and Lait (1996) found that in hospital wards where there was no standardized regimen of wound management, patients were statistically more likely to develop complications, thereby increasing length of stay and cost. Therefore, a trust-wide policy would be recommended with increased education for those professionals involved in giving wound care.

Any product used on a surgical wound should offer non-adherence, warmth and trauma-free removal. Any dressing can be removed within 24–48 hours and either replaced or the wound left without cover.

Scarring

Foetal wound healing has a greater regenerative process with little inflammation and no scarring within the first two trimesters. This has been related to higher levels of hyaluronan-stimulating factor found in the foetus and the amniotic fluid that surrounds the foetus. Wound healing in adults is a complex process and growth factors, including hyaluronan, holding responsibility for promoting the healing process, only remain within the wound in the early stages of healing. Therefore, scarring in adults does not have the excellent regenerative properties found in the foetus. Nevertheless, hyaluronan is now being used in dressings (Hyalofil) and research and experience will identify the potential in surgical wound healing and scarring. There is some evidence that hypertrophic scars have significantly higher levels of apoptosis than flat scars, suggesting that selected fibroblasts in keloid and hypertrophic scars undergo apoptosis (cell suicide), which may play a role in the process of pathological scarring (Akasaka et al. 2001).

Hypertrophic and keloid scarring occur in 5–15 per cent of wounds (Alhady and Siavanatharajah 1961) with treatment involving surgery, corticosteroid therapy, laser, cryosurgery or, more importantly today, silicone gel sheets (Cica-Care). Keloid is Greek for 'claw-like' and is the responsibility of an overproduction of collagen and this overproduction can continue for 10 years post scarring.

Conclusion

Scott et al. (1999a), argue that peri-operative nursing is a complex arena that involves various roles and procedures and the main key to success is good multidisciplinary communication. That involved the entire multidisciplinary team.

Treatment of surgical wounds relies on a multidisciplinary team approach with each professional providing care that is based on researched evidence. With pre-operative nutritional assessment, a wound care formulary, excellent pre-operative cleansing and appropriate wound assessment, surgical wounds will heal with few problems.

Activity

Interview a patient who has recently undergone surgery. Discover the following:

1 How long was the patient starved pre-operatively?
2 What pain rating would the patient consider they experienced? (1–10 pain analogue scale)
3 What analgesia were they given for the pain?

Write 250 words reflecting on the care of this patient post-operatively either in hospital or in the community. Describe it as a critical incidence – reflecting on commendable aspects of the patient's care and the care that could have been improved. Describe how you could have cared for the patient in ideal circumstances.

CHAPTER 8

Fungating tumours

This speciality is so unique that the chapter will be organized separately to the rest of the book. The aim is to inform the reader about a wound that is unlikely to heal and the chapter looks at dressings and treatment as a stand-alone section. There are sections that are repeated in earlier chapters and the author does not try to excuse this but suffice to say that a healing wound will be viewed in a different light to a fungating, non-healing wound.

The appearance of a wound generally leads the nurse to select a dressing based on knowledge and experience of wound healing, although this experience is unlikely to benefit the nurse when faced with a fungating tumour. Wound management objectives require different assessment criteria and treatment to that of a wound that is likely to heal. Care is often palliative, addressing uncomfortable and distressing symptoms rather than offering the aggressive treatments that strive for an optimum healing environment. Control of pain, odour, bleeding and exudate become the first consideration and removal of necrotic tissue becomes low priority.

Unfortunately, much of the care of patients with fungating tumours is based on trial and error, rather than research (Hastings 1993). This is unacceptable today when clinical governance and audit are becoming increasingly important and care must be based on clinical evidence. Each clinician is expected to provide a rationale for the care given in any situation and it would be difficult to rationalize why different types of wounds are dressed with similar products when each patient's needs are different.

Care of a fungating wound requires excellent communication skills and an understanding of the grieving process along with a first-rate knowledge of relevant anatomy and physiology, the wound healing process, related microbiology, an understanding of dressing interactions, scientific approach to treatment and an ideal holistic assessment.

Care of the patient with a fungating wound often requires remarkable patience as the symptoms being treated are sometimes difficult to manage.

Fungating lesions

A fungating lesion is a malignant infiltration of the skin (Hastings 1993). Cooper (1993) describes it as:

> A malignant ulcer is defined as a break in the epidermal integrity because of infiltration of malignant cells. This may be due to primary skin malignancy, including basal cell carcinoma, squamous cell carcinoma and malignant melanoma, or because of metastatic deposits or extensions of malignancy from deeper structures that may result in fungating carcinomas.

Although the locations of fungating wounds can vary greatly, the most common site is the breast (62 per cent) (Hallett 1993).

Treatment for control of the tumour is beyond the scope of this book and may include radiotherapy, surgery, laser, hormone therapy or chemotherapy. Treatment of the wound will require a nurse experienced in wound healing to manage the problems that may be caused by the cancer treatment, particularly when tissue regeneration is prevented and there is extensive skin damage.

Tumours can rapidly increase in size with a 'cauliflower' appearance, can quickly ulcerate and the ulceration can bring symptoms, which then become the patient's primary problem. The pain, malodour, excessive exudate and the large amount of dressings required, which show through or under clothes, can be distressing and embarrassing for the patient.

Tumours that arise from a bacterially contaminated surface (such as skin or gut) tend to become ulcerated. An every day example of skin tumour would be the basal cell carcinoma of the face. This carcinoma grows slowly but relentlessly (Majno and Joris 1996). An example of this was a patient with a basal cell carcinoma that had eaten away the eye and exposed the inside of the skull (Figure 8.1). This patient was in complete denial of the problem, did not appreciate that

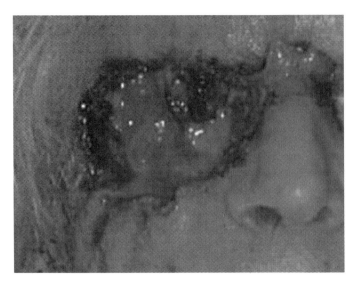

Figure 8.1 Basal cell carcinoma (see Plate 32).

other patients may be repulsed by her wound and had a tendency to unwittingly remove the dressing and to walk around the ward. The dressing considered most suitable in this case, was Cavicare, a foam that composes of two catalysts, which, when combined, froth up and then set solid. When poured into a wound, this foam takes on the shape of the wound, absorbs fluid but does not enter channels (nose or tear ducts, etc.) where harm may be caused. The foam cast can be removed from the wound, washed, soaked in chlorhexidine for ten minutes and reused in the same wound. Hydrogels and similar dressings may have blocked the delicate channels within the cavity or may have entered the throat and been swallowed.

Cancer cells proliferate and can effect tissues within a local area causing a hypoxic environment and necrosis. The most common emergency experienced in fungating tumours, is haemorrhage due to erosion of the blood vessels by the malignancy itself, secondary necrosis or the sloughing of tissues following radiotherapy (Brunner and Suddarth 1975). The abnormal conditions of the wound can also lead to poor drainage of interstitial fluid leading to oedema and collapse of capillaries and lymph vessels, thereby further reducing fluid drainage and supply of nutrients to the damaged area. Tissue, deprived of oxygen and nutrients, will eventually become non-viable and take on a black leathery appearance when exposed to air, or yellow/grey appearance when moist. The length of time this takes to occur will be different in each individual and depends largely on underlying pathology.

The harmful influences of devitalized tissue on the body's defences are without question; moist, devitalized soft tissue acts as a culture medium promoting bacterial growth and inhibits leucocyte phagocytosis of bacteria (Haury et al. 1978). However, natural debridement is the only option open to fungating wounds for obvious reasons. Surgical debridement will either cause excessive bleeding or could 'seed' the malignant cells.

Treating symptoms

Malodour

For the patient and relatives, malodour can be the most distressing symptom of a fungating tumour and is most generally caused by bacterial colonization of the wound. The hypoxic environment within the ulcerated tissue is a microbiological heaven to anaerobic bacteria (which require an oxygen-free environment to survive). Fatty acids, released as an end product of the action of anaerobes, produce the characteristic odour within necrotic tissue. As blood supply is likely to be poor to the area, leucocytes are unable to attack the anaerobes, leaving them free to proliferate and so increase malodour.

A by-product of all bacteria, is excessive exudate production. The colour and odour produced by the bacteria can be recognized and identified by an experienced nurse. Antibiotics are unlikely to reduce the bacterial count unless there is a clinical infection present. Therefore, bacterial colonization must be addressed by the selected dressing and knowledge of the action of dressings become essential to the nurse.

Green exudate often signifies a *Pseudomonas* colonization, which has a sweet, musty smell. This is a Gram-negative, aerobic bacteria (requires oxygen to survive) and the colour can often be startlingly green, almost florescent. *Pseudomonas* produces large amounts of exudate and the musty smell can be very embarrassing for the patient. Gram-negative bacteria respond very well to silver found in silver sulphadiazine cream (Flamazine) and within a charcoal, silver-impregnated dressing (Actisorb silver 220). Silver sulphadiazine should be used for a short period when the green discharge is first noted and discontinued when green has disappeared – probably after two or three applications. Continued use of the cream appears to lead to *Pseudomonas* remaining in the wound as low grade colonization (anecdotal evidence only). Actisorb silver 220 is an excellent alternative choice, although this dressing should be used as a primary dressing because it has two actions:

1 The charcoal filters the odour.
2 The silver residues in the dressing reduce the bacteria through interfering with the electrical charge in the bacterial cell. An ideal alternative would be Acticoat which again contains silver to destroy bacteria.

An increase in pain of those wounds colonized by *Pseudomonas* has been noted and a reduction of pain when the bacteria are controlled. However, to date, this is purely anecdotal and requires research.

Red/brown exudate can often be associated with *Staphylococcus* or (more likely) *Streptococcus* colonization and particularly with haemolytic streptococci as this microorganism destroys red blood cells. These bacteria often have an 'old blood' malodour and it is Gram-positive bacteria which is often easily controlled by use of iodine cadexomer dressings (Iodoflex, Iodosorb). Iodine is rapidly deactivated by contact with pus and so, although iodine has a rapid kill rate, its value is very limited in wounds. The iodine cadexomer dressings allow slow release of iodine into the wound in exchange for exudate. This has three values:

1 The iodine 'bathes' the wound, killing bacteria.
2 The cadexomer dressing absorbs large quantities of exudate.
3 The dressing is excellent for wound debridement.

These values offer a rationale for the usefulness of cadexomer dressings in malodorous, high exudate, necrotic wounds.

Anaerobic bacteria are partly responsible for the dreadful odour associated with gangrene, often described as 'the smell of hell'. Anaerobes survive in necrotic tissue because oxygen is not found in non-viable tissue. Hyperbaric oxygen may be a way forward for the future but, at present, dressings are relied on to address the problem.

Sugar paste creates a hyperosmotic environment by forcing bacteria to give up fluid through osmosis. Bacteria cannot survive this osmotic 'pull' and malodour will decrease, along with exudate production, as bacterial count is reduced. It also has a debriding action (Topham 1996) which makes it ideal in treatment of sloughy wounds. The problem associated with sugar paste (particularly thin paste) is that it can be messy, therefore, use of a commercial glycerine dressing (Novogel) may be appropriate. However, care should be taken in painful wounds when introducing a hyperosmotic or hydrophilic dressing as the 'pull' of these dressings can increase pain.

Metronidazole gel is effective against malodour (Newman et al. 1989) although systemic Metronidazole is often given for the same reason. However, systemic administration is less likely to be effective as poor blood supply, to the local tissues, will prevent delivery of the treatment at the wound site particularly as anaerobes survive in necrotic tissue; the amount that is delivered to the wound bed will have small effect on these bacteria. Long-term use of oral Metronidazole may cause neuropathy and patients who are receiving systemic therapy must refrain from consuming alcohol (Thomas 1992b). Metrotop is a hypromellose gel containing 0.8 per cent Metronidazole (licensed for wound care) which is useful against the aerobic and anaerobic organisms that cause odour within the wound (Thomas 1992b).

Other dressings to be considered are homeopathic treatments with tea tree oil controlling bacteria, and aloe vera and many of the essential oils controlling the malodour and pain. Included on the list of natural treatments will be larvae therapy – available through the Surgical Material Testing Laboratory (SMTL) at Bridgend. However, maggots should never be applied to bleeding wounds and may encourage angiogenesis. This may increase the proliferation of the tumour.

Natural myiasis (the infection of wounds with larvae) is seen commonly in hot climates, occasionally in this country and is often greeted with horror when the dressing is removed to expose the infestation (Flanagan 1997). Nevertheless, maggot therapy has been used for many centuries as a natural debrider of wounds and there is evidence that the benefits of maggots were noted in 1557 (Morgan 1997a). Later, in the American Civil war (Thomas et al. 1996a), Morgan (1997a) relates anecdotal reports of Malay Indians using maggots to remove superficial malignancies.

The most commonly used fly in biosurgery is *Lucilia sericata* or greenbottle fly (Thomas et al. 1996b). Maggots will not pupate in the wound and so the patient and the nurse can be assured that the dressing will not be taken off to find flies. This method of debridement is increasing in popularity, particularly in difficult wounds requiring palliative management, such as fungating tumours, as a reduction of odour and exudate can be achieved by the treatment (Thomas et al. 1996a, 1996b). However, larvae therapy is contraindicated in bleeding wounds as it can increase the potential of haemorrhage and this limits the usage in fungating tumours. Maggots are also associated with death and may be inappropriate for a dying patient.

Dressings containing carbon can filter odour and can, therefore, be very useful as primary or secondary dressings.

Methicillin-resistant *Staphylococcus aureus* (MRSA) is now endemic in hospitals and is the cause of life-threatening infections in patients (Irizarry et al. 1996). Antibiotics are used with caution now and antiseptics and disinfectants are becoming more widely used in hospitals to control infections (Irizarry et al. 1996). Wound management, too, will look increasingly to antiseptics to prevent infection. However, the law of 'survival of the fittest' means that there may only be limited time before bacteria mutate and become antiseptic/disinfectant resistant. Therefore, use of general antiseptics (e.g. chlorhexidine) and topical antibiotics are no longer acceptable in wound management. Iodine is one of the few antiseptics to which bacteria have so far developed resistance.

Pain

McCaffery's (1983) work led to the belief that 'Pain is what the patient says it is and exists when he/she says it does'. If the patient claims to have pain then the problem must be addressed. Use of a visual analogue scale (Hill 1991) can be useful, particularly when assessing whether treatment is effective.

Included in the assessment of pain should be an appraisal of the dressing. Any dressing that has adhered to any wound and proves difficult to remove, should never be used on that wound again. Certain dressings are more prone to adhere than others; impregnated tulles (iodine, paraffin), gauze, non-adherent dressings (excluding

NA Ultra) have all, at some time, adhered to wounds. This does not detract from their usefulness as a dressing but should be reconsidered in individual cases when adherence is noted.

Pain in fungating tumours may be related to size or site of the lesion, pressure from other organs (Hastings 1993), the type of bacteria present within the wound or a psychological pain caused by the presence of the lesion. Pain control is a medical problem, addressed through finely balanced analgesia. However, this chapter will review how pain may be reduced with appropriate selection of dressings.

The cause of the pain can often be exposed nerve endings and reduction of pain may be achieved by 'bathing' the exposed nerves with the wound dressing. Hydrocolloids and hydrogels can soothe this type of pain and can be very useful. However, before they can be successfully applied, the amount of exudate and odour often requires treatment. Gels and hydrocolloids are water donating to some extent and when applied to highly exuding wounds, the amount of exudate and malodour may well increase.

Exudate

Exudate is often the bi-product of bacterial colonization. Reduce colonization and the exudate will also lessen in amount. Iodine cadexomers are obviously an ideal choice as this controls the exudate whilst killing the bacteria and can be moulded to the wound shape. However, it is unwise to continue using iodine over long periods and, on the occasions when high exudate problems have not been addressed by cadexomers, an alternative must be selected. These cadexomers can also be very painful, particularly in an already painful wound.

Gauze is inappropriate for use as a primary dressing in any wound as cotton can donate fibres and can increase the possibility of clinical infection (Wood 1976). Gauze can also adhere to the wound bed, causing pain, bleeding and distress on removal. Therefore, suitable alternative dressings would be a non-adherent, high absorbency dressing.

Once the exudate is controlled, there are many, inexpensive dressings, that can be used to support the wound. The optimum dressing type would be one that can support the symptoms without misshaping the patient's clothes.

In highly exuding wounds, it would be unwise to use dressings that increase 'wetness' within the wound (an example is hydrogels). A general rule of thumb would be, if the wound is wet, dry it and if the wound is dry, moisten it. If this rule is ignored, a problem of peri-wound skin maceration can occur, particularly as the fatty acids, produced as a bi-product of metabolism of anaerobic bacteria, create profuse exudate which can damage the good skin. This problem can be exacerbated by the use of inappropriate dressings and any wound that has the appearance of maceration on the peri-wound skin, should lead the nurse to question the type of dressing that is being used. Also, a dry dressing on a dry wound may cause adherence and potential bleeding and is therefore inadvisable for fungating wounds.

Although the aim is to reduce damaging exudate, some exudate can support the wound environment. Maceration continues to be a difficulty in wound healing and few studies have addressed the problem (Hampton 1997b, 1998a). Wound exudate and 'wet' dressings such as hydrogels, can exacerbate the problem, particularly when the secondary dressing promotes the 'wetness' on the peri-wound skin. The treatment of the wound should be appropriate and suitable for the peri-wound area.

Maceration occurs when the tissues are kept over-moist for long periods of time. The cells become 'waterlogged', softened, fragile and easily damaged and this can lead to excoriation. Macerated tissues have the appearance of white or pink, softened skin and can easily become excoriated. There are significant differences in structure and characteristics of skin of various people of all ages. Skin that is oily, dry, moist, papery or normal will react differently to any mechanical insult applied to it. Therefore, patients' wounds may be treated in identical ways with one having a reaction to a dressing (causing maceration) and another will remain clear even though the dressings are similar. Tissues, softened and macerated in this way become easily damaged and have the potential for grazing (excoriation) to occur offering an entry for infection. There are excellent products on the market today, which prevent and/or treat maceration. Cavilon, no-sting barrier film is the first of a new type of treatment that will not cause pain on application providing a clear barrier that holds the dressing firmly *in situ* and protects the viable skin in the peri-wound area (Hampton 1998a).

Exudate, is a shared problem between nurse and patient as it is distressing for the patient and increases nurse workload. It is particularly problematic when the peri-wound areas deteriorate because of exudate 'over-spill'. It is important to understand exudate so that dressing selection is appropriate for the wound and treatment for the peri-wound area is relevant.

Purpose of exudate

Metalloproteinases break down collagens and help to remodel extra-cellular matrix in healing (Vickery 1997). Exudate promotes the rate of growth of fibroblasts (Vickery 1997) and contains growth factors that promote tissue regeneration (Kreig and Eming 1997). Exudate also facilitates the migration of cells involved in tissue repair and acts as a transport medium for white cells whilst assisting in the process of autolysis (Dealey 1997).

The potential for exudate to cause tissue damage

Exudate can exacerbate skin damage (Cameron and Powell 1996) through irritation of the surrounding tissues and bacteria can produce proteolytic enzymes, which delay healing and also damage peri-wound areas. The amount of exudates produced can require large amount of nurses' time in changing dressings. There is also a potential for the loss of exudate to led to lowered serum proteins.

Staphylococci easily replicate in exudate (Vickery 1997) and that could lead to an increased risk of MRSA. Therefore, dressing selection relies on reducing the bacterial count in a wound but will allow exudate to continue with support from the dressing (moist but not wet).

The recommended dressings for absorbency are:

* foam dressings (all types);
* alginates (all types);
* hydrofibre dressings (e.g. Aquacel).

Bleeding

Haemorrhage should be dealt with quickly by local pressure and the application of an alginate dressing. Alginates are produced from seaweed with a high calcium content. Alginates exchange sodium ions for calcium ions in the wound bed and encourage the clotting cascade within a bleeding wound; this has led to alginates being widely used in theatres and in dental treatment. Therefore, alginates are particularly useful in bleeding fungating tumours. All alginates transform to gel in the presence of exudate, are hydrophilic and are useful in highly exuding wounds but are best avoided in low exudate wounds (Miller and Dyson 1996). Apart from alginates, all dry dressings are best avoided in fungating wounds that are likely to easily bleed. All dry dressings have the potential to adhere to the wound and removal could initiate bleeding. Dressings that will keep the wound moist, gels, hydrocolloids and pastes, are best used in the friable wound.

Calcium alginates were first used in the 1940s (Thomas 1992a) and are extracted from the brown seaweed harvested off the coasts of Scotland (Williams 1994). Alginate dressings are made from different parts of the seaweed plant and can be composed of galuronic and mannuronic acid units linked together (Williams 1994) with the proportions of these units determining the gel forming properties of the final fibre (Thomas and Loveless 1992). The high galuronic acid alginates (e.g. Kaltostat) are slow to gel and produce firmer gels. This gives the gelled fibres strength, retains the shape in the wound bed and can generally be lifted out of the wound in a thick gel form. The alginates high in mannuronic acid (e.g. Sorbsan) are weaker and the gel from these can easily be rinsed out of a wound with normal saline. The value of both these types of alginates is very similar. Sorbsan plus and Kaltostat plus are highly absorbent alginates and are very useful in high exudate fungating wounds.

Alginates are best used in moderate to highly exuding wounds (Miller and Dyson 1996) as the fibres are hydrophilic and cause an osmotic 'pull' on the fluid within a wound. If the wound bed is dry, the fibres may 'pull' fluid from the cells, thereby, drying the wound out – this goes against researched evidence that recommends a moist healing environment (Winter 1962). When applied to a highly exuding wound, the hydrophilic fibres form a gel. When a film or hydrocolloid dressing is used as a secondary dressing, the alginate gel provides warmth, moisture, occlusion (through the secondary dressing), absorption and trauma-free removal, all of which are requirements of the optimum wound environment (Torrance 1983).

Alginates can be obtained in sheets of various sizes, rope and extra thick (Sorbsan plus or Kaltostat extra), which are very useful in highly exuding fungating wounds.

Silver sulphadiazine (Flamazine) has been found effective in controlling capillary bleeding (Fitzgerald and Sims 1987). Fitzgerald and Sims believed that the silver acts as a haemostat although they recognize that this is based on experience, not on researched evidence (Flamazine, and many alginates, are available on the drug tariff).

Treating fungating wounds

Nurses were traditionally taught to always clean a wound with sterile saline or antiseptics. Today, research has shown that cleansing wounds may actually be harmful and in some instances, use of saline unnecessary and use of antiseptics inadvisable (Morgan 1993). Bacteria can rapidly become resistant to antiseptics and use should be limited, as should the use of antibiotics (Hampton 1997a). Therefore, before cleansing a wound it is important to ask the question 'does the wound require cleaning?' Wound cleansing must have a rationale. The fact that it makes the practitioner feel better to have performed a certain ritualistic task is not enough (Flanagan 1997). The only rationale for cleaning a wound is when there is something that can be physically flushed out of the wound (dressing residue, debris or removable slough). If the wound is clean or has unremovable slough, then it is best left to be redressed.

Debridement

Debridement will be difficult to achieve as poor vascularity of the wound will continually produce further necrotic tissue. If debridement of the wound is the overall aim then use of a dressing that promotes autolysis is the route of choice. Hydrogels, cadexomers, hydrocolloids and sugar paste all promote natural autolysis. When the wound becomes moist through the natural rehydration of necrotic tissue, the wound can be exposed to bacterial colonization, causing increased malodour and exudate.

Hydrocolloid dressings consist of a mixture of pectins, gelatines, sodium carboxymethyl cellulose and elastomers. Hydrocolloids are available in a number of forms, as wafers, extra absorbent wafers, extra thin wafers, granules, powders, gels and pastes. On contact with wound exudate, the hydrocolloid material dissolves into a gel. This gel provides many of the favourable conditions of moist wound healing. But, as it mixes with exudate, it has a particular 'yellow' appearance and can exude a characteristic odour. Although this is normal and to be expected with these products, those handling the dressing and also the patient being treated, need to be aware (Flanagan 1997), particularly when the wound is a fungating lesion and malodour an identified problem.

Care should be taken to ensure that the correct size of dressing is applied, i.e. one large enough to cover the wound with an overlap of at least 5 cms. Hydrocolloids can reduce dressing change intervals to around five days when exudate is low. Hydrocolloid paste is easily used and is an effective desloughing agent. It is excellent for small cavity wounds and can reduce pain through moistening the nerve endings. However, the odour produced by the action of the hydrocolloid may well be unacceptable to patients with fungating wounds.

Hydrogels are available in sheets or as a gel. The sheets are made up of gelable polysaccharide agarose, cross-linked with polyacrylamide. This material provides a moist environment for fungating lesions and dry to slightly exuding wounds. The gels are suitable for cavities and are effective for desloughing and debriding wounds (Bale and Harding 1990). Hydrogels have a high water content, are useful in rehydration of hard eschar, promote autolysis and are useful as a cavity dressing.

Nutrition

Nutritional assessment (see Chapter 6) will be part of the holistic assessment and associated problems must be addressed. Malignant wounds require large amounts of carbohydrates to grow and this is taken from patients who may well be debilitated through loss of appetite and possible vomiting. This will drive the body to use its own protein as energy and this depletion of body protein, along with loss of protein through exudate production, will cause a low serum albumin. Therefore, a high calorie and high protein diet is to be encouraged and food supplements considered (see Chapter 6).

Chocolate bars are an excellent way of taking proteins and vitamins and release endorphins which provide a 'feel good' factor.

The patient

It is important that the patient is given the opportunity to be involved in the overall management of their wound and its associated problems. However, it is possible that denial will disassociate the patient from the treatment and this will require a supportive and understanding approach from the nurse.

A holistic assessment of the patient will help to make decisions for wound management. However, it is helpful to write down the patient's identified problems in priority order and then to address each problem in turn. For example, if the identified problem is malodour, then dressing treatment will rely on removing the bacteria causing the malodour. If the problem is pain, this would require a multidisciplinary approach when the pain specialist nurse, physiotherapist, pharmacist and doctor will be involved in reducing the symptom to a level acceptable to the patient. There seems little point in measuring the wound size if this is likely to distress the patient as the wound enlarges. Nevertheless, some patients may welcome the opportunity to follow the changes that are occurring and may find that it helps them to come to terms with disease. Whether to measure or not, should be based on the individual patient's needs.

It is vital to continually update the patient on the treatment aims and evaluations and to use comments, made by the patient on their treatment, to form further objectives.

A fungating, offensive tumour, can socially isolate a patient and, therefore, the treatment or management of a wound is vitally important to the well-being of the patient both psychologically and physically. A nurse who is well educated in the use and application of dressings can be the most important link for the patient. Development of wound management protocols will assist the nurse in selection of dressings.

Consequences of radiation therapy

Radiotherapy skin reactions are unique, primarily due to the biological consequences of radiation which effects normal skin maturation (Noble-Adams 1999). Reproduction of keratinized epithelium will be most likely effected as it is the development of the new cell that is interrupted and it is within the epidermis that the fastest cell reproduction occurs. Because of this, the greatest damage from radiation will be seen within the basal and supra-basal layer of the epidermis. The basal layer is particularly sensitive and damage to these cells can produce a wide spectrum of reactions (Noble-Adams 1999). The damage to the basal layer may not be apparent for four weeks post radiation therapy. As the basal cells mature they are expected to rise to the surface layer where they are shed as dead cells. If the cells do not mature in the normal way, due to radiation interference, the cells may rapidly shed and expose the dermis. This becomes sore and oozes, causing further distress and discomfort for the patient.

Treatment of radiation therapy burns is difficult. Application of creams may increase the potential problems from radiation therapy. When the treatment is complete, an excellent cover is a no-sting barrier film (such as Cavilon), which would act as the surface epithelium, covering exposed nerve endings and reducing pain.

Patients are often told they cannot shower or bathe the irradiated site (Thomas 1992b) although the reasons for this are not entirely clear but may be related to the potential of damage caused by the use of towels or soap. Being unable to shower or bathe may cause the patient to feel unclean or socially unacceptable.

Thomas (1992b) reports a pilot study where a control of cotton gauze, coated with lanolin was used to cover the irradiated tissue of a randomized group of patients and compared with a semi-permeable film (Tegaderm). Healing rates were five days sooner in the group with film than in the control group and those with film experienced less discomfort than the control group. Thomas also reports a second study using polyethylene oxide hydrogel dressing (Spenco 2nd skin), which appeared to relieve discomfort and reduced healing time. Cavilon liquid film is a useful protection for irradiated skin. However, with all dressings and creams, the effect on the radiation therapy must be first consideration and any protection or soothing creams may need to be post treatment.

Conclusion

Caring for a patient with a fungating tumour is both challenging and particularly satisfying when the symptoms abate because of expert care. Certainly, quality of life can be greatly affected by the careful consideration of wound management by a knowledgeable nurse and this is of paramount importance to the patient suffering from the malignant lesion. The value of a skilful, knowledgeable and supportive nurse is without question.

CHAPTER 9

Pressure ulcer prevention

Infarction of tissue can occur anywhere on the body. However, the greatest risk is to the skin and subcutaneous tissues, which bear the brunt of exogenous pressure on the body (Bliss 1993). A pressure ulcer is defined as a 'lesion caused by unrelieved pressure that results in damage to underlying tissue' (US Department of Health and Human Services 1992) and the formation of an ulcer is a complex mixture of extrinsic and intrinsic variables.

The responsibility for the formation of ulcers has been traditionally placed on nurses' shoulders and the expression 'bad nursing' (Norton et al. 1962; Dealey 1992) is a term that has been applied to any ward with an incidence of ulcers. This view risked leaving nurses with a sense of guilt leading to a potential of denial or in danger of minimizing the problem (Warner 1986). Pressure ulcers are not a new issue but are an ancient problem and have been identified in the remains of a mummified Egyptian priestess (Burton 1995). However, traditionally, prevention of pressure ulcers has relied on 'two-hourly-turns', where nurses went from immobile patient to immobile patient, turning them onto the alternate side. This task often took two hours to perform in a 'Nightingale' ward (many beds in long lines) and results showed a reduction in pressure ulcer formation and the ritual 'two-hourly-turn' was formed. This method of prevention relied on custom rather than clinically based evidence and only reduced pressure ulcer incidence. To prevent pressure ulcers, individual turning times are required.

Patients within orthopaedic wards are particularly at risk of tissue damage, especially among the elderly. Incidence in these wards may be as high as 42.7 per cent (Department of Health 1993). However, much of this is the result of being found on a floor or road prior to admission, or partly due to extended ambulance journeys, poor trolley surfaces or a period of immobility prior to administration of pain-control drugs. Theatre tables and length of time taken during surgery will only contribute to the potential of ulcer development, particularly if more than eight hours are spent on the table (Hoyman and Gruber 1992).

Bridel (1992) believes that most pressure ulcers can be prevented if an active preventative plan is initiated and implemented. As long ago as 1987, Hibbs stated that pressure ulcers were '95 per cent preventable'; the five per cent that were not preventable were possibly due to being admitted to hospital with a fractured neck of femur following a fall and the possibility of having been lying on the ground for some hours. Other than a slight redness, pressure areas may not necessarily show signs of pressure damage on admission. It can take up to 3–5 days before the pressure damage begins to be manifest and patient may develop a necrotic area over a bony prominence. This is often, mistakenly, thought to be the result of poor nursing, particularly when the patient is discharged to a nursing home or community where the carer may believe the pressure ulcer to be the responsibility of the hospital. After some time, the patient may be readmitted to hospital and the pressure ulcer development may then be seen as the responsibility or fault of the carer/nursing home. This finger pointing exercise is a waste of time and does not increase the quality of patient care. Quality care may never be truly applied until hospitals and communities work together to provide seamless care.

Aetiology of pressure ulcers

There are many complex contributory factors in the formation of pressure ulcers (Table 9.1), but only one true cause and that is unrelieved pressure. Understanding of the physiological response of the tissue to sustained pressure, knowledge of contributory factors and of how to address the problems they present will enable practitioners to make informed decisions in prevention of pressure ulcers.

There are two forms of loading, pressure and shear (Bliss 1993). Pressure is the force applied vertically to a surface and shear is the force that is applied tangentially or in parallel (Bliss 1993). An imaginary line being drawn through the body can demonstrate vertical force and offer a reason why pressure exerted on the lower part of the body depends greatly on the position of the body. The seated

Table 9.1 Factors effecting pressure sore formation

Immobility	Occlusion of the blood vessels will produce localised tissue damage leading to necrosis if pressure is not relieved.
Tissue distortion	Caused by gravity 'pulling' the body down in the bed or chair. The tissue remains static whilst the bone slides against the surface. This pinches the tissues, occludes capillaries and exerts much greater damage than direct pressure.
Vasomotor failure	This affects the delivery of blood to the tissues. Multiple sclerosis victims may be at greater risk than most patients with other diseases.
Peripheral vascular disease	Heels and toes are a very high risk. Even air mattresses do not always prevent pressure sores in these instances.
Sensory loss	Diabetic neuropathy, hemiplegia, paraplegia are all high risk factors.
Hypotension	Normal blood pressure will potentially keep the tissue viable up to 33 mmHg of pressure. Low blood pressure will be unable to keep the tissues viable at such high pressures.
Malnutrition	Without a diet high in calories, proteins and minerals, the tissues will be unable to recover from slight damage and are, therefore, at greater risk.

position would exert higher pressures because of the mass from the head pressing onto a small area (see Chapter 10). A prone body would have less mass pressing onto a larger area and will be less likely to develop a pressure ulcer. Shear cannot exist unless pressure is present. Therefore, although the prime cause of pressure ulcers is immobility, both should be considered together as the combination of the two, pressure and shear, is very damaging (Bliss 1993).

Capillaries form a network within subcutaneous tissues, dividing and sub-dividing as arterioles, forming capillaries, through to venules and finally feeding into minor then major veins. This system is collectively known as the microcirculation, which provides the tissues with nutrients and performs metabolite exchange, thereby keeping the tissues viable. Blood pressure within the arterioles is controlled by the heart and by the release of vasodilator substances. Osmotic pressures from blood albumin and hydrostatic pressures all have a role to play in the exchange of nutrients, fluids and waste products. Pressure will occlude the vessels and will disrupt the necessary exchange process, leading to inflammation within the tissues, the formation of micro-thrombi and, finally, death of the surrounding tissues. If this action is interrupted prior to destruction of the tissues, reactive hyper-aemia will occur and this reaction is proportional to the duration of the occlusion. Bliss (1998) states that 'reactive hyperaemia is the vital process by which the body increases the blood flow to tissue which has been deprived of oxygen to restore levels to normal as quickly as possi-ble'. Therefore, tissues will be flushed red with blood when vasodila-tion occurs and metabolite removal and oxygen supply will be replenished. The red mark seen over bony prominences when a patient is repositioned, is a visible sign of this process.

Pressure ulcers nearly always develop internally over a bony prominence and are due to a 'squeezing' and distortion of tissues (and microcirculation) between bone and a hard surface; this 'squeezing' is measured in millimetres of mercury (mmHg). Capil-lary closure occurs when the pressure between the bed surface and the bony prominence exceeds 16–32 mmHg (Landis 1930), thereby starving the tissues of oxygen and nutrients. This pressure increases (and can be up to five times greater) as it approaches the bone surface. This is known as the 'cone of pressure' and can explain why a surface redness can hide extensive tissue damage nearer the bone (Figure 9.1). It also explains why a small ulcer can open into a large,

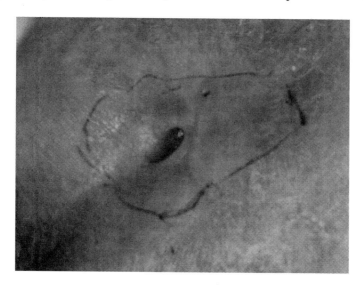

Figure 9.1 Pressure ulcer with evidence of undermining (see Plate 33).

undermined ulcer with overhanging edges and sinus formation. Bliss (1993) identifies that the formation of undermined tissues and sinuses are not due to infection but are produced by lysis of necrotic tissue produced during the original ischaemic episode.

The argument for reactive hyperaemia

Hyperaemia is the process by which the body adjusts blood flow to meet the metabolic needs of its different tissues in health and disease (Bliss 1998) and reactive hyperaemia can be seen in daily life. For instance, a person who crosses their legs for some time will note a reddened area when the legs are uncrossed and this is a natural response to occlusion of the blood vessels. Bliss (1998) described this as 'the local vasodilation which occurs in response to oxygen debt and accumulation of metabolic waste products due to interruption of blood flow'. Therefore, reactive hyperaemia is an important process in the prevention and treatment of pressure ulcers. The process occurs when the arterioles and venules in tissues have been occluded by pressure over a period of time. When the insult (pressure) is removed, vasodilation occurs, promoting rapid reoxygenation of the tissues and removal of metabolites. The reactive hyperaemia response in human subjects has been shown to vary with the temperature of the anatomical area involved with higher temperatures leading to a faster response (Collier 1999). This could, perhaps, provide an argument for mattress or seating design with inbuilt warming devices.

A literature review, completed by Bliss (1993) found that the hyperaemic response is associated with the release of three endothelial factors followed by chemical and hormonal release of, for example:

- endothelin (a vasoconstrictor);
- prostacyclin (a vasodilator);
- endothelial-derived relaxing factor (a vasodilator);
- nitric oxide, triggered by hypoxia, which inhibits contraction in adjacent smooth muscle and works with prostacylcin to limit thrombus formation;
- platelet aggregate products;
- adrenocorticotrophic hormone (ACTH).

The action of reactive hyperaemia, leads to the flushing of damaging metabolites, removal and destruction of bacteria at the site of insult and provision of extra oxygen and nutrients. Therefore, reactive hyperaemia (EPUAP grade 0 pressure ulcer or blanching hyperaemia) can be seen as a positive benefit to those patients with an established pressure ulcer. If the patient's ulcer is placed onto a high-grade air mattress and the blood vessels occluded for no longer than 10 minutes, the resultant reactive hyperaemia could be beneficial for healing the ulcer. The toxins will be removed and oxygen and nutrients provided to the damaged tissues promoting healing of the ulcer.

Any neurological disease will have an effect on the microcirculation and this will reduce reactive hyperaemia and lead to poor reperfusion of the occluded blood vessels, thereby increasing the potential of ischaemic changes in the tissues. Bader (1990b) found that $TcpO_2$ improved in the able-bodied following repetitive loading through a dynamic air cushion whereas, in the neurologically compromised patient, the $TcpO_2$ deteriorated. Chronic spinal injury patients who have a high resting skin blood flow have impaired reactive hyperaemia (Bliss 1998), which increases the risk of pressure ulcers. Therefore, even on an air mattress, the neurological patient's tissues may be jeopardized.

The argument against reactive hyperaemia

There are arguments against the theory of reactive hyperaemia. When occlusion of the blood vessels occurs (as in pressure) then restoration of the blood flow becomes of prime importance and is instantaneous (Bliss 1998 cites Lewis and Grant 1935). When occlusion occurs over a few seconds or minutes, restoration of blood supply is simply achieved by removing the pressure. There would be an initial phase of increased activity with the blood supply overreacting (reactive hyperaemia) due to metabolic products acting on the arterioles and causing vasodilation. Adenosine triphosphate (ATP) provides energy for active transport of substances from a low concentration to a high concentration. However, ATP of ischaemic tissues, cannot be regenerated but is degraded until it becomes adenosine, a powerful vasodilator (Majno and Joris 1996) and as such can to correct the ischaemia caused by pressure. The tissues flush red and any potential harm has been corrected.

However, prolonged pressure of longer than five minutes causes plateauing of the hyperaemic response. Bliss (1998) cites Michel and Gillott (1990) and states 'Cardiologists studying the effect of ischaemic lesions in the heart have observed that tissue damage can sometimes be worsened by reperfusion'. This finding has recently been confirmed by Niitsuma (2001), who found that ulcers may deteriorate further during reperfusion during repeated compressions.

It is believed that the ischaemic endothelium breaks down when blood flow returns and plasma escapes from the vessels, which remain filled with a sludge of red blood cells that cannot be pushed along. Tissue pressure rises and the veins become compressed. Thromboplastin is released by all the dead cells and whatever plasma is left in the vessel clots, thereby permanently blocking the path to any reflow (Majno and Joris 1996). Once this occurs, the surrounding tissue dies of starvation and Majno and Joris point out that reperfusion of dead tissue is impossible; therefore, a pressure ulcer is formed.

When pressure is of short duration (five minutes) the ischaemic tissues suffer incomplete reperfusion due to obstacles (at capillary level), such as granulocyte plugging, compression due to cellular swelling and endothelial damage that develops within the vessels. Tissue reperfusion can potentially cause damage due to congestion, inflammation and resultant oedema. This is due to metabolites that accumulate in the cells during a phase of ischaemia ready to cause osmotic swelling as soon as blood flow provides further fluid. Therefore, the theory that reactive hyperaemia may increase wound healing could be questioned.

The relation of bacteria to pressure ulcer formation

Sample biopsies from tissues reddened through pressure would show an increase in bacterial loading within the tissues. Freeman, as long ago as 1906 (cited by Bliss 1993), identified that bacterial poisonings and poor nutrition caused alterations in the vascular intima, resulting in hypostasis and increased the liability of small vessels to thrombosis under pressure. Once a wound is established, the bacteria will centralize in the wound bed and will continue to destroy the tissues. Barton (1983) identified bacteraemia and endotoxins as the most important cause of full-thickness ulcers.

Given that the standard NHS contract mattresses can exert pressures of 150 mmHg (Medical Devices Directorate 1993), it is unsurprising that any patient who does not, or cannot, reposition themselves will develop a pressure ulcer within a short period of time if nursed on a standard mattress. Ek et al. (1987) found that pressure of 11 mmHg caused capillary occlusion in some patients with hemiplegia. In an acutely ill patient, particularly those in shock, with possible low blood pressure, capillary occlusion can occur as low as 6 mmHg. Linked with malnutrition, neuropathy, immobility or poor mobility, the firm NHS contract mattress can be seen as a disaster and a pressure ulcer waiting to occur.

Landis's (1930) work was completed on healthy medical students and he used their nail beds to assess capillary closure. He found that the average capillary closure occurred at between 16 and 32 mmHg. However, this was an average figure and does not reflect all capillary closure pressures. Some of the students had much higher closure pressures and some much lower. It was also performed on healthy subjects and does not reflect capillary closures in ill or elderly patients, particularly when shock is present. The final problem with this study was that it was performed on the nail bed and this does not reflect the action that occurs over a bony prominence in soft tissues.

The duration of pressure is an important factor in whether the localized tissues become ulcerated. Repositioning the patient regularly will reduce pressure ulcer incidence and two-hourly turns are now almost ritualistic practice (Collier 1993). However, pressure ulcer formation is multifactorial and for many reasons (drug therapy, low blood pressure, etc.) acutely ill patients may require turning hourly or even more often and failure to do so will increase the risk of pressure ulcer formation. Agate (1972) believed that frequent turning as a method of pressure ulcer prevention merely caused disorientation in elderly patients. It also places a high demand on nursing time and, in a time of nursing shortage, an improved method of prevention is required.

Prevalence and cost

Pressure ulcer prevention is properly receiving high profile attention from the government, particularly as costs may be as high as £200m to £321m per year (Department of Health 1993). Collier (1995) found the cost to be £40 000 for one patient with an established pressure ulcer and litigation costs can run as high as £250 000 for one patient with a pressure ulcer. However, monetary settlements do not reflect the pain and suffering that can affect patients for many years following discharge from hospital.

Pressure ulcers and leg ulcers together cost £800 million per annum (Thomas 1994). Thomas writes 'No other figures are available for treating wounds such as surgical infected wounds, fungating wounds, traumatic wounds etc, but it is not unreasonable to assume that together these would cause the total cost of wound management to exceed £1 billion per annum'. However, pressure ulcers that do not heal can be painful, become necrotic, infected and malodorous or can even be the cause of death of the patient and this misery cannot be calculated in monetary terms.

Estimates of hospital prevalence of pressure ulcers vary between five per cent and 10 per cent (Davies et al. 1991) although in certain specialities, the actual figure may be as high as 60 per cent (Verluysen 1986). In acute care, prevalence of pressure ulcer formation ranges from three per cent to 14 per cent and in long-term care it is as high as 15–25 per cent. National average of pressure ulcers was nine per cent in 1987 (Bergstrom et al. 1987) and Waterlow (1988) found an incidence of 15 per cent in acute settings with another study showing an incidence of 40 per cent in ITU. If Hibbs (1987) is correct and pressure ulcers are 95 per cent preventable, even taking into account pre-existing pressure ulcers, even nine per cent would be an unacceptable level of prevalence. Within Eastbourne Hospitals NHS Trust, audit has shown that the introduction of appropriate pressure-relieving/reducing equipment has reduced pressure ulcer prevalence to an average of three per cent. However, prevalence can be used and adapted by each trust and a direct comparison is not helpful. One trust may use incidence to assess pressure ulcer problems, whilst another may use prevalence. The two measurements cannot be compared. One trust may use a break in the skin, whereas another trust may use reddened areas to identify pressure ulcers. These two trusts will have completely different prevalence results.

Mortality of patients with pressure ulcers is between 22 per cent and 37 per cent (Davies et al. 1991). Of those patients developing a pressure ulcer, 90 per cent of patients die within four months (Bader 1990a).

Equipment and repositioning as prevention

The rationale for turning patients should be given consideration as turning side-to-side will not prevent pressure ulcers. There is, at present, a general reduction in staffing levels within hospitals and these low levels may mean that two-hourly turning regimes cannot always be applied. Pressure ulcers are, almost always, found on bony prominences and turning patients onto their sides ensures that bony prominences are always in contact with a pressure-generating surface. There is also a potential that repositioning may increase pain in patients with painful illness or wounds.

Two-hourly turns can increase the risk of shearing and friction, even when a hoist is used and heel tissues can be damaged through friction when slides are used to assist with turning unless a full-length slide is used. However, relieving pressure over the bony prominence is a vital part of nursing. Hussian (1953) found that sustained pressure of 100 mmHg over two hours caused irreversible changes in the muscles of rats; if this relates to humans then two hours without change of position is too long.

Work completed by Exton Smith and Sherwin (1961) demonstrated that the number of movements elderly patients made, during the night, directly correlated with the formation of pressure ulcers. Johnson et al. (1930) showed that the normal number of movements through the night were 20–40 full turns with small position changes every 5–10 minutes. This would be for the normal healthy adult and the situation would be different for those who were sedated or immobile.

Assessment

Waterlow (1988) refers to assessment as the 'key to pressure ulcer prevention'; certainly, the use of an assessment tool will assist the practitioner to make decisions on required resources (Figure 9.2, page 266). The purpose of a risk assessment tool is to predict which patients are liable to sustain pressure damage and, as such, are very useful.

Nevertheless, there are many debates about which risk assessment tool is 'safe' to use, even though the risk assessment tool should only be a guide to the practitioner and is not a definitive answer. Clinical judgement must still be the mainstay of the art and science of nursing, and risk assessment tools, of any kind, should only be used to confirm clinical diagnosis rather than replace clinical judgement. It is preferable, even important, to select a tool, such as the Waterlow risk assessment score, the Norton score or the Braden score, to use as an argument for provision of mattresses for individual patients or to develop resource requirements through audit. The scoring systems are also useful throughout the clinical area to give a universal language between practitioners from different specialities, hospital to community or nursing homes. However, it is important to remember that these systems may over- or under-predict the risk to the patient and this can lead to either an increased risk of pressure ulcer development or to increased and unnecessary use of scarce resources.

When the practitioner is not assisted by a risk assessment tool and is unable to identify risk through clinical judgement, prevention can become a reactive process rather than a proactive one. A reactive process is still reliant on assessment but reacting to an obvious deterioration in the patient's pressure areas rather identifying the potential for tissue damage and preventing that damage in a proactive way. Full physical risk assessment allows the practitioner to provide the appropriate equipment before the damage is established in the tissues.

Identifying risk through physical assessment is easily accomplished through a pressure ulcer classification system and use of blanching hyperaemia (EPUAP 2001, grade 0) as an indication of potential tissue damage.

Risk assessment tools

There are various risk assessment tools to choose from and selection depends on the needs of the patients within any particular speciality. Categorization of a patient as 'at risk' through use of a risk assessment tool justifies mobilization of costly pressure-relieving equipment (Shakespeare 1994). It is, therefore, important to ensure that the risk assessment tool is reliable and does not over- (or under-) predict. When a risk assessment score is being considered for use, the specificity and sensitivity of the tool will provide information on the reliability of the tool to predict the development of pressure ulcers.

Interrater reliability

For many years, the route to excellent assessment was through the use of scoring systems such as the Waterlow, Norton and Braden risk assessment tools. However, knowledge and techniques continually evolve, providing new analytical tools and the research that looks at these scoring systems is beginning to look dated (Ratcliffe 1998). Edwards (1996) claims that many risk assessment tools achieve high sensitivity through gross over-prediction with serious implications for efficient targeting of resources.

FLOW CHART FOR THE PREVENTION AND TREATMENT OF PRESSURE ULCERS

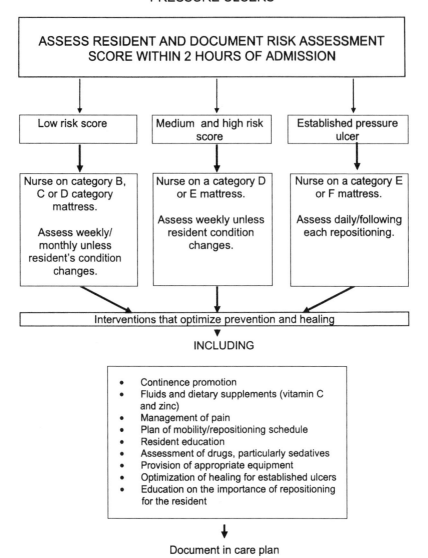

Figure 9.2 A sample algorithm for mattress selection.

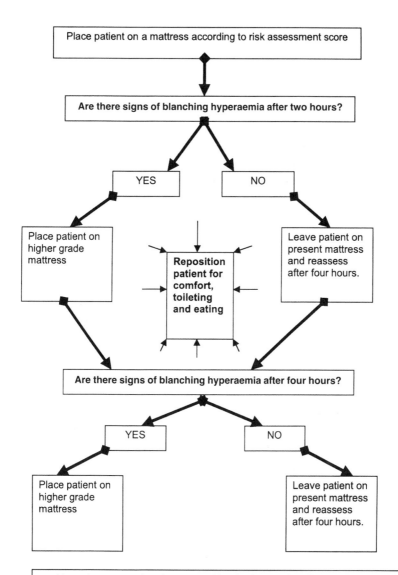

Figure 9.2 (contd).

Sensitivity

This is a test that looks at the amount of people – declared to be 'at risk' who go on to develop a pressure ulcer. An accurate risk assessment scoring system will correctly identify the patients who go on to develop ulcers.

Specificity

This test looks at those patients considered to be 'not at risk' and identifies how many of these go on to produce a pressure ulcer. An accurate risk assessment scoring system will correctly identify those who will not develop a pressure ulcer.

The Waterlow risk assessment tool is a popular choice for many areas. However, this is one tool that over-predicts the potential of an ulcer (Hopkins 1998). Although patients treated according to the Waterlow score are less likely to develop ulcers, the system tends to use vital resources on patients who may not have gone on to develop ulcers. This is costly and there is a risk that, if equipment is not readily available, patients may be admitted without the possibility of being given an appropriate mattress and, therefore, may go on to develop an ulcer. Nevertheless, reliability tests are difficult to undertake as pressure ulcer formation is dependent on so many different factors. A specificity test will look at how many patients, identified 'at risk', go on to develop a pressure ulcer. However, a scoring system would recommend appropriate pressure reducing equipment for 'at risk' patients and this would immediately reduce the risk. These patients are then unlikely to develop a ulcer and this would affect the reliability of the risk assessment tool.

Reliability will also be affected by:

* individual nurses' interpretations of the scoring system;
* unqualified staff may be asked to undertake the follow-up assessments;
* a tendency/temptation to follow the scoring system of the day before;
* lack of understanding of the tool that is used.

It would be impossible to analyse the true validity using markers of sensitivity and specificity as that would involve NOT placing patients on pressure-relieving equipment to see whether they develop pressure ulcers and that would be unethical. Therefore, risk assessment tools can never be completely validated.

Waterlow risk assessment score

The Waterlow scoring system is a comprehensive tool that covers 10 risk factors (Figure 9.3) and includes time spent in theatre and medication. The higher the score, the greater the risk for pressure ulcer formation and the assessment rating differentiates between at-risk, high-risk and very high-risk status and makes recommendations for appropriate equipment to reduce potential of pressure ulcer formation. Although this system does tend to over-predict and sometimes uses resources unnecessarily, it does help to reduce pressure ulcer formation and used in conjunction with excellent physical assessment, it is a useful tool and one that can be presented at times of litigation threat. Figures 9.3, 9.4, 9.5 and 9.6 can be used as part of a strategy for the prevention of pressure ulcers.

Body Mass Index (BMI)	★	Skin Type Visual Risk Areas	★	Sex Age	★	Special Risks	★
BMI 20–24 (average)	0	Healthy	0	Male	1	Tissue malnutrition	★
BMI 25–29.9 (medium)	1	Tissue paper	1	Female	2	Terminal cachexia	8
BMI 30–</>>40 (large)	2	Dry	1	14–49	1	Cardiac failure	5
BMI </<>20 (obese)	3	Oedematous	1	50–64	2	Peripheral vascular	
Continence	★	Clammy (temp↑)	1	65–74	3	disease	5
Complete/		Discoloured	2	75–80	4	Anaemia	2
catheterized	0	Broken/spot	3	81+	5	Smoking	1
Occasionally incontinent	1	Mobility	★	Appetite	★	Neurological deficit	★
Cath/Incontinent		Fully	0	Average	0	eg diabetes, MS, CVA,	
of faeces	2	Restless/Fidgety	1	Poor	1	Motor/sensory	
Doubly incontinent	3	Apathetic	2	NG tube/		Paraplegia	5
		Restricted	3	fluids only	2	Major surgery/trauma	★
		Inert/traction	4	NBM/		Orthopaedic -	
		Chairbound	5	Anorexic	3	Below waist, spinal	5
						on table </>>2 hours	5
Score						Medication	★
10+ At Risk						Cytotoxics	
15+ High Risk						High dose steroids	
20+ Very High Risk						Anti-inflammatory	4

Figure 9.3 The Waterlow scoring system.

Initial assessment on admission																	
Date	Time		Score		Frequency of assessment												

Date and time																	
Build/weight for height																	
Continence																	
Skin type, visual risk areas																	
Mobility																	
Sex																	
Age																	
Appetite																	
Special risks																	
Tissue malnutrition																	
Neurological deficit																	
Major surgery/ trauma																	
Medication																	
Total for the date																	

Figure 9.4 A scoring sheet which can be used for recording Waterlow risk assessment findings.

USE OF THE WATERLOW SCORING SYSTEM
I.   Any risk assessment system is merely a tool to assist the trained nurse in assessment of the patient, it is not a replacement for clinical judgement and should only be used to support clinical decisions.
II. Responsibility for assessment, and choice of assessor, goes to the qualified nurse who is accountable for the patient's care. Initial assessment must always be completed by a qualified nurse.
III. The risk score should be entered on the patient's record along with the name of the support system the patient is nursed on and the suggested frequency of assessment.

Figure 9.5 Using a scoring system.

IV.   Assessment will be completed in accident and emergency department and wards advised of the score before transfer.

V.   The patient should be discharged to community/nursing home with a Waterlow risk assessment score when appropriate.

VI.   Pressure ulcers should be graded using a pressure ulcer classification.

VII.   Theatre should be informed of the patient's Waterlow score prior to surgery and consideration will be given to supplying pressure-relieving mattress / heel supports, during surgery and recovery.

VIII.   Initial assessment: ring appropriate areas on the Waterlow score sheet. All subsequent assessments should be made without ringing the scores. This is to ensure that the initial assessment remains and any changes can be identified by referring to the original score.

IX.   There are 10 boxed categories within the Waterlow scoring system. Each box may contain more than one problem for the individual patient; each problem should be scored, therefore, more than on selection can be made in each category.

Figure 9.5 (contd).

Documenting mattress type			
Type of mattress on admission:	_____		
After first assessment:	_____		
Score <10: assess weekly/monthly >11 to <20 assess twice weekly. >21 assess daily	Date when mattress changed		
<u>OR</u> as patient condition dictates	Type of mattress		

Suggested Criteria for Pressure Area Assessment

RISK CATEGORY	MATTRESS CATEGORY	MATTRESS TYPE
</<>15 at risk	B, C & D	Pressure redistributing foam or cut foam overlay
15+ high risk	E	**Dynamic air overlay (visco-elastic foam mattress)**
20+ very high risk	F	Dynamic / static mattress replacement system

Patients with established pressure ulcer grade </>>4 should always be nursed on a category C mattress.

Decisions should be based on clinical judgement using above criteria as a guide to assist in choice of mattress.

Ensure that patients sitting in chairs have appropriate cushions.

Consider electric beds as part of pressure ulcer prevention plan.

Figure 9.6 Selecting and documenting mattress types, according to needs.

Norton risk assessment score

The Norton score (Figure 9.7) is a popular risk assessment tool but, as a predictor of pressure ulcers, there are discrepancies with a tendency to over-predict in 64 per cent of cases and under-predict in 14 per cent of cases (Flanagan 1993). The scoring system looks at five risk factors and is very simple to use. The final score indicates the risk with a high score not at risk and low score at high risk. The scoring is limited in that it is not related to short-term potential problems such as enforced immobility on theatre tables, and is probably best used in long-term elderly care where the risk remains fairly static.

Score	Physical condition	Mental condition	Activity	Mobility	Incontinence
4	Good	Alert	Ambulant	Full	Not
3	Fair	Apathetic	Walks with help	Slightly limited	Occasionally
2	Poor	Confused	Chair-bound	Very limited	Usually urine
1	Very bad	Stuporous	Bed-fast	Immobile	Doubly
A score of 14 or less indicates that a person is at risk of pressure ulcer development					

Figure 9.7 Norton scoring system. A score of 14 or less indicates that a person is at risk of pressure ulcer development.

Braden risk assessment score

The Braden score (Figure 9.8) was originally developed in the USA for use in nursing homes and primarily identified malnutrition as a marker for the development of pressure ulcers. The scoring system has six risk factors: sensory perception, moisture, activity, mobility, nutrition and friction and/or shear. Each risk category scores from 1 to 4 with 4 as low-risk. The Braden score can over-predict pressure ulcer formation by as much as 36 per cent (Flanagan 1993). However, Braden and Bergstrom (1988) found this scoring system to have a greater specificity and sensitivity than other scoring systems and may therefore be a useful predictor.

SCORE	SENSORY	MOISTURE	ACTIVITY	MOBILITY	NUTRITION	FRICTION and SHEAR
1	Completely limited	Constantly moist	Bed-bound	Completely immobile	Very poor	Problem
2	Very limited	Very moist	Chair-bound	Very limited	Probably inadequate	Potential problem
3	Slightly limited	Occasionally moist	Walks occasionally	Slightly limited	Adequate	No apparent problem
4	No impairment	Rarely moist	Walks frequently	No limitations	Excellent	

A score of 16 or less indicates that a person is at risk of pressure ulcer development

Figure 9.8 The Braden score.

Classification of pressure ulcers

Healey (1995) found there were at least 14 grading or classification systems in use within the UK in 1995. In 1992, at a consensus conference held in Stirling (Reid and Morison 1994), the role of the invited group was to develop a grading system for pressure ulcers and the chosen classification gave five stages with sub-classification in each of the stages (Table 9.2). Torrance's (1983) grading system uses five stages and both grading systems are similar (Figure 9.9, p. 275). Healey (1995) found that none of the scales demonstrated great reliability, especially for some of the less severe grades. To achieve a universal language, the new European classification for pressure ulcers (EPUAP 2001) was devised. It has four simple stages and is expected to become the future universal assessment for pressure wounds.

Unrelieved pressure will lead to pressure ulcers which develop over a period of 4–5 days and pass through the various stages during this time. A black ulcer will not become noticeable on day one but will present on days 3–6. However, the damage that leads to the necrosis will begin within a few hours of immobility and recognition of stage 1, blanching hyperaemia, will lead the practitioner to make an accurate prediction of risk. If any redness exists, the patient requires either increased repositioning or a higher grade mattress.

Table 9.2 Stirling pressure ulcer grading

0	No clinical evidence of a sore
0.0	Normal appearence intact skin
0.1	Healed with scarring
0.2	Tissue damaged – not assessed as a score
1	Discoloured, intact skin. Non-blanching with light finger pressure
1.1	Erythema non-blanching with increased local heat
1.2	Blue/purple/black discolouration
2	Partial thickness skin loss
2.1	Blister
2.2	Abrasion
2.3	Shallow ulcer
2.4	Any of the above with underlying blue/purple/black discolouration/induration
3	Full thickness skin loss involving damage or necrosis of subcutaneous tissue but not involving underlying bone, tendon or joint capsule
3.1	Crater without undermining of local tissue
3.2	Crater with undermining
3.3	Sinus the full extent of which is not certain
3.4	Full thickness skin loss but wound covered with necrotic tissue (hard/black/brown or softer/creamy slough). Not possible to fully assess damage until debrided
4	Full skin thickness tissue necrosis, bone, tendon, joints involved
4.1	Visible bone/tendon at the surface capsule
4.2	Sinus extending to bone/capsule/tendon

First stage pressure ulcer or grade 0

The first stage ulcer (blanching hyperaemia, grade 0) is a useful physical assessment tool. When a patient rests on a bony prominence, the tissues between the bone and the support surface will be almost certainly occluded leading to a blanching of the tissues. When the pressure is removed from the area, through turning the patient or through use of alternating air mattresses, the capillaries overreact and flush bright red. This is known as reactive hyperaemia and is a healthy counteraction to the occlusion, which can be noted in healthy subjects who sit for a period of time with their legs crossed and the tissues appear red when the legs are uncrossed. The tissues are not damaged by this flush of blood but it can be used as a warning that pressure has been sustained over too long a period. This means that any patient with a reddened area over a bony prominence has

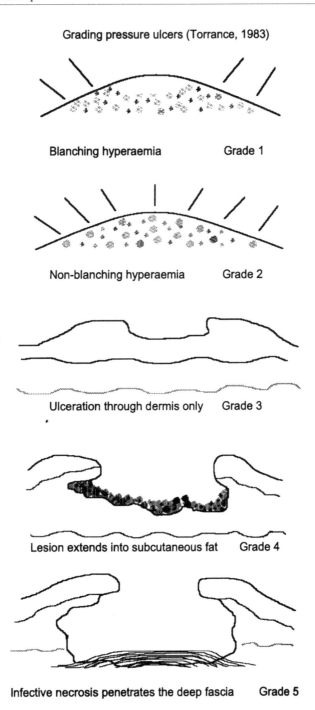

Figure 9.9 Torrance pressure ulcer grading system.

been left in that position too long and requires either a higher grade mattress or more frequent repositioning. However, should this warning be ignored, then the first stage pressure ulcer may well progress to the second stage (non-blanching hyperaemia).

Second stage pressure ulcer, grade 1

This stage has inflammation in progress within the tissues and the first stages of damage are occurring. Micro-thrombi will be forming within the capillaries; bacteria will gather around the threatened area and metabolites will be present. The reddened area may feel firm or hard and hot to the touch. Although non-blanching hyperaemia demonstrates that damage is occurring, it is still reversible at this stage; prompt action in placing the patient on an appropriate air mattress will help to reduce the tissue damage. Kosiak (1961) demonstrated the benefits of alternating pressure relief compared with continuous pressure in the prevention of tissue damage. Stage 2 is an indication that a break in the skin is inevitable if the patient is not given urgent pressure relief through the use of repositioning or an appropriate mattress.

Third stage pressure ulcer, grade 2

The third stage is a break in the skin and the pressure ulcer is now a wound (blister, 'scraze' or small ulcer) that will take nursing time and effort to heal. A small ulcer may belie the amount of damage in the dermis. The cone of pressure (Figure 9.10) ensures that the highest pressure, and damage, is close to the bone and the tissue destruction can be very difficult to classify. This can lead to misinterpretation of the patient's resource requirements and may guide the practitioner to use a lower grade mattress instead of an air mattress.

Fourth stage pressure ulcer, grade 3

The fourth stage is a deep ulcer, involving muscle destruction. This ulcer is often filled with hard necrotic tissue and is difficult to correctly classify until fully debrided (Figure 9.11). Patients with this grade of ulcer are prone to clinical wound infections and loss of proteins through exudate can produce hypoproteinaemia, which leads to delayed healing and/or further tissue destruction.

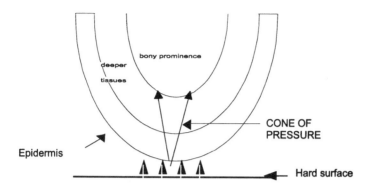

Pressures increase as nearer to the bone and pressure ulcers develop close to the bone and appear on the surface as a redness or small ulcer. This can later develop into a much larger cavity and, as the damage is already established, nursing care will not prevent the deterioration.

Figure 9.10 Cone of pressure.

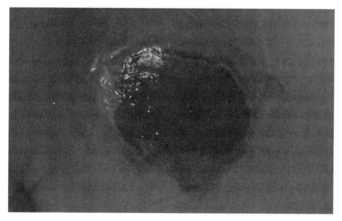

Figure 9.11 Pressure ulcers are often difficult to classify until fully debrided (see Plate 34).

Fifth stage pressure ulcer, grade 4

The final and fifth stage is a deep tissue injury with bone exposed (Figure 9.12). An ulcer at this stage often involves infective necrosis and the patient may be moribund; death can be a consequence of this stage. The patient in Figure 9.12 died as a consequence of his pressure ulcers. Bliss and Silver (1988) found that 90 per cent of patients with deep ulcers die within four months.

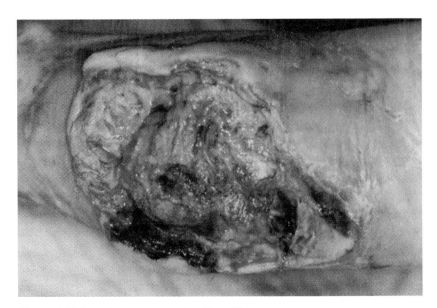

Figure 9.12 Stage 5 pressure ulcer (see Plate 35).

Groth (cited by Bliss 1993), in 1942, identified two types of pressure ulcers: superficial 'benign' and deep 'malignant'. Another way of describing this could be ulcers that are 'inside out' or those that have formed next to the bone and are developing from the deeper tissues, appearing as a small outer ulcer with large undermining. Alternatively, they could be referred to 'outside in' or those ulcers caused by friction and shear that are often superficial but can increase in size and depth.

This can be often be seen in heel ulcers where there is a necrotic area, often following the formation of a blister, the roof of which, if left alone, will break away within a few days leaving healed tissue. The deep ulcers will require debriding or they will never heal. The difference between superficial and deep is often difficult to assess, particularly with inexperience. There are often markers however with deeper ulcers often having a reddened induration surrounding the necrosis. This is an indication of further damage beneath the surface and may lead to an increase in depth and area of necrosis.

Pressure ulcers take many weeks or months to heal, leading to distress for the patient and the use of expensive resources. Therefore assessment and prevention is vital.

Prevention

The Kings Fund Centre (1988) identified three main factors involved in improving pressure ulcer prevention and management:

1   the patient;
2   the resources;
3   the knowledge required for improvement in standards of care.

The patient

Patients can be malnourished, debilitated, moribund, immobile, unable to control urinary or faecal continence or depressed and these factors must be taken into consideration if prevention, or treatment, is to be achieved. Nourishment is vital to repair of tissues or in maintaining tissue viability and can easily be neglected. Community nurses rely on carers to report difficulty with eating and hospital nurses may be busy at mealtimes and so miss meal trays being taken away with the food untouched.

Patients who are moribund or immobile may require a mattress that either mimics movement for them or reduces pressure as with a dynamic air mattress or overlay, Vicair mattress, De-cube mattress, Repose overlay or Care bed mattress overlay. Patients who are able to move can be asked to reposition themselves every half hour. Electric profiling beds are also an excellent way of allowing the patient independence of movement and the patient can again be asked to sit themselves up or down every half hour (Hampton 1998b), giving regular repositioning and reducing pressure ulcers. Assessment of each individual patient is the key to providing appropriate care. Education of the patient and/or carer is the 'icing on the cake' giving independence and control of their own individual circumstances.

Incontinence is thought to be a high contributory factor with 39 per cent of patients with urinary incontinence developing pressure ulcers compared with only 7 per cent of continent patients who developed ulcers (Norton et al. 1975). Lowthian (1970) claimed that sodden skin has greater adhesion and is at greater risk of frictional or shearing damage and, therefore, incontinence is an immense risk factor.

The resources

Mattresses and chairs can be expensive and arguments for provision of equipment can remain ignored by financial departments and supply departments, particularly when the potential risk is unrecognized by non-medical personnel. Collins (1998b) demonstrated that patients on an acute medical ward would stay for five days longer if a pressure ulcer developed and, when the patient, with a pressure ulcer, is transferred to a rehabilitation ward, their stay can be lengthened by as much as 12 weeks (North West Thames Regional Advisory Committee 1989). Collins also demonstrated that hospital acquired pressure ulcer incidence could be reduced from 5.2 per cent to 0.3 per cent on a medical elderly ward by the use of appropriate resources. Therefore, selection of cost-effective and clinically effective resources is a vital part of pressure ulcer prevention for hospital or community trusts.

Excellent individual assessment and knowledge of how pressure ulcers are prevented can lead to inexpensive selection of mattress types. Over many years, manufacturers have completed excellent work, looking at air mattresses and pressure ulcer prevention. The results have led nurses erroneously to believe that the only type of mattress that prevents pressure ulcers in high-risk patients is an expensive air mattress. This is not true. Dynamic air mattresses are an excellent resource in the prevention of pressure ulcers, but they are not the only resource that can be used in prevention. The author would claim that an air mattress is undoubtedly required to treat a pressure ulcer, but prevention can be achieved through use of a new generation of static foam mattresses. These mattresses are discussed under grades of mattresses, later in this chapter.

Heel pressure ulcers

The heels sustain greater pressures when the patient is prone and, if the skin is of poor quality or the blood supply is poor, the patient will develop pressure ulcers on the heels, even when the sacrum remains free of damage. There is a tendency to blame the air mattress or foam mattress when pressure ulcers are noted on heels or feet. However, it is unlikely to be the fault of a pressure-relieving or reducing mattress, but is more likely to be related to patient condition or that the patient is sitting out of bed, with the heel on the floor or stool, for several hours a day. It may be useful to bear the following questions in mind:

1   Is the mattress a pressure-redistributing foam mattress or an air mattress?

2   Does the foot of the foam mattress have a specially adapted foot area for lowering interface pressures?

3   Is the patient diabetic? Diabetes will cause micro-vascular changes; could this be the cause of the ulcers?

4   Is there evidence of arterial disease? To answer this, a Doppler assessment will be required (see Chapter 5).

5   Does the patient sit out of bed and could the ulcer relate to heels being rested on the floor?

6   Does the patient have restless legs? Could friction and shearing, related to movement, be the cause of the ulcer?

7   Does the patient cross their legs when in bed? If one foot is pressed against another foot or a shin, there is likely to be two marks (and possibly two ulcers) on both areas experiencing the pressure.

8   Does the patient press one foot against the other foot?

9   Is the assessment score a low to medium score for foam mattresses or a medium to high score for air mattresses?

10 When was the ulcer noted? Was it after the skin damage became apparent or when redness was first noted? The two conditions are very different as a pressure ulcer can be developing deep within the tissues for many days with only a slight redness on the surface. Often, when the skin shows signs of damage, the occult damage will be extensive.

11 If it was noted after the ulcer formed, why was the patient not provided with a higher grade mattress when erythema was first noted?

12 Has the patient been given an epidural? If so, they will be unaware of any pressure stimulation. Women in labour and those patients having had orthopaedic surgery may be susceptible to pressure damage following an epidural analgesic (Roche and Walker 2000; Hughes 2001).

13 Was it some time before the patient was admitted to the ward/nursing home (or have they been away from home) within the last five days. Pressure ulcers are occult in the first stages and often will not show broken skin until the internal damage has completed and become visible on the skin.

14 Is there a bed cradle in place? If not, the weight of bed clothes can significantly add to the amount of pressure applied to the heels (Donnelly 2001).

15 Does the patient have congestive cardiac failure (CCF)? The
    oedema from CCF prevents nutrients and oxygen from reaching
    the tissues and the tissues become vulnerable to injury. CCF, by
    its very nature, also causes poor delivery of blood to the lower
    limbs and, thereby, increases the potential risk of pressure ulcers.
16 Is the patient depressed? They may appear to be fully mobile but
    depression may lead them to sit or lie for many hours without
    moving.

All the above factors will have an impact on pressure ulcer formation,
regardless of the type of mattress that is used. If these questions are all
answered fully, and the answer to each is 'no', then the mattress may
be at fault. However, with assessment and reassessment, pressure
ulcers should never develop beyond the first stage.

Knowledge of pressure ulcer prevention and management

The management of pressure ulcers has, for many years, relied on
two-hourly turning and repositioning. Despite an accumulation of
a vast amount of literature on the subject of pressure ulcer management, prevention and the importance of pressure-redistributing
and relieving mattresses, this particular aspect has seen little or no
change (Preston 1988). Anecdotally, nurses will continue to turn
patients 'two-hourly' even when being nursed on excellent
dynamic equipment and will continue to 'turn' the patient from
side to side on bony prominences. It is the bony prominences
where pressure ulcers are formed. Therefore, side-to-side repositioning could be considered a contributing factor in the formation
of ulcers. This ritualistic practice is reminiscent of the 'back round'
when pre-nursing assessment, nurses would work from bed to bed,
washing patients buttocks and creaming or rubbing them to
'prevent pressure ulcers'. This approach to prevention of pressure
ulcers was passed from one nurse to another without rationale or
research and was an unquestioning tradition of obedience inherited
as part of the Victorian legacy with which nursing is still struggling
today (Walsh and Ford 1989). Hopefully, nursing has moved on
from a task-orientated approach and is developing an individual
patient assessment approach.

Sheets and incontinence pads as factors in pressure ulcer formation

Incontinence pads are large paper squares with plastic backing, which are used to protect bed sheets and chairs from incontinent patients. They can vary in quality, size and thickness and each of these elements have the potential to influence the formation of pressure ulcers. Within nursing homes, washable, material incontinence pads (also with plastic backing) are commonly used for incontinent presidents. The potential for these paper and material pads to produce pressure ulcers is high as the paper linings often 'pill', which means the material will roll into small balls within the pad and create 'hot spots' of pressure. Many pads will reflect urine onto the skin and the contact with the air produces an ammoniac reaction, which can damage good skin. The pads can also wrinkle under a patient when there is movement, and this also will create hot spots of pressure with the thickness of the pads detracting from any pressure-relieving resources that are being used. Added to this, the waterproof backing of the pads will increase the possibility of the patient perspiring, leading to moistened tissues and increasing the risk.

The author names the pads the 'just in case pads', because whenever a nurse is asked why the patient has an incontinence pad, the nurse will reply 'just in case'.

Patients who are incontinent and require support would be better served with body-worn pads. These pads generally have a stay dry liner, which will not allow urine to be reflected onto the skin and are held firmly in place by pants/knickers, preventing the movement that would cause 'hot spots' of pressure.

Drawsheets can be equally damaging to at risk tissues. They are often placed over plastic sheeting, causing the patient to perspire, and they wrinkle as the patient moves, leading to large areas of sheet rolled under vulnerable areas. The softness and smoothness of fabrics can be altered by laundering (Alberman 1992) and drawsheets are generally a thick and hard material before they are washed. This is compounded by the use of caustic washing chemicals and, if a patient perspires or is incontinent in a sheet, there may be an exchange of chemicals for urine leading to increased potential for tissue damage and pressure ulcer formation.

The plastic sheeting beneath the drawsheet will increase the risk of macerated tissues. Therefore, it is important to assess the patient's individual requirements and to supply body-worn incontinence pads that are appropriate for their need. Excellent assessment offers greater dignity and comfort to the patient.

Equipment in prevention

It is important that nurses understand how pressure ulcers are formed and how static and dynamic air mattresses can achieve either excellent pressure redistribution or periodic relief of pressure. It will be these two factors combined with physical assessment of the patient that will prevent pressure ulcer formation and these factors will be part of the practitioners' knowledge. It may also be obvious that only a knowledgeable practitioner will be able to identify and address the issue of blanching hyperaemia.

Pressure ulcers are due to unrelieved pressure. Other factors such as friction and shear, incontinence and nutrition, may contribute to the formation of a ulcer, but the primary cause is sustained pressure on a bony prominence (Young 1992). Unrelieved pressure on a bony prominence creates different levels of pressure. This varies according to the surface providing the pressure – a hard, ungiving, surface will create high pressures and a soft surface that redistributes the body weight, will give low pressures.

A normal NHS mattress can generate interface pressures of over 150 mmHg and is 30–50 per cent higher than modern pressure-redistributing foam mattresses (Medical Devises Directorate 1993). If a patient, with a capillary closure of 12 mmHg, is nursed on a normal NHS mattress, they would almost certainly develop a pressure ulcer. Even healthy subjects are at risk of pressure formation on NHS mattresses. Interface pressure is assessed through the use of a pressure monitor, such as the Talley hand-held monitor or the Tekscan. The Talley monitor is useful for demonstration purposes or for simple assessments. However, it depends greatly on the positioning of the patient and accuracy of placement of the pad. Tekscan is, on the other hand, expensive and complex to use and has greater use in research.

Kosiak (1961) wrote 'Since it is impossible to completely eliminate all pressure for a long period of time, it becomes imperative that the pressure be completely eliminated at frequent intervals in order to allow circulation to ischaemic tissues'. This could be achieved by repositioning with the 30° tilt or through the use of equipment such as dynamic mattresses.

Traditionally, nurses have used two-hourly turns to provide pressure relief and to restore tissue integrity. However, because patients who are moribund require increased turning to prevent pressure ulcer formation, two-hourly turns are no longer adequate. There are also the patients who are in pain, dying or require sleep through the night, and these would experience discomfort and sleep deprivation and, therefore, their pressure relief should be through the use of appropriate equipment. Provision of a pressure-redistributing mattress, according to the patient's holistic assessment, will negate the need to reposition for anything other than comfort or treatment. Toileting, sitting up for food and normal mobilization would, along with good assessment and a suitable mattress, provide enough repositioning to prevent discomfort. Those patients who are unable to eat or get out of bed for toileting, must be repositioned for comfort.

There is a myth that patients do not require repositioning on an air mattress. Air mattresses are designed to prevent pressure ulcers and represent the body's natural movement, thereby preventing the occurrence of pressure ulcers. However, if a patient is left in one position for too long, the joints become stiffened and the patient feels uncomfortable along with an increase in risk of airway infections. Given that the patient is provided with an appropriate mattress, repositioning should be for comfort and treatment and not for pressure ulcer prevention. A patient with chronic obstructive airways disease may find difficulty with repositioning as changing position may interfere with breathing. Providing these patients are nursed on appropriate air mattresses and sacral areas are checked every time they use the toilet or are sat up, they will be safe from pressure damage when they maintain a stable position such as sitting up in bed.

Repositioning for prevention

Barrett (1987) suggested that measures taken to prevent pressure ulcer development, that is two-hourly repositioning, can cause the patient distress and discomfort. Therefore, the highest quality treatment would be the use of a dynamic air mattress to reduce both risk of ulceration and risk of causing distress.

Two-hourly turns were initiated during wartime when orderlies were employed to provide 24-hour care to servicemen with spinal injuries. The orderlies would proceed from bed to bed, washing and 'log-rolling' patients and, because of the 'Nightingale' design of the ward it would take the orderlies two hours to complete the task. They found it reduced pressure ulcers and the myth of two-hourly turns was born. Norton et al. (1975) looked at two-hourly turns and found that they truly did reduce pressure ulcers. Today we seek, not just to reduce pressure ulcer formation, but to prevent their formation altogether. This can only be achieved with appropriate use of foam and air mattresses or sensible and individualized repositioning regimes.

When repositioning cannot be avoided, the 30° tilt is the simplest method of repositioning and places the patient off any bony prominence. This reduces the potential of pressure ulcer damage. A study by Defloor (2000) demonstrated that the 30° semi-Fowler position and the prone position resulted in the lowest interface pressures. The aim of this investigation was to determine which positions resulted in the lowest pressures to the skin of persons lying in bed. Pressures were recorded in 10 different lying positions on two mattresses in 62 healthy volunteers. The 30° laterally inclined position had lower pressure readings than the 90° side lying position; the latter gives the highest pressure readings and thus should be avoided.

The 30° tilt was introduced following investigations in a Young Disabled Unit where the researcher had carefully monitored positions and interface pressure (Preston 1988). The 30° tilt position removes the patient from all bony prominences, where the tissue damage normally occurs, and places them on the fatty areas of their back and buttock. Passing a hand underneath the sacrum demonstrates there is a space between the bone of the sacrum and the bed. This allows the patient to remain in that position up to three times longer than when lying directly on a bony prominence. The 30° tilt technique can provide a useful alternative system of repositioning which, in some cases, obviates the need for specialized equipment and may be readily adopted in community and nursing home settings. As the patient can be left in this position longer than any other position, repositioning times may be increased, thereby increasing sleep periods.

A study undertaken in Japan (Arao et al. 2001) clarified the morphological differences in the blood capillaries and elastic fibres and confirmed that blood capillaries were more numerous in the sacral skin than in the gluteus maximus, whilst elastic fibres were more dense in the gluteus maximus. The conclusion of the study suggested that the thick elastic fibres in the gluteus maximus may contribute to rapid tissue recovery and reduce tissue distress. This may explain why pressure ulcers occur over the bony sacrum and rarely over the gluteus maximus and why the 30° tilt may be considered successful.

Nurses have used the 30° tilt for many years without a rationale. The use of this position was probably to offer comfort to some patients; other patients were traditionally placed onto their sides and onto a bony prominence, and, as pressure ulcers are prone to form between bone and the hard support surface, this increased the risk of tissue damage.

The 30° tilt would be recommended as it reduces risk of back injury for the nurses, offers painless repositioning for the patient who would also have180° view around the room (turning side to side greatly limits the patient's view). They can also be left in the new position 3–5 times longer than if placed onto a bony prominence. There is an added advantage that repositioning is quickly and simply achieved.

A hospital in Cape Town, South Africa, successfully uses the 30° tilt position as the primary treatment for established grade 4 (EPUAP) pressure ulcers and this has proven to be a very effective method in a country that is unable to obtain dynamic systems.

When repositioning is unavoidable (when equipment is unavailable or when the provided equipment allows erythema to occur), the 30° tilt is an excellent alternative method to use. This makes four-hourly turning appropriate in patients who are not on an appropriate mattress. Extended periods of eight hours or more are possible for some, allowing a complete night's sleep. As sleep favours anabolic processes, wound healing will be facilitated (Preston 1988). Physical repositioning of patients will soon become outlawed because of the damage that can be caused to nurses' backs and patient's tissues. A 30° tilt allows the patient to be repositioned safely and use of appropriate mattresses reduces the risk of pressure ulcers. Leaving patients in this position, undisturbed, for longer periods does not mean that they receive less time and attention for their needs (Preston 1988) and in fact, the contrary is true.

The 30° tilt method

For this manoeuvre, two extra pillows are required:

- As with all procedures, the patient should be informed.
- Two nurses are required (A and B) one on each side of the bed.
- Raise the bed to waist level.
- Ask the patient to turn their head in the direction they will be turned. Ask them to cross their arms across the chest.
- Nurse A will have two pillows prepared.
- Nurse A will untuck the long bottom sheet and pass the edge over the patient to nurse B.
- Nurse B folds or rolls the edge of the sheet to form a hand-hold. The rolled edge of the sheet will be halfway across the patient.
- Nurse B grips the sheet in line with the patient's shoulder and hip.
- With arms straight, nurse B rocks back onto one foot, using the body weight to roll the patient. The patient will be at an angle of approximately 40° and will be comfortably cocooned in the sheet. Nurse B will be in a non-stressful position.
- Nurse A places a pillow from the patient's shoulder (with the pillow end under the top pillows) to waist.
- The patient is relaxed back onto the pillow and the sheet is arranged over the top.
- The patient is now at an angle of 30° and the head pillows can be arranged for comfort.
- Nurse A will lift the leg on to a second pillow which is placed lengthways. The long edge of the pillow should be between the patient's legs to ensure that knees and ankles do not connect and cause pressure.
- A third pillow, placed lengthways, can be used to support the other leg if required.

Physical assessment

The weight of the patient is an important factor, particularly in underweight and obese patients. The underweight patient will not have enough fatty padding to protect the tissues form being pinched between the bone and the bed/chair surface. Conversely, the over-weight patient's weight will cause higher pressures between the bone and the hard surface, thereby increasing the risk of pressure ulcer formation.

Selection of appropriate mattresses can be achieved through the use of physical assessment.

As previously mentioned, non-blanching erythema is an area of redness that is usually over a bony prominence. The redness is caused by occlusion of the capillaries. When the pressure is relieved, through removing the pressure, the occluded area overcompensates and flushes red. This redness can be identified, as the tissue is viable and will turn white under a finger pressure. If this redness is identified, at any time, then the patient is on an inappropriate mattress and must be given a higher grade mattress. Redness that does not turn white under finger pressure indicates tissue damage and there will be inflammatory changes with a collection of micro-thrombi and bacteria, deep within the tissue and close to the bone. Removing this patient to a higher grade mattress is an emergency as two-hourly turns will not prevent the formation of an ulcer on the mattress that has allowed the tissue to become occluded.

John Bull (1930) recommended rubbing pressure areas with a little cotton wool soaked in some stimulant of skin such as eau-de-cologne or methylated spirit. This method became, for many years, the favoured prevention of pressure ulcers. However, an important study completed by Dyson (1978) compared two groups of patients; those who received massage of pressure areas as part of their preventative treatment and those who did not. Post-mortem examinations showed a marked difference between the two groups with the non-massaged group having a lower incidence of pressure ulcers and the massaged group showing macerated and degenerated tissues.

Anecdotally, nurses can still be heard to say 'we never had pressure ulcers when we used to rub the patients with spirit'. However, the development of pressure ulcers today cannot be compared with that of yesterday. An increase in the elderly population has resulted in an increase in disease, which requires increased nursing care, and an increase in knowledge brings an expansion in technology and increase in treatment requiring a further increase of nursing care. There is also the potential for the extended role of the nurse to take more time with technological tasks and previously held doctors' roles. There are also fewer nurses in ratio to patients and the reduction of staff on the wards can lead to one or two qualified nurses being responsible for often as many as 45 patients.

During the 1980s, patients would be given a place on a ward quite quickly. Today, it is not uncommon for patients to be found in corridors on hard trolleys several hours after admission. Also, in the 1980s, patients would remain on a ward until they had recovered from their illness or operation. This gave a fair balance of patients who were acutely ill and those who were recovering. Today, these patients are returned home very quickly and this can leave a ward full of acutely ill patients. Therefore, the balance no longer exists and fewer nurses are expected to take responsibility of all of the physical, technological and psychological needs of each acutely ill patient as well as the responsibility of physical repositioning.

Patients with established pressure ulcers should be nursed in bed as much as possible, providing they have been assessed for an appropriate piece of equipment, preferably a high grade air mattress. This is particularly important because adequate pressure relief is more difficult to achieve in a chair than in bed (Bliss 1993). One reason that is often anecdotally given for insisting that a patient is placed in a chair is the risk of deep vein thrombosis. However, the pressure of the chair on the back of the leg and the fact that the legs are dependent increases the difficulty for blood returning to the heart and this can increase the risk of thrombosis when the patient is sitting out. Deep vein thrombosis is a medical problem and must be addressed through the prescription of anti-embolic stockings and appropriate anticoagulant therapy. However, prior to the application of anti-embolic stockings, it is important to establish whether there is arterial disease and this can only be achieved through Doppler assessment. If anti-embolic stockings are fitted to a patient with arterial disease, there would be a potential for heel or foot necrosis.

Providing an appropriate mattress for each patient need not be expensive and, if pressure ulcer incidence is properly audited, can be both cost-effective and efficient.

Selecting appropriate mattresses

Pressure redistribution on static mattresses occurs through the foam distributing around the bony prominence, thereby, spreading the load or weight. An analogy would be the diver who is deep under the sea. The pressure from the surrounding waters at 90 feet will be intense, possibly as high as 2050 mmHg, far higher than any mattress can produce. However, he does not develop pressure ulcers because pressure is evenly (or uniformly) distributed over the body. This redistribution of pressure is the aim of placing a patient on a soft foam mattress which can mimic the action of the diver's water and the foam will 'flow' around the hard prominence. If pressure is redistributed over the wide area of the body, the patient is less likely to develop ulcers (Hussian 1953).

For many years nurses were led to believe that only high grade mattresses could prevent or treat ulcers but tissue viability nurses have since had years of experience showing this to be untrue. If the mattress is an appropriate selection for the individual patient, the patient's tissues will remain (or become) viable.

An easy way to distinguish the types of mattresses is to place them in seven grades:

Grade A   NHS mattresses and fibre-filled overlays
Grade B   Pressure-redistributing foam overlays
Grade C   Pressure-redistributing foam mattresses and gel-filled mattresses
Grade D   Static air overlays
Grade E   Dynamic air overlays
Grade F   Dynamic air mattress replacement or low-air loss mattress replacement
Grade G   Air-fluidized beds

Grade A

The NHS mattress is a solid block of low-grade foam, which is deliberately made larger than the cover to prevent 'wrinkling' in the material (thought to cause 'hot spots' of pressure). Therefore, the cover stretches tightly over the block of foam creating a hard surface for the patient to lay on (Santy 1995). The cover is not vapour permeable and, therefore, the patient will perspire, creating a potential for damp tissues (Young 1992) over bony prominences with the potential for reducing tissue viability. The cover will slowly 'give' in the area where the patient sits and a brown stain often appears with a 'dip' in the mattress. The brown stain indicates that the cover is allowing bodily fluids through to the sponge and removal of the cover would show a brown stain in the foam and, probably, a strong malodour. The 'dip' in the mattress can be pressed with a closed fist and it is possible that the fist will come into contact with the solid bed base. In this case, the patient will be at very high risk of a pressure ulcer as they will be sitting on the solid bed base, not the foam. This was confirmed by the work undertaken for the Medical Devices Directorate (1993) when the NHS mattress showed indentation in the foam with the 130 mm mattress being withdrawn from the evaluation on week 17 as a result of marked indentation. Santy (1998) found that NHS mattresses often had to be condemned after 6–12 months use. However, visco-elastic foam will never perform well under a fist test due to the softness of the foam and the method of its action. The warmth of the patient's body creates a 'well' in visco-elastic foam. This redistributes the weight, removing pressure from bony prominences (see section on grade C mattresses). There are two methods of testing visco-elastic foam. The subjective method is to press the fist into several areas along the sides of the foam to obtain a 'reference'. Then when the fist is pressed on the area where the patient sits, any bottoming out will be evident. However, the objective method is to use a special tool that may be provided by some of the companies. This accurately assesses the depth to which the foam can sink.

The standard hospital mattress produces areas of high pressure, potentially as high as 150 mmHg (Lindon et al. 1961) reducing still further the blood supply to potentially ischaemic tissues. The Medical Devices Directorate (1993) evaluated the NHS mattress and found: 'At best it is uncomfortable, and at worst it is potentially dangerous' and, due to the high interface pressures, they were unable to place the mattress on a ward for evaluation.

Flame retardation has reduced life expectancy of the mattress to a matter of months but, despite this, many hospitals go on using such mattresses for years (Burton 1995). The problem of NHS mattress purchase is compounded by their low cost – potentially as low as £25–30 each. Purchasers may argue that not every patient requires a pressure-redistributing mattress and this is true. However, within hospitals, the problem remains and speed of admission leads to the inevitability of patients who are at risk of being placed on an NHS mattress (unless all beds in the hospital are covered with appropriate pressure-redistributing foam mattresses). It is therefore, important to provide excellent pressure-redistributing base mattresses as a first line of defence in pressure ulcer prevention.

Fibre overlays are excellent when new and will give good pressure relief. However, with washing and through compression from use, the fibres begin to clump together making the fibre overlay reliable for six months (Medical Devices Agency 1994) when it should then be replaced. The fibre overlay is more appropriate for comfort only and will require the patient to be repositioned (potentially) more often than two hourly.

Grade B

The foam overlay is commonly referred to as 'the chocolate box' or 'egg box' overlay because of the foam cut into squares or blocks across the overlay surface. These overlays are made by several companies and provide good pressure redistribution. The cut foam 'squeezes' down over bony prominences, providing pressure redistribution. These provide an alternative to purchasing foam mattress replacements although this method of purchase can sometimes be as expensive as a full mattress, particularly when covered with vapour permeable material.

Grade C

Pressure-redistributing foam mattresses are the fastest selling pressure-relieving resource. This is due to tissue viability specialists and companies' realization that provision of an excellent base mattress can reduce the need for expensive air mattresses. However, there have been concerns about the mattress covers with some covers delaminating, permitting fluids to pass through and contaminate the foam. This is thought to be related to the use of strong fluids for cleaning, although this has never been proven. The problem appears (at present) only to effect UK produced covers and there are several mattress companies that claim to have covers now that will last. Six-monthly audit of mattresses is important if this breakdown is to be identified and any cross-infection risk eliminated.

The covers of most of these new pressure-redistributing foam mattresses are vapour permeable; this reduces the potential of the patient perspiring. The covers are also two-way, or multistretch to allow the bony prominence to sink into the foam, thereby redistributing the pressure. The foam is designed to redistribute the pressure (often with chocolate box/egg box cut foam squares as a part of the design). These mattresses should be placed onto a mesh-based bed (not solid) and care must be taken to clean the covers with soap and water only. Each mattress must be turned at least monthly according to manufacturer's instructions as not complying with this demand negates any claim on the guarantee. Without care, the covers may continue to delaminate and allow fluids to enter.

Visco-elastic polymer foam is becoming a popular alternative to the soft foam mattresses. Visco-elastic has little memory so that when it is pressed, the foam maintains a 'well' and does not try to push back against the bony prominence as normal foam would. The foam reacts to heat and the hardness of the mattress on initial contact gives way to soft conformability through the heat of the patient's body.

The mattress is comfortable and excellent for pressure relief as it redistributes the body weight throughout the mattress. However, because there is little memory, people with rheumatoid arthritis may find difficulty with sitting up in bed as they cannot get lever for their hands and they sink into the mattress. Also, patients who have difficulty moving may find it a little difficult to turn in bed as the mattress forms a 'well', which can appear mountainous as they attempt to turn over. One company produces Pressurease mattresses which contains a visco-elastic gel that has a faster response time.

A study completed in Eastbourne (Hampton 1999) demonstrates that visco-elastic mattresses can provide for high-risk patients (often >25 Waterlow score) without developing pressure ulcers. However, assessment would be individual for each patient, and any patient developing a sustained redness on any mattress should lead to an upgrade of mattress type.

Visco-elastic cushions may have a tendency to compress when patients are sitting for long periods, although this remains anecdotal at present. Prior to purchase it would be wise to enquire whether evaluations have been completed using both pressure mapping and clinical studies.

The authors (Hampton and Collins) undertook a project on visco-elastic mattresses. They used a nursing home with a prevalence of 53 per cent pressure ulcers of grade 1 and 2. The mattresses within the nursing home were a variety of types but the largest amount comprised NHS standard (pink marble cover) mattresses. A baseline audit was completed and every resident with a pressure ulcer was photographed. New visco-elastic mattresses (Pressurease) were placed on every bed and each resident was provided with a visco-elastic cushion. A data collector (untrained in tissue viability) went weekly to photograph the ulcers. No education that may have effected the outcome was provided to the nursing home. The aim of the work was to demonstrate a reduction in pressure ulcers over a two-year period and to assess the durability of the mattress over a three-year period. The residents with pressure ulcers actually improved within two weeks and at the end of a three-week period, all pressure ulcers had resolved. This was a remarkable and unexpected result.

A new type of mattress, produced in America, is now on the UK market – the 'De-cube' mattress. This mattress is ideal for nursing homes as pressure can be relieved over bony prominences at very low cost. There are cubes throughout the foam that can be removed to provide pressure relief without causing loading around the hole produced by removal of the cube. The mattress is guaranteed for 15 years and is slightly more expensive than most other mattresses but can offer excellent pressure relief. The cover is not made of the commonly used vapour permeable type material and is guaranteed for 10 years against normal wear. Hofman et al. (1994) undertook a randomized controlled trial with 44 patients, admitted with grade 2 pressure ulcers, randomized to either a standard NHS mattress or a De-cube mattress. At 14 days, 68 per cent on the NHS mattress were found to have grade 2 ulcers compared with 24 per cent on the De-cube mattress. The difference between the two mattresses, and the effect on pressure ulcer development, were so significant that the trial was discontinued. However, all patients are at risk on the NHS standard mattress and it would have been more useful to compare the De-cube with air mattresses or pressure-redistributing foam mattresses rather than a NHS mattress.

Grade D

The Repose mattress is inexpensive, for single patient use only and is sold with a cushion at approximately £150 for the two. Bale et al. (1998) completed a randomized controlled trial comparing the static Repose mattress with a Nimbus 2 and found no difference in the number of patients developing pressure ulcers on either system. Either system can be highly recommended for pressure relief. However, the Repose is disposable and will possibly need replacing within six months to one year. This would still be a cost-effective and clinically effective method of pressure ulcer prevention. The Repose mattress provides an inexpensive mattress for discharge of patients.

The Vicair mattress is an unusual and unique design. The centre of the mattress is filled with small tea-bag shaped, air-filled sacks which are covered in a silicone covered material. The silicone allows the units to slide together so that when the patient moves (or is moved) the units readjust to the new position.

The Carebed, a static air-overlay, is easy to use, inexpensive and clinically effective. It can be a cost-effective solution to the prevention of pressure ulcers in high-risk patients. The manufacturers claim that pressure ulcers can even be healed when patients are nursed on these mattresses.

Grade E

Dynamic air overlays are generally two-cell cycle with alternating cells inflating and deflating over a 10-minute period. This means that pressure is relieved for the 10-minute periods and then reapplied for no longer than 10 minutes. There are different designs of air overlays, some with alternating cells and some with the appearance of 'bubble' cells. These mattresses are generally excellent for pressure ulcer prevention, even in high-risk patients, and can also assist with healing established pressure ulcers. Patients would require assessment whenever they are repositioned for toileting or food, etc. Any blanching hyperaemia requires the patient to be placed on a higher grade mattress. They are highly recommended and most companies will provide mattresses that are equal in pressure relief. The choice of mattress should rely on excellence of service and reliability of machinery.

A new type of dynamic overlay now available is the disposable mattress. A compressor is purchased and then mattresses can be purchased and disposed of as required. This will offer a cost-effective way of reducing cross-infection.

Grade F

Dynamic air mattress replacement systems and low-air loss (LAL) mattresses are the 'cream' of air mattresses – although all systems are thought to support healing of established ulcers. Most dynamic systems have a three-cell cycle where the cells are in sets of three with each third cell inflating for 6–10 minutes giving a cycle with a wave effect that constantly flows from feet to head. This means that the patient's tissues have pressure for no longer than 6–10 minutes at any time. Some systems provide a static section for the head, mainly to prevent the feeling of 'sea sickness' that may be experienced by some patients. This static section often allows for a bed headrest to lay on the top of the static section. If the top three cells were alternating, the headrest would gradually slip backwards and would offer discomfort for the patient. The headrest can be left open under the air mattress; however, this will mimic a 'slide' effect and the patient may slip down the bed.

A new type of mattress (Airform) provides a mixture of dynamic air cells and visco-elastic foam. The foam 'dampens' the movement of the cells but continues to provide a reduced potential for pressure ulceration.

Low-air loss mattresses can be described as a large bag of air, which successfully redistributes pressure over the body. The LAL system has warmed air, which escapes through minute holes in the system and can warm and comfort the patient. It has certain advantages over the dynamic systems, such as providing lower interface pressure because the method of pressure reduction relies on pressure redistribution rather than pressure relief. There may be increased comfort because the patient 'sinks' into the 'bag of air'. The mattress can be programmed to judge the patient's weight and readjust the air support to give the optimum pressure redistribution.

The disadvantages of the dynamic systems are the hardness of some cells (not Airform) and that the movement of the cells may be disorientating for the patient. Indeed, some patients may have difficulty repositioning independently or they may find mobilization from the bed difficult because of the softness of the mattress. On the other hand, an advantage may be the initiation of reactive hyperaemia in patients with established pressure ulcers as this may aid healing. Certainly, the firm support and ridges would aid movement, allowing the patient some independence of repositioning.

Grade G

Air-fluidized beds. These beds are expensive (hired at £68–85 per day plus VAT at the time of writing) and are really for critically ill patients in ITU, burns units or with highly exuding wounds. Healing of pressure ulcers is generally excellent on these beds and they offer comfort to the immobile patients. However, these are unsuitable for patients wishing to mobilize as lifting from the bed must be by hoist. Air-fluidized beds use a solution of warm air and glass beads (or microspheres) to provide support to enhance wound healing (Lockyer-Stevens 1994). The beads are 80 microns in diameter through which air is blown (Ryan 1990) and the result of the air, passing through the beads, is a 'fluid' appearance and sensation.

There is a concern about the safety of air-fluidized beds because of reports of contamination (Ryan 1990) particularly as the bed is non-autoclavable. Ryan identified four potential problems; transmission of infection by airflow, cross-infection by the filter sheet, retention of organisms on the microshpheres and the possibility of a reservoir of organisms in the clumps found on the diffuser board at the bottom of the bed.

These beds are very heavy and difficult to manoeuvre around wards, and normal household floors are less likely to be able to support such a heavy object. Therefore, these beds are not generally recommended for nursing homes or home use.

Selecting the appropriate equipment

Pressure 'relief' is a term wrongly used to describe most equipment used in pressure ulcer prevention; pressure 'relief' can only truly be achieved by complete suspension in the air. Some air mattresses do offer temporary periods of relief from pressure, but other types of equipment generally give pressure redistribution, not pressure relief. Understanding the two types of mattresses and how they effect the formation of pressure ulcers will lead the practitioner into confident selection of appropriate mattresses for prevention. This experience, combined with clinical evidence of efficacy, will greatly reduce incidence and prevalence of pressure ulcers. There are few randomized trials completed in the use of air mattresses (Young 1992) and clinical evidence is still sparse. Each manufacturer will claim their mattress is the very best and will prevent pressure ulcers, and they are possibly correct in their claims. However, there is little work completed comparing dynamic air mattresses with dynamic, or static, air overlays. A small amount of work is completed on the Repose static air overlay compared with a dynamic system and this found that prevention was equal to that of a Nimbus 2.

It is possible that the future for pressure ulcer prevention will be very different to the methods of today. Overlays, such as the Repose (£150), can be very inexpensive compared with the £2000–5000 cost of a dynamic system.

Foam mattresses must be at least 12.5 cm thick with a middle surface that conforms to the patient's weight. The sides of the mattress should be firm enough to support a patient when mobilizing as a too soft foam will be unstable when the patient is trying to stand. The mattress must also have covers that will withstand normal wear and tear experienced on a busy ward; without excellence in cover protection the mattresses will quickly become worn, allowing the entry of bacteria into the foam. Ndwadula and Brown (1990) report an outbreak of MRSA with 82 mothers and 28 babies infected or colonized. The outbreak only ended when all mattresses were incinerated.

To test for a dangerously worn mattress cover:

1 Place an absorbent tissue between the cover and the mattress foam. Hand towels are ideal.
2 Pour water onto the mattress cover.
3 Press the fist into the water and rub the surface of the mattress cover.
4 Remove the absorbent tissue.

Any dampness of the tissue shows that the mattress is allowing fluid through to the foam. However, the inability of the cover to hold fluid should be evident from the state of the foam when the cover is unzipped as the foam will be evidently contaminated. Alternatively, inspect the foam inside the mattress. If any staining is apparent, hold a torchlight to the area where fluid is likely to have entered and any pinholes will be clearly seen through the material.

Many of the decisions for equipment selection relies on anecdotal tales, representatives' persuasiveness, advertising, the availability of the product and individual nurses' personal likes or dislikes. Lockyer-Stevens (1994) believed decisions could be largely cost driven with supplies and finance departments influencing final decisions.

Decisions for purchase are formed on clinical evidence such as cinical evaluations prior to purchase and ease of maintenance. Purchase could also follow discussions with physiotherapists, occupational therapists, infection control nurses, resuscitation officers and the experience of the purchaser.

Cost is the least important part of the decision, but is, nevertheless, a vital part of the overall picture. If a £100 mattress will prevent pressure ulcers as effectively as a £3000 mattress, then this should be considered. The cheaper mattress may require replacing within a few months and this will have a long-term cost implication. However, the more expensive mattress has a maintenance requirement that can cost up to £400 per year and may require periodic cleaning at a cost of £70 each time. It may be cheaper, long-term, to continually replace a cheaper mattress each time a patient is discharged.

Alternatively, on busy wards, nurses might not have the time to pump up an air overlay for each patient at risk, and the wrongly inflated mattress could lead to development of ulcers. Nevertheless, purchase of cheaper equipment means that more equipment can be purchased. This is an altruistic view with the 'needs of the many' the consideration, with a higher number of patients benefiting from purchase of cheaper mattresses; conversely, less people will benefit if one expensive mattress is bought.

The decision to place a patient on a mattress must stay with the primary or responsible nurse and that decision must be based on clinical and physical evidence. The clinical efficacy that is found in some of the small studies completed by a few manufacturers is best collected and collated by a tissue viability specialist nurse. The recommendations may be placed in the form of an algorithm or chart and may be made available for all staff to follow as required (see Figure 9.2, p. 266). Selection is then a mixture of clinical judgement, expert advice and clinical evidence.

It is important to include reassessment as part of any pressure ulcer prevention policy. Without reassessment, it is possible that a patient can remain on a high-grade mattress long after their need for it has been eliminated. This deprives other, more needy, patients and increases the potential for high incidence of pressure ulcers.

Mattress replacement policies

A recognized and properly conducted mattress replacement programme is a vital part of a pressure ulcer prevention policy. Flanagan (1991) cited DHSS Management of Equipment (1982):

If replacement policies are not implemented, standards of reliability will fall, leading to a gradual deterioration in equipment performance and safety. It is good practice to identify such equipment in good time so that appropriate financial arrangements can be made for the purchase of its replacement.

Identification of faulty mattresses is simply accomplished. The general foam mattresses are often given the 'fist' test (described earlier) and air-beds can be checked six-monthly by electrical engineers. The fist test is not an accurate method of assessing foam, particularly in the case of visco-elastic foam as this is a softer foam with a unique action and will not perform well under the 'fist test'.

Foam mattresses should be turned according to the manufacturers' instructions. If the mattresses are not turned according to recommendations then a guarantee becomes worthless. The situation would be the same if cleaning instructions are not adhered to, with chemicals used when only soap and water is recommended. Mattresses should only be cleaned when soiled or following contamination from an infected patient (Flanagan 1991).

Mattresses are a hidden problem and one that is often seen only by housekeeping staff and, without being informed otherwise, they cannot be expected to understand the implications of a worn mattress. Mattress care must be taken very seriously and regular audits (3–6 monthly) undertaken to evaluate the chosen mattresses for wear and efficacy.

Six-monthly audits were made of mattresses and pressure ulcer prevalence. This reviewed the size of the pressure ulcer problem, identified the rate that mattresses were deteriorating and whether the patient was nursed on an appropriate mattress for the Waterlow score and this shaped and developed future audits through change as problems were identified. It was decided not to 'put all the eggs in one basket' and all types of mattresses were purchased from different companies over a four-year period. This allowed decisions to be made for the future as each mattress was included in the audit every six months and problems with individual mattresses could be identified and addressed at an early date. It also began to shape decisions for the future as some mattresses performed better than others. During this time, pressure ulcers reduced from 10.8 per cent to 2.4 per cent, demonstrating the importance of assessment.

Prevalence and incidence of pressure ulcers

Point prevalence is the total number of patients (population) with established pressure ulcers at a particular time with measurements usually taken on one day. The simplest method of point prevalence is to take midnight on one day to midnight on the next. Any patient present (not admitted or discharged on that day) is included in the numbers and each patient is examined for pressure damage. The final figures will give the total population number and the total population with established pressure ulcers. This can give a very accurate picture of pressure ulcer prevalence and can be used to audit standards of pressure area care, identifying risk scores and correlating this with the type of mattress supplied to 'at risk' patients.

Prevalence measurement is likely to be higher than incidence measurement as incidence only accounts for new ulcers developing whereas prevalence includes every ulcer. The final percentage figure will also vary from trust to trust as there is not a standardized way of monitoring pressure ulcer grading systems. One trust may use EPUAP grading and include blanching hyperaemia in the prevalence, and another trust may only include a break in the skin and above (EPUAP grade 2). This will greatly effect the overall figures with one trust having high prevalence and the other trust showing a low prevalence. Anecdotally, there are some trusts that will only use grade 3 as a pressure ulcer and act on this stage. This is a reactive process rather than a proactive one. The patient will only receive the correct mattress when an ulcer develops instead of preventing the ulcer completely.

Incidence is the rate at which new ulcers develop and the measurement is taken constantly (usually either daily or weekly). The final figures for incidence will be lower than prevalence and cannot be compared. There are difficulties with data collection for incidence as it relies on the reporting honesty of the nurses involved and also takes time. On a busy ward, the reporting could easily be missed (Hampton 1997d). Bridel (1993a) recognized that difficulties with reliability and validity measures meant that reported rates require careful interpretation. David et al. (1983) found under-reporting in pressure ulcers and this is probably related to a belief that pressure ulcers are a result of 'bad nursing'. With prevalence, an independent assessor physically examines every patient on one day; therefore prevalence audit achieves higher accuracy. However, as prevalence is generally taken every 3–6 months, it can miss many important pressure ulcers during that time.

Equipment availability

The importance of provision of pressure-relieving or reducing equipment combined with education must never be underestimated. However, an increase in education and increase in availability of resources will inevitably lead to an increase in demand. This, in turn, leads to higher usage of equipment and lower availability. Air mattresses can be part of a 'black hole' with an increasing range of resources and a reducing amount of money available. Providing greater supplies of air mattresses does not relieve the situation as nurses become increasingly educated in pressure ulcer prevention and demand increasing amounts of mattresses. Raised expectations of receiving requested equipment raises the demand for mattresses and this can be compounded by the use of a risk assessment score that over-predicted requirements. This means that the demand will always exceeded supply. The only answer to the problem is to increase education in assessment with recommendations that nurses use physical assessment as an accurate indication of requirements and risk assessment scores to support their physical findings. There is always a risk that assessment scores either do not give an accurate picture of individual patient requirements or may over-prescribe, thereby using up vital resource. Another scenario would be the patient who is placed on an air mattress when the risk is high during acute illness, but is never reassessed for a lower grade mattress. This will also use up vital resources both in hospital and in community.

One trust decided to set up a scheme where nurses could hire mattresses from a pre-selected list. They would telephone the (selected) company for a mattress each time that a patient was considered at risk. This had a very large financial implication for the trust for two reasons:

1 The company had marketed their product extremely well, and the nurses felt neglectful if their patient was not supplied with a mattress, even when the patient was recovering or at a risk level that would not produce a pressure ulcer when nursed on a pressure-redistributing foam mattress.

2 The ease of availability meant that mattresses were hired whilst the trust's own purchased equipment remained in the store.

An excellent way of funding and providing equipment is through an equipment loan store. This can easily be set up in hospitals or community and leads to accurate provision of suitable equipment and excellent maintenance of the beds and mattresses. An equipment store co-ordinator can also control cleaning of mattresses after each use.

Setting up an equipment loan store can be achieved in several ways as the store can be for mattresses only or for all equipment; stock control can be through infrared bars and the co-ordinator of the equipment can be a qualified nurse with full knowledge of tissue viability who acts as a support to a tissue viability specialist nurse. Alternatively, the co-ordinator could be unqualified and could act under the direct control of a tissue viability specialist nurse. The stock could be controlled through a 'virtual reality' stock room (controlled by computer) but held on wards and collected as required by the co-ordinator. The stock could be held in a main store where it can be checked for maintenance and cleaning requirements before being reissued and this ensures some control over infection control issues.

A second system is total bed management. One company that is selected by the individual hospital supports this system or community trust. The chosen company would be contracted to supply all the mattress and electric bed requirements. This would involve repair, cleaning and replacing. This may initially appear an expensive alternative. However, the cost of mattress repairs, the reduction of mattress use whilst the repairs are carried out, cost of cleaning mattresses and replacement mattresses are hidden costs and total bed management negates much of these hidden costs. It also allows a trust to replace all mattresses and necessary beds at an affordable rate.

Whichever type of control is used, each system offers large cost savings to a trust by reducing expensive individual hiring requirements through efficient use of equipment and is to be recommended as part of any development in pressure ulcer prevention policies.

The selection of equipment may be based on a two-type system such as a clinically effective static pressure-redistributing mattress and a dynamic air mattress. The recommendation would be that every patient without a pressure ulcer would be placed on a static

A personal view

Work completed by the tissue viability nurse in Eastbourne hospital (Hampton) provided information on air mattress provision and healing of pressure ulcers. During a three-year period, every patient who entered the local general hospital with a grade 3 or 4 (EPUAP 2001) pressure ulcer, was provided with a dynamic mattress replacement system. Mattresses were supplied to 100 patients and remained with the patient until the patient died or the ulcer healed. The hospital photographer and the tissue viability nurse visited the patients weekly to measure and to photograph the progress of the wounds. The recommendations to carers were to place the patient with the wound against the mattress to promote reactive hyperaemia within the wound. As air mattresses have alternate cells that inflate and deflate, this gives pressure relief under the deflated cell, thereby ensuring that the wound is free of pressure for a large percentage of the day. Of the 100 patients assessed in this way; six died and 94 healed; of the six patients who died, only one wound deteriorated in condition prior to death. This led the author to recommend, within her own trust, that patients with pressure ulcers should be nursed on a high grade air mattress with the ulcer to the mattress when possible.

A further recommendation was that patients should be moved regularly for comfort, toileting and treatment but not for pressure ulcer prevention. A report completed by NHS Executive in November 1999 (Hibbs 1999) highlighted tissue viability as an area of excellence in Eastbourne, indicating that the tissue viability nurse had correctly identified pressure ulcer prevention techniques.

Although this work was an important part of development of a policy, the authors' personal view is that many less expensive pressure-redistributing mattresses will offer a reduction in the formation of pressure ulcers. Nevertheless, it is also the authors' personal opinion that patients with an established pressure ulcer, must be nursed on a higher grade mattress such as a dynamic air mattress. This leads to a positive argument for providing the appropriate equipment prior to the development of any tissue damage.

system. Pressure areas of high-risk patients would be examined very 2–4 hours. Those patients forming a reddened area (blanching hyperaemia) would be placed on an air mattress immediately. Those being admitted with an established pressure ulcer would be placed directly onto an air mattress. Patients with high Waterlow risk scores, will not develop pressure ulcers on basic mattresses providing assessment is carried out and appropriate action taken as required. This method has the potential to reduce pressure ulcer formation and to greatly reduce cost.

Inadvised methods of pressure ulcer prevention

* *Rubbing pressure areas*: Dyson (1978) divided a ward of elderly, long-stay patients into two groups. The control group received normal treatment involving vigorous massage over bony prominences which, at the time, was thought to stimulate the blood supply. The experimental group were not given massage. The study was for a six-month period involving 200 patients. On death, the tissues were examined for signs of pressure damage and there was a 38 per cent reduction in pressure ulcers for the non-rubbed group compared with the control group. This was thought to be due to the fact that vigorous massage encouraged blood flow on the surface tissues. As the greatest damage will occur next to the bone, the greater blood supply is required in that area – not on the surface.
* *Turning side to side on bony prominences for pressure relief*: Pressure ulcers nearly always form on bony prominences and turning side to side placed the patient onto the prominence. This increases the risk of pressure ulcer development.
* *Placing 'at risk' patients on NHS standard mattresses*: Although this was not necessarily thought to be a method of prevention, the actual damage caused by these mattresses was not appreciated at the time. It is now considered poor practice to place an at-risk patient on one of these mattresses and it is now to be totally avoided.
* *Use of water- or air-filled latex gloves*: There is a popular practice of filling latex gloves with water and placing them under heels in an attempt to prevent pressure ulcers from developing (Williams 1993). This practice is dangerous and will actually increase the risk to the patient by increasing interface pressure by an average of 12.5 per cent and the practice should be discouraged (Williams 1993).

- *Sitting patients out of bed as a method of pressure ulcer reduction*: It is now known that a large number of pressure ulcers are caused through sitting in the chair. This increased risk does not justify sitting patients out for hours on end and this practice must stop. If the patient is to sit out, they must be given an appropriate size chair (see Chapter 10) with a suitable cushion and should not sit out for more than two or three hours at a time.
- *Use of sheepskins in pressure ulcer prevention*: Marchant et al. (1990) identified genuine sheepskins as, at best, of some use for low-risk patients and, at worst actually contributing to pressure ulcer development. Nevertheless, there is a new move to the use of these genuine sheepskins as they prevent friction and shearing and urine passes through the oily wool, keeping the tissue dry. This is, however, an unproven theory.

Pressure ulcers in intensive therapy units

Patients in intensive therapy units (ITU) are particularly at risk of developing pressure ulcers due to periods of immobility on a road following an accident, several hours on a theatre table prior to admission to ITU and possible instability of condition which prevents repositioning.

There is also a risk that a pressure ulcer may be established on the main wards prior to ITU admission.

Other reasons for the increased risk could be low blood pressure, drug therapy or use of inotropes, poor perfusion, sedation and muscle relaxants, which prevent natural movement of the patient and physiological effects of shock and stress. Pre-operative fasting could also contribute to the increased risk. Torrance (1981) found that half-an-hour anoxia caused by shock, surgery or a result of anaesthesia, could be enough to cause irreversible tissue changes within the tissues.

Tubing used in ITU for respiration purposes may also cause pressure ulcers due to the potential for tubing pressure on the mouth or face. Prevention of this pressure could form part of an ITU assessment.

Treatment of established ulcers

The nurse can place any modern dressing onto a pressure ulcer but unless pressure is removed the wound will never improve. The old adage is 'the nurse can put anything on a pressure ulcer EXCEPT THE PATIENT!' (Convatec 1993).

Treating the wound is simple, as the prime consideration must be to provide appropriate equipment, to form a plan of care and to outline methods of prevention, with 30° tilt a priority for immobile patients. The patient must be reassessed within 2–4 hours and an assessment made for any blanching erythema. If any notable erythema is found, a further plan of care would be required and this requires the patient to have a higher grade mattress and or more frequent repositioning. The patient must also be observed for potential occurance of shearing forces. Patients who are sitting in the chair are potentially at a greater risk (see Chapter 10).

Any concern about the nutritional status of the patient requires a plan of care to increase nutritional intake. An assessment of the patient's weight, compared with ideal body weight is a useful method of assessing both nutritional status and risk as any deviation from the 'norm' increases risk. A thin patient will require a soft mattress to allow the bony prominences to 'sink' into the foam, thereby redistributing pressure. The overweight patient will require soft foam to allow the body weight to sink into the mattress, thereby redistributing the body weight within the foam.

The oxygen status of the patient is important and if hypoxia is suspected, it is vital to increase oxygen provision. Anaemia, chronic obstructive airways disease, poor tissue perfusion caused through heart disease will all contribute to hypoxia. Low oxygen combined with localized pressure is a recipe for disaster.

Transcutaneous oxygen ($TcpO_2$) monitoring records the product of an equation relating oxygen supplied to the soft tissues minus a combination of the amount of oxygen consumed by the tissues and any resistance to oxygen diffusion (Mani and White 1988). Clark (1994) identified that a decrease in $TcpO_2$ may result from either a decrease in supply of the amount oxygen or an increase in consumption of tissue oxygen. Clark also identifies that any $TcpO_2$ measurement relies on an excess of oxygen supply in the tissues and does not reflect the oxygen debt that would cause pressure ulcer formation. Therefore, measurement of $TcpO_2$ may not have value in pressure ulcer risk identification. However, Bliss (1993) reports that $TcpO_2$ has a value as the measurements have identified that subcutaneous tissue pressure is of greater importance to the formation of pressure ulcers than surface loading.

Administration of drugs may be a potential risk factor. Sedatives will reduce mobility during sleep, whilst chemotherapy will increase the risk to tissues as will steroid therapy. Inotropes reduce the delivery of blood to heels.

Safe repositioning techniques must be employed. Patients are safer if nursed on electric profiling beds where the knees can be raised prior to sitting the patient up through electrically profiling the top section of the bed. The knee raise will prevent the patient from slipping down the bed and will reduce potential for friction or shearing damage.

Perspiration caused by vinyl mattress covers and cushions or moist tissue caused through incontinence will also contribute to the formation of pressure ulcers. Therefore, if the patient is on NHS mattress they should be removed and placed on a higher grade mattress.

Debridement of necrotic tissue is the fastest way to initiate healing. However, unless the pressure is completely eliminated, the necrotic tissue will continue to form even after debridement.

The use of vacuum therapy in grade 3 to 4 (EPUAP 2001) pressure ulcers and has been found to be one of the most successful methods of treating the ulcers. Possibly because it creates a negative pressure which is opposed to the positive pressure that formed the ulcer.

Wound imaging

Guys Nuffield Hospital Tissue Viability Research Unit are in the process of developing a machine that will reflect tissue damage that occurs as deep as bone. When the machine is fully developed it can be produced as a hand-held device that nurses will be able to use to identify the risk of pressure ulcer development.

Conclusion

The importance of appropriate equipment cannot by emphasized highly enough. Nevertheless, holistic assessment leading to an increased nutritional status and improved mobilization, has the larger part to play in prevention. As shown by the South African hospital, pressure ulcers can be prevented and healed with simplistic methods and prevention does not necessarily equate with expensive equipment. Experience and knowledge will lead to improved services in prevention of pressure ulcers although managers of hospitals, community and nursing homes will need to support the nurses in offering high-quality care and this will require a commitment to education.

The obvious importance of education, audit and use of preventative measures also cannot be overemphasized. There is overwhelming evidence that pressure ulcers are largely avoidable and, therefore, refusal to provide equipment and education in order to reduce pressure ulcer formation is an unnecessary and expensive means of trying to save money. Each hospital and community trust MUST work toward a cost-effective policy of prevention.

Activities

1 Examine a dynamic, alternating air mattress and compare it with a dynamic overlay.

What are the differences?

2 Question a patient who is nursed on a dynamic air mattress.
   Is it comfortable?
   Is it easy to move over the surface?
   Does the action of the mattress cells create nausea?
   What do they like or dislike about the mattress?

Use the results of this mini audit to write a 250-word reflective essay about what you learned in this exercise and how that may change your practice.

CHAPTER 10

The relationship of seating to pressure ulcer prevention

Why is seating so important?

A disproportionately low quantity of published literature on pressure ulcer aetiology refers to seating as a major causative factor, despite pressure ulcer incidence being frequently attributed to this (Lowry 1989). Work undertaken by Dealey et al. (1991) and Collins (1999) has found that suitable pressure-relieving/reducing sitting surfaces are essential to maintenance of skin integrity in the at-risk patient, and that pressure ulcers can be reduced in this population by such provision. Barbenel et al. (1977) found that chair-bound patients had consistently more pressure ulcers than bed-bound patients of a similar age and disability.

Seating is a complex issue for the simple reason that it is impossible to position a person in one constant place for any significant period of time, due to both functional requirements, gravity and to the anatomy of the pelvis. Unlike lying, sitting is a dynamic not static behaviour (Mayall and Desharnais 1995), because we change our seated position in order to carry out a specific functional activity. For example, in order to work at a desk we must tilt our pelvis anteriorly, which allows our upper body to lean forwards. When we relax, we frequently tilt our pelvis posteriorly and rest our upper body against the back of the chair (Collins and Shipperley 1999). However, neither of these positions can be maintained for any length of time due to fatigue, the forces of gravity, and the shape of the pelvis as we are simply not designed to sit down! Many factors contrive to disrupt an optimum sitting position, and these include gravity, time, pressure, shear forces and friction. The downward forces of gravity place great strain on the seated person. If

311

they are unable to counteract these to any great extent (for example if they have poor trunk control), they will slump in the chair, especially if the person is required to sit for unrealistic periods of time. If the patient is unable to reposition himself, then these factors are increased (Krasilovsky 1993). Whilst abdominal and spinal muscles help to maintain an upright position in a seated position for short period, it will be difficult to counteract the gravitational force over any length of time. It has been widely documented that prolonged periods of time spent in one position may increase the risk of pressure ulcer development (Bridel 1993a; Gebhardt and Bliss 1994).

The position within a chair will directly affect the seated person's posture (Collins 1998a). If positioning in the chair is poor, it will disrupt optimum pressure distribution, and will increase shear forces and friction, which may predispose the person to develop pressure ulcers and fixed postural changes. Certainly if a person is allowed to adopt a poor position within the chair, the comfort will be reduced. The dimensions and design qualities of a chair will also influence the position adopted by a person. Provision of suitable seating will directly enhance the functional potential of a patient (Presperin 1992).

The pelvis

When providing seating equipment for a client, it is vital to consider the position of the pelvis before concentrating on any other aspect of the human body. This is because the pelvis is the major interface with the seat surface (Mayall and Desharnais 1995), and therefore any change in position of the pelvis will result in a change of overall posture. The pelvic bones form the intermediary between the spinal column and the lower extremities, and as such they play a crucial role in the load transfer mechanism from the trunk to the legs and vice versa (Dalstra 1997). The anatomy of the pelvis makes it difficult to remain seated in one position for any length of time. In healthy individuals this poses no great problem. In fact, it is an important feature of human function that the pelvis is able to move freely in order that a number of different activities can take place; indeed if the pelvis was not able to move our function would be severely inhibited. Posture will constantly change as movement occurs, and the efficiency of our posture can be perceived by the amount it loads the skeleton and the skeletal or postural muscles (Asatekin 1975). It is also important to consider that a person's sitting posture, spinal posture, pressure distribution, comfort, fatigue and energy expenditure are all interrelated (Zacharkow 1984).

The anatomy of the pelvis

The pelvic girdle (Figures 10.1 and 10.2) attaches the lower limbs to the axial skeleton, transmits the weight of the upper body to the lower limbs, and supports the visceral organs of the pelvis (Marieb 1998).

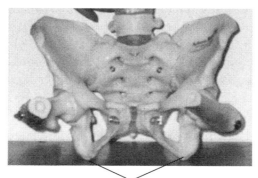

Ischial tuberosities
These take weight evenly in normal sitting

Figure 10.1 Anterior view of pelvis.

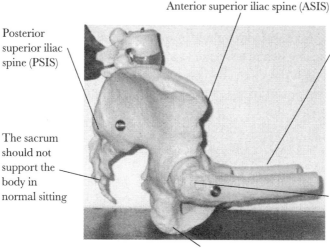

Anterior superior iliac spine (ASIS)

Posterior superior iliac spine (PSIS)

The femurs sit 4cm above the ischial tuberosities in normal sitting

The sacrum should not support the body in normal sitting

Pressure ulcers on the greater trochanter are often attributed to prolonged side lying, whereas in fact, many are due to poor sitting posture

The rounded ischial tuberosities act as 'rockers', making sitting an unstable activity

Figure 10.2 Lateral view of pelvis.

The pelvis is constructed from two irregular shaped coxae or innominate bones (Martini et al. 1999). These are joined together at the anterior aspect by a cartilaginous joint called the pubic symphysis. Posteriorly, the coxae attach on either side of the spinal column at the sacrum, forming the sacro-iliac joint. Consequently, any movement of the pelvic girdle will also affect the position of the spinal column. On the lateral aspect of the pelvic girdle the acetabulum of the hip joint can be located. At this point the femurs attach to the pelvic girdle, forming the hip joint, and this provides the main axis of rotation between the pelvis and the lower limbs. Again, it may therefore be assumed that any change of position of the pelvis will also affect the subsequent position of the lower limbs. The aspect of the pelvic girdle, which forms the main interface with the seat surface is the ischial tuberosity, one of which is located on the distal portion of each innominate bone.

The ischial tuberosities are the main culprits of poor sitting posture due to their shape and location. With respect to shape, they are rounded, which creates difficulty for any healthy individual to sit in one position for any length of time, as there is no flat surface on which to stabilize the rest of the upper body. Consequently, the body tends to rock forwards and backwards in an attempt to find stability. This poses no great problem for a healthy person, as their trunk muscles will enable them to deal with this perpetual movement, and allow them to reposition when necessary. However, a less healthy or able person will experience considerable difficulties in maintaining such an upright sitting position. The ischial tuberosities are also located approximately 3–4 cm lower than the thighs in a seated position, which necessitates them contacting with the seat surface before any other part of the lower limbs can get close. In a flat seat this causes major problems, as the thighs are prevented from contacting with the seat and therefore sharing the load of body weight. Inadequate loading of the thighs will contribute to an unstable sitting position, which will result in poor posture, as the person becomes fatigued. With the shape and position of the ischial tuberosities in mind, one can very quickly understand that it is crucial for any seat surface to accommodate both the shape of the ischial tuberosities, and to control the rocking motion, in order to maintain a comfortable and stable sitting position.

Two important landmarks of the pelvic girdle should also be located, and these are the anterior superior iliac spine (ASIS) and posterior superior iliac spine (PSIS). Each side of the pelvic girdle has an ASIS and a PSIS. It is important for the clinician to be able to locate both of these points, as they will give a crucial indication of the position of the pelvis when in a seated position.

The ASIS locating points are found on the anterior aspect of the pelvis, below the iliac crests. In a neutral sitting position the ASISs are level with each other when viewed / palpated from an anterior position. They can be located by either palpating anteriorly and inferiorly from the iliac crests, or by palpating the area where the pelvis and thighs meet. The shape of the ASISs is slightly hooked, which gives the clinician an indication that he or she has located the correct point.

Activity 1

1 Locate the ASISs of your own pelvis by running your fingers anteriorly along the superior surface of the iliac crests and then downwards until your fingers move under a hooked bony prominence. This is the ASIS.
2 Locate the ASISs on a colleague – ask them to sit in a chair with their feet flat on the floor. Kneel down and face their knees. Run your fingers along the top of the thighs until they reach the anterior aspect of the pelvis and move under a hooked prominence on each side – these are the ASISs.

The PSISs are located on the posterior aspect of the pelvis, either side of the sacrum. They are more difficult to pinpoint than the ASISs as they are less prominent. In a neutral sitting position the PSISs sit at the same height as the ASISs. They can clearly be seen in a standing position once clothing has been removed, as each one forms a small dimple on either side of the sacrum.

Activity 2

1 Locate your PSISs. First sit upright, locate your ASISs and then run your fingers round to the posterior surface of your pelvis. Your PSISs sit at the same height as the ASISs, and feel like two small subtle 'lumps'. They are much closer

together than the ASISs as they sit only one 2–3 cm either side of the spine.

2 Locate the PSISs of your colleague – ask them to sit in an upright position. First repeat the above method of locating the PSISs with your colleague. To confirm that you have found the correct position you can also use another method to find the PSIS: find your colleague's coccyx. Place four fingers horizontally onto the sacrum, above the coccyx. The PSISs should be just above the top of your fingers.

Movements of the pelvis

The pelvis is able to move in a number of different planes: anterior/posterior, medial/lateral rotation, and oblique. All of these movements enable the human being to function normally both in a seated and standing position. Futhermore, a healthy person is able to readjust the position of the pelvis when any activity carried out over a length of time becomes uncomfortable. This maintains the flexibility of the joints involved at the pelvic girdle. However, some people are frequently unable to change their position, either because they do not perceive discomfort or because they are unable to change their position independently. This inability to realign the position of the pelvis places the person at risk of developing postural changes, which if left uncorrected, will result in postural deformity.

Pressure, shear forces and friction

As discussed in previous chapters, pressure ulcers are caused by a number of intrinsic, extrinsic and external factors. Intrinsic factors such as nutrition, poor sensation and loss of consciousness (Birchall 1993) will all impact on the seated person, and may obviously influence the clinical decision as to whether to sit a person out of bed at all. However, the extrinsic factors related to pressure ulcer development can be influenced by appropriate provision of seating equipment, which maximizes pressure distribution, posture and stability. These factors are pressure, shear forces and friction (Birchall 1993); they can, to some extent, be controlled by suitable seating provision, and methods of achieving this will be discussed later in this chapter.

Pressure, shear forces and friction are discussed below. External factors are further influences that contribute to pressure ulcer development. They include aspects such as inappropriate moving and handling techniques, poor positioning, time, gravity, moisture (for example incontinence or perspiration caused by a vinyl seat cover), and imposed immobilization (for example, traction). These factors will, when added to aetiological factors, increase the person's risk of pressure ulcer development. For example, the effects of friction and shear forces will be increased if moisture is present (Torrance 1983).

Pressure

Unrelieved pressure or 'interface' pressure is the most common cause of pressure ulcers (Clarke 1997). It can be calculated by dividing the body weight by the surface area. Seated pressure is caused by gravity forcing the weight of the body against a hard seat surface. The soft tissues surrounding the buttocks become compressed, and the capillaries occluded. If this force is not relieved, then tissue necrosis will occur (Bridel 1993b). Pressure is a concern in the seated client, as such a small surface area of the body supports the majority of body weight (Crow 1988). Interface pressures are therefore always high in a sitting position, and whatever pressures may be measured at the interface between the seat and the skin, pressure is known to be greatest deep in the tissues, directly next to the bone (McClemont 1984; Le et al. 1984). Interface pressure in the seated position is invariably higher than the average capillary closing pressure (Souther et al. 1974), due to the small surface area of the body being supported. There has always been debate as to what pressure is required to occlude the capillaries (Landis 1930; Bridel 1993a), and interface measurement can form only a part of client assessment for seating, due to the differing integrity of clients' skin. It is therefore essential that as much of the lower half of the body is supported by the seat surface (Burman 1993), so that pressure may be distributed as widely as possible.

Shear

Shear forces are a major contributor to pressure ulcer development in the seated client, due to the position of the body within the chair. Shear stress is caused by a force which acts on the tissue in a direction parallel to the plane of the support surface (Ham et al. 1998). When seated, even for a short period of time, gravity attempts to force the body downwards in the chair. At first the soft tissues remain static, whilst the skeleton slides down within the tissues, rubbing the tissues and distorting and kinking the shape of the capillaries, which in turn increases occlusion (Jay 1995a). It is the combination of shear forces and unrelieved pressure which presents the most danger with regard to pressure ulcer development (Collier 1994b; Jay 1995b). Shear forces give little indication that internal tissue damage is occurring until the skin breaks to reveal a large cavity. When providing seating for clients, it is essential that shear forces are minimized by the use of appropriate positioning.

Friction

Friction is the resistance of one surface to another that moves over it. Once the impact of shear forces has taken full effect, the body weight of the person will cause them to slide downwards in the chair. Friction occurs as the skin moves over the seat surface. Friction will be minimized if shear forces are addressed. However, the chair upholstery or cushion cover will influence the frictional properties of the seat. For example, many cushions are covered in vinyl in order to ease cleaning. Vinyl offers no frictional properties and allows the body to slide freely over it, reducing sitting stability. Conversely, other upholstery materials such as velour offer frictional properties, which reduce the tendency to slide, thereby increasing seating stability. However, it should also be appreciated that when friction does occur on materials offering increased frictional properties, then more damage may potentially occur to the skin surface.

Normal seated posture

Any posture adopted whilst sitting in order to carry out a functional activity may be described as normal. However, normal sitting describes the position that may be considered 'optimum' when sitting persons out of bed for any length of time, whether they are using an armchair or a wheelchair.

In normal sitting (Figure 10.2), the buttocks and thighs take 75 per cent of body weight. The ischial tuberosities are the major

Activity 3

Sit in a normal upright sitting position. Concentrate on your ischial tuberosities. Try rocking backwards and forwards to see if you are able to gain better stability in any particular position. Try and sit still. How long are you able to maintain this for?

You should find that you cannot obtain stability unless you lean back onto the sacrum – where you will gain temporary respite! You should also find that you cannot still for any length of time – you will tend to rock forwards and backwards and feel fatigued.

contact between the pelvis and the seat, and it is important that they share the body weight equally. This requirement has a major implication on cushion design, as it must allow contouring of the body. The pelvis is positioned in a slight anterior tilt, and if viewed from a lateral aspect the ASISs and PSISs will be at a level height. The sacrum or the pubis should take no weight in normal sitting.

The head is positioned directly over the pelvis in normal sitting, allowing the spine to maintain it's normal anterior and posterior curves. This in turn allows the body to manage the forces of gravity as it falls in front of the nose, down through the chest and through both ischial tuberosities. NB The head will always prefer to be positioned directly over the pelvis. Therefore, should the pelvis adopt any change of position, the head will naturally realign itself over the pelvis, requiring the spine to compromise its position.

A normal sitting position will enable the lower limbs to be placed in a neutral alignment, with the knees facing forwards. The angle of flexion at the hip and knee should be 90°. The feet should be placed flat on the floor or on some form of support, for example footrests. This is of great importance, because in a seated position, the feet support 19 per cent of the body weight. Adequate foot support is also crucial to ensure sitting stability (Medical Devices Agency 1997a).

It is important to state here that even the healthiest person will be unable to maintain a normal sitting position for a sustained period of time, due to the effects of gravity and upper body fatigue. It is therefore unreasonable to expect anyone whose health and/or function is compromised to do so either. Any client who is sat out of bed and into a chair should be positioned as optimally as possible initially and then repositioned as frequently as required. Failure to do this will result in the person sliding down in the chair, and experiencing general discomfort. Whilst many patients are frequently repositioned in bed, few have chair repositioning schedules.

Suitable sitting dimensions

In order to assist someone to sit in a normal sitting position it is essential to ensure that the dimensions of the seat are correct (Collins and Shipperley 1999) (Table 10.1). An incorrect seat size will cause them to adopt a poor sitting posture which will in turn lead to pressure ulcer development, if the person is required to sit for any length of time. NB When a client complains of discomfort whilst sitting, it is tempting to simply provide them with a pressure-relieving cushion in order to relieve their discomfort, without first examining the chair itself. Very often this is an unnecessary and expensive

Table 10.1 Optimum sitting dimensions

Seat height	The height of the chair must be the same measurement as the length of the client's lower leg with the person wearing their normal footwear such as slippers (back of knee to floor)
Seat width	The optimum seat width allows for approximately 2cm either side of the client's thighs, which can facilitate easier transfers, and allows for heavy clothing, such as a coat, to be used occasionally.
Seat depth	The correct seat depth is from the back of the buttocks to 2cm behind the back of the knee. The thigh should be fully supported, with no pressure being placed on the popliteal fossa.
Backrest height	There are no firm guidelines as to the optimum backrest height, as each client will need a different height according to medical needs. However, in general terms, a higher backrest is more supportive, and is recommended for persons who sit for long periods of time or who fatigue easily.
Armrest height	Armrests should be at a height to allow the shoulders to rest in a neutral position, neither elevated or depressed. In some instances it will be important for armrests to be adjustable in height, particularly if a person is using a wheelchair to take part in sporting activities.

exercise, as it may well be the chair dimensions which are causing the problem, and the provision of a pressure-relieving cushion could further enhance the problems (Banks and Bridel 1995). Therefore always examine the chair prior to providing equipment. Remember that both the dimensions of the chair and the overall condition of the chair will influence posture and therefore pressure ulcer risk (Collins 2000). The recommended chair dimensions are as follows:

Seat width

An appropriate seat width should allow 2 cm of clearance on either side of the person's thighs and buttocks. The assessor measures this by sliding his or her hands, thumbs upwards along the outer margins of the patient's thighs. If the hands cannot be placed comfortably, then the seat is too narrow, and conversely, if there is additional space once the hands are in position, then the chair is too wide.

If a chair is too narrow for a person, it will cause a number of problems. Firstly, it will prevent the person sitting back into the chair, as the hips become stuck. This restricts the person from utilizing the whole of the seat surface. When the person leans against the backrest, his pelvis will rotate into a posterior pelvic tilt, effectively reclining him, and placing a large percentage of the body weight onto the sacrum and spine. This increases the risk of pressure ulcer development both in the sacral and spinal region, but also in the thigh area, potentially causing a pressure ulcer over the greater trochanters of the femurs (Collins 2001c). Moving and handling is also compromised, as the person will be less able to reposition himself and will experience difficulty sitting forwards in order to stand. Furthermore, this will also cause problems in those people who require hoisting, as positioning the slings adequately would be extremely difficult, and could cause tissue trauma. In such instances only the provision of a larger chair is acceptable, as no other inter-vention will solve such a problem. For some wheelchair users it is possible to 'outrig' the armrests by several inches. Outrigging can provide up to two or three inches extra space in the seat area but it is important that a wider cushion is also provided, in order to prevent the person from sitting directly over the seat rails of the wheelchair.

If a chair is too wide, then the person will tend to lie across the seat rather than sit in it. However, the majority of the body weight is then supported by one half of the body only, causing a pressure ulcer risk on the supporting ischial tuberosity and the greater trochanter on the same side (Collins 2001c). The elbow on the supporting side may also develop pressure trauma. It is possible, as a short-term measure, to make an armchair's seat width narrower, by using pillows on either side of the person. This gives them added support and stability. It may be preferable to place several pillows down one side of the seat only, thereby allowing the person to utilize one of the armrests. For those patients who are using self-propelling wheelchairs, this is not a suitable measure, as a wheelchair that is too wide also inhibits the person from propelling the chair adequately, as reaching the wheel rims can be difficult (Collins 2001a). This can place increased strain on the shoulder girdle.

Seat depth

Appropriate seat depth should support the whole of the person's buttocks and thighs, allowing a small gap of 2 cm behind the back of the knee, which avoids damage to the popliteal fossa (Collins 2001a). Inadequate seat depth will lead to some of the thigh being unsupported in taller people and, as a result, interface pressures increase under the buttocks and thighs. A seat depth that is too long for the person will cause discomfort behind the back of the knee and consequently, he repositions himself by sliding forwards in the chair in order to increase his comfort, adopting a posterior pelvic tilt.

Occasionally, the environment of a wheelchair user may not allow for the provision of a larger sized wheelchair, as turning space can be limited. For those people who require a longer seat depth this can be achieved, in some instances, by the provision of a cushion that is longer than the wheelchair canvas. In this way, both the wheelchair user and the environment can be accommodated. However, it is essential to use a cushion that has a firm base, such as plywood, in order to prevent the cushion from folding over the edge of the canvas, and such provision brings its own risks (Collins 2001a). For example, the use of plywood will increase interface pressures (Medical Devices Agency 1997a).

If the seat depth is too long for a person, then pillows may be placed behind his back, to reduce the depth of the seat. However the pillows must also be placed high enough in the seat to provide suitable back support, and this may entail the use of two or three pillows.

Seat height

The height of the seat is perhaps the most crucial measurement, as it will affect the person's ability to reach the floor, thereby having a fundamental effect on whether the person will develop a pressure ulcer or not. Correct seat height is ascertained by measuring from the back of the person's knee to the floor. It is important that the person is wearing normal footwear at the time, as this will affect the measurement (Collins 2001a).

If a seat is too low for a person, the thighs will be unsupported by the seat and this increases interface pressures on the buttocks and sacrum. Provision such as this will cause the person to slide downwards in the chair in order to search for comfort. If however, the seat is too high, then the person will not be able to reach the ground and place his feet flat on the floor or footrests. The weight that should have been taken by the feet is then transferred onto the thighs and buttocks, decreasing comfort and resulting in poor sitting stability. In order to increase stability and comfort, the person will slide forwards in the chair so that he can place his feet on the floor. However, this postural compromise causes the person to adopt a posterior pelvic tilt, taking weight on the sacrum. It is unlikely that the feet can be placed flat on the floor, and more likely that the heels support the weight of the feet, which could account for many of the pressure ulcers observed on heels (Collins 2001c). Providing the correct seat height by provision of suitable foot support can reduce pressure ulcer development (Medical Devices Agency 1997a).

Backrest

Most people who have to sit for long periods of time require a backrest that is supportive. As such the backrest needs to be higher rather than lower in most instances. When providing seating for elderly or neurologically impaired patients, a high backrest is essential in order to provide appropriate sitting support. The height of the backrest should therefore reach the top of the person's shoulders or even the top of their head if possible. Some client groups can cope with a lower backrest, such as people with a low spinal cord lesion. In such instances a high backrest may inhibit the shoulder girdle movements associated with self-propelling.

Armrests

When sitting the arms only support two per cent of the person's body weight. However, the arms do need to remain in a comfortable resting position when seated allowing the shoulder girdle to rest in a neutral position. In some more active wheelchair users, height-adjustable armrests may be indicated, particularly if the person is taking part in sporting activities.

Development of poor sitting posture

Poor sitting posture occurs for several reasons. Firstly, the chair itself may be inappropriate for the person's needs, either in size or in support. Secondly, the person's illness or disability may result in poor posture (Letts 1991), for example, due to reduced trunk control or extensor spasm. Thirdly, the sitting posture will automatically be changed due to the effects of gravity over a period of time; if the person is unable to reposition himself, then postural changes will occur. If sitting posture changes, the surface area for weight bearing is often reduced, and pressures experienced over bony prominences increased (Ham et al. 1998). Such postural changes are flexible in the short term, allowing for repositioning by means of seating systems. However, in the longer term, these changes will become fixed, due to muscle contractures and soft tissue accommodation. Fixed postural changes cannot be altered, other than by the use of surgery, and therefore in these instances seating provision can only provide accommodation of the posture rather than alteration of it.

Posterior pelvic tilt

This position is also known as the 'sacral sitting position', and tends to be the most commonly encountered poor posture associated with sitting. There are a number of reasons for the position occurring; however, the position itself is first described.

Posterior pelvic tilt (Figures 10.3 and 10.4) occurs when the person leans back onto the sacrum, rather than taking weight through the ischial tuberosities only. At first this position seems stable, as the sacrum offers a flat surface to lean against; however, within a short time, the pelvis slides forwards on the chair. Weight is taken on the sacrum, and this increased loading accounts for many incidences of pressure ulcer development in this area (Brienza et al. 1996).

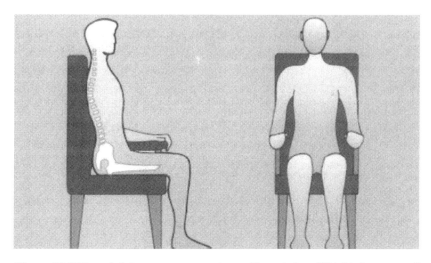

Figure 10.3 Normal sitting posture – anterior and lateral view. With kind courtesy of Karomed Seating.

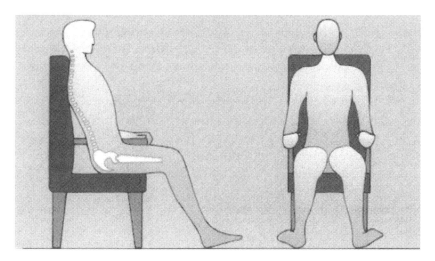

Figure 10.4 Posterior pelvic tilt – anterior view and lateral view. With kind courtesy of Karomed Seating.

In posterior pelvic tilt, the sacrum supports a proportion of the body weight. The ischial tuberosities still support some of the body weight, but as the pelvis tilts posteriorly, they push forwards, creating shear forces (Ham et al. 1998). The PSISs tilt downwards posteriorly, whilst the ASISs tilt upwards, and this can be noted from a lateral aspect when palpating both prominences.

The change in position of the pelvis alters the position of the whole body within the chair, and has a particularly damaging impact on the lower limbs and on the spine. As the pelvis slides forwards, the lower limbs lose the majority of their contact with the seat surface. This results in increased interface pressures at the buttocks, as a smaller surface area of the body is expected to support the same body weight. The angle at the hip joint widens, causing the person to slide down further in the chair. Should the person in question suffer from extensor spasm, the effect of this open hip angle will exacerbate the problem, potentially increasing the speed at which the sliding occurs. This can make sitting extremely difficult for people who suffer from neurological conditions for example. The effect of the posterior tilt also causes lateral rotation at the hip joint and abduction, the angle at the knee joint increases, and the result is that the feet can no longer be placed flat on the floor. The heels consequently take the weight of the lower limbs, frequently accounting for the development of pressure ulcers. It is often assumed that many pressure ulcers, which have occurred on heels, have occurred in the bed, whereas in fact poor seating in as many as 65 per cent of cases may have caused them.

As discussed earlier in this chapter, the head positions itself over the pelvis. Therefore when the person assumes a posterior pelvic tilt, the head will eventually position itself forwards over the pelvis. The spinal column must therefore compromise in order to facilitate this position, and this results in a kyphosis. The lumbar lordosis is lost as a result of the spinal changes. If no attention is paid to the development of the kyphosis, it will result in the person being unable to utilize the seat surface, as only the apex of the kyphosis will contact with the backrest, preventing the rest of the body from sitting back into the seat. Furthermore, the kyphosis results in the person's head being tilted forwards, which prevents him from being able to look forwards to watch television or eat, etc. In order to achieve this, the person has to hyperextend at the cervical spine, which in time, also becomes fixed in this position. This can create difficulties with swallowing.

Activity 4

Sit in your armchair in an upright position with your feet flat on the floor. Lean over to the left as far as you can. Repeat this exercise with your feet off the floor. How easy is this? Would your patients find it as easy as you? This exercise is designed to demonstrate the importance of foot support in providing sitting stability

Long-term consequences of posterior pelvic tilt

The resultant position of posterior pelvic tilt is extremely uncomfortable for the client; it also places many aspects of the body at risk from developing pressure ulcers. In addition to the heels, both the sacrum and ischial tuberosities are at increased risk from developing pressure ulcers due to the effects of shear forces and friction, with additional reduced thigh support. Furthermore, the kyphosis also places the spine at risk from developing pressure ulcers.

A fixed kyphosis creates many problems when planning seating for a person. The spinous and transverse processes of the spine open, allowing rotation to occur. The changed shape of the spine also results in weight being taken over a small surface area of the spine, resulting in a pressure ulcer. As the person is positioned into the chair, the kyphosis immediately contacts with the backrest, preventing the person from being able to gain much contact with the seat surface. It results in the pelvis being placed on the edge of the chair, with no contact achieved by the thighs. Specialist equipment has to be considered for clients with fixed kyphoses in order to support the maximum surface area of the body, to increase comfort and to maximize function.

Causes of posterior pelvic tilt

The effects of gravitational forces over time will frequently result in a person adopting a posterior pelvic tilt. However, poor seating provision and the person's physical condition will also play an important role in causing this position.

Poor or inappropriate seating provision can cause a posterior pelvic tilt in several ways. The dimensions of the chair are one major influence: if the seat depth is too long, it will cause discomfort behind the back of the knee. In order to increase comfort the person will shuffle forwards in the seat, effectively reducing seat depth. Unfortunately, once he then tries to lean against the backrest he immediately adopts a posterior pelvic tilt.

If the seat height is too high, the person's feet will not touch the floor. This will be uncomfortable because the buttocks and thighs will take all body weight. The feet will be unable to share this load. Furthermore, the person will feel unstable in the chair; he will therefore slide forwards in the seat in his attempt to reach the floor with his feet, and this will cause him to adopt a posterior pelvic tilt.

If the seat height is too low, then the thighs will be raised off the front of the seat surface, increasing the weight taken by the buttocks. The person will also experience increased hip flexion, which will reduce comfort and potentially increase heat and moisture in the groin area. If left in this position, the person could potentially suffer from flexion contractures at the hip joint. In order to compensate and to increase comfort, he or she will slide forwards in the chair, increasing the angle of flexion at the hip joint. However in order to achieve this, he or she adopts a posterior pelvic tilt.

If the backrest is inadequate for the needs of a person with poor trunk control or fatigue, he or she will seek appropriate support by sliding downwards in the chair, in order to rest the scapulae against the backrest. This has the effect of increasing the level of support for the spine. However, in order to achieve this the person has to adopt a posterior pelvic tilt.

Other aspects of inappropriate seating which cause posterior pelvic tilt include a chair with a saggy seat surface and backrest. This often applies to old armchairs and to wheelchairs with stretched seat and back canvases. Any chair or cushion with a slippery cover such as vinyl will cause the person to slide forwards and therefore adopt a posterior pelvic tilt. Providing a chair with a reclined backrest will almost certainly cause the client to sit in a posterior pelvic tilt as the angle at which he or she sits automatically opens up the hip angle. It may be more appropriate to select a chair that is able to tilt in space rather than simply reclining (Collins 2000), although in some instances a reclining chair is the only suitable option for some clients, and tilt-in-space chairs, whilst more versatile, are generally more expensive to purchase.

Aspects of the person's physical condition that result in the development of a posterior pelvic tilt include: low tone and weakness of lumbar extensors (Letts 1991) and contractures of the hamstrings. Contractures of the hamstrings as they attach to the pelvis and cross the knee joint affect the position and movements of the hip and knee joints and compromise either pelvic or lower limb positions. Extensor spasm, as previously discussed, will lead to posterior pelvic tilt, and people who have conditions such as multiple sclerosis and cerebral palsy frequently experience this problem. It is also common in people who have had spinal cord injuries. Any person in a poor state of health who is required to sit for any length of time will adopt a posterior pelvic tilt.

In addition to the risk of pressure ulcer development, a posterior pelvic tilt may also cause other associated physical problems, such as chest infections, as many of the internal organs become compressed as the spine rounds in order to compensate.

Activity 5

Ask a friend to sit in a comfortable chair in front of the television. Make a note of their initial position. Ask your friend to watch the television for about half an hour, and during this time observe their position. Make a note of how often they move, and what happens to their posture when they move. What is their final posture like – are they still in a 'normal sitting position'?

Activity 6

Sit in an upright position. Take a deep breath. Sit in a posterior pelvic tilt, with a rounded spinal position, head over your pelvis. Try to take another deep breath. Notice how much more difficult it is to expand your lungs. All your internal organs will be similarly compromised!

Assessment

A detailed seating assessment involves a number of different aspects, some of which are complex to perform if not suitably trained, in order to define the person's needs. These components include risk assessment, assessment of the person in his existing seating, some definition of the existing problems, a full physical assessment, pressure mapping or interface pressure measurements, and the person's needs and wishes for future seating provision (Collins 2001a).

In a ward environment, several of the more simple assessment components can be utilized by nursing staff in order to attempt to solve the seating problem. If the problem proves to be more complex than this, specialist advice should be sought from an occupational therapist or physiotherapist, with a potential referral to the wheelchair service for a specialist seating service. (Specialist seating for non-wheelchair users in the UK is frequently difficult to obtain, as budgetary responsibility for such equipment is often unclear. Therefore, anyone requiring any seating equipment other than pressure-reducing cushions may encounter difficulty with regard to who accepts responsibility for payment.)

Risk assessment

A risk assessment score is a tool, which determines the client's risk status of developing a pressure ulcer, by quantifying a range of the most commonly recognized risk factors affecting the patient at a given time (Flanagan 1995). Risk assessment tools should not be used in isolation of other seating assessment methods. Bennett and Moody pointed out in 1995 that risk assessments 'are an aid, not a substitute for good management and prevention'. Prior to carrying out a seating assessment, the person's risk assessment score should have been calculated, and this will indicate their overall risk of pressure ulcer development. However, a risk assessment score will give little information on the person's risk with respect to postural threats. Risk assessment scores should be used to enhance, not replace clinical judgement, and are most useful when combined with other assessment methods such as interface testing.

Interface pressure testing and pressure mapping

It is possible, to an extent, to test the interface pressures of the seated client, although no pressure measuring tool will be entirely accurate, as they cannot conform exactly to the skin (Clark 1994). Small hand-held pressure monitors such as the Talley Hand Held Pressure Monitor can provide the clinician with an indication of the interface pressures existing between the buttocks and the seat surface. This may therefore enable the clinician to test several products in order to choose which one is the most acceptable pressure-reducing or pressure-relieving cushion for the client. However, several aspects should be considered when using such monitors. Firstly, they only work well when they are positioned directly under the client's ischial tuberosities; in the hands of an inexperienced user, it is possible for the sensor to slip away from the bony prominences as the person sits onto the cushion, and this will directly affect the readings. Secondly, whatever measurement is observed at the skin surface may be up to 3–5 times greater deep within the tissues, directly next to the bony prominence (Le et al. 1984; McClemont 1984). Thirdly, it is important to bear in mind that whilst certain products appear to offer increased pressure redistribution, their true capability will only be seen by observation of skin integrity after the person has sat on the cushion for approximately half an hour. This is because the exact amount of pressure required to occlude the capillaries will vary from individual to individual (Landis 1930). It may be found that one cushion offering apparently superior pressure readings to another in fact causes more skin erythema than the alternative (whose readings suggest that it offers less pressure reduction). Finally, comfort is essential to everyone. A cushion may be provided with the greatest of care following a detailed assessment. However, if the client finds it cold, uncomfortable or unstable, then he will be reluctant to use it.

Assessment of the dimensions and positional qualities of the chair

It is important to observe the dimensions of the person's chair. The assessor should note whether the dimensions are suitable for the size of the person, or whether this aspect needs adjusting, if possible. For example, it is possible to effectively make a chair smaller by providing an all-in-one hollowfibre back and side support.

Activity 7

Sit in your favourite armchair. What makes it so comfortable? Is it the size that is comfortable, or is it the materials that it is constructed from? Analyze what makes a good chair from your perspective.

In addition to the dimensions of the chair, the clinician must ascertain whether the actual shape of the chair is suitable for the person. For example, some hospital chairs have backrests with a slight angle recline. For many people a backrest angle above 12° is too great, and potentially places the person into a posterior pelvic tilt. Other chairs have a ramped cushion, which transfers body weight onto the sacrum rather than the ischial tuberosities, creating friction and shear forces. These can be particularly dangerous if used without an integral pressure-relieving cushion, and must therefore be used with care. There are increasing numbers of tilt-in-space armchairs on the market. These chairs enable the user to be positioned either in a normal upright position, or tilted backwards. At all stages, the angle of the hips and knees remain at 90°, and the spinal column retains its natural curvature. These chairs allow long-term sitters to be re-positioned, for example tilted backwards to alleviate fatigue; this in turn alters pressure distribution. However, no one position should be adopted for any length of time, and clinicians should maximize such a chair's potential by frequently repositioning their clients.

Less common postural changes

As discussed previously, the posterior pelvic tilt is perhaps the most common postural change associated with long-term sitting. However, other positions do occur, as outlined below.

Anterior pelvic tilt

In this position the pelvis tilts forwards. The body weight is trans-ferred onto the thighs, and in rare instances, taken through the pubis. The cause of an anterior pelvic tilt is often associated more with the client's physical condition and less with the qualities of the seat. For example, people with spina bifida and muscular dystrophy are known to often adopt this position.

In the anterior pelvic tilt the following body position is adopted: the pelvis tilts forwards, lowering the anterior superior iliac spines and raising the posterior superior iliac spines. The sacrum is suspended in mid-air. The ischial tuberosities are forced posteriorly, creating shear forces and friction.

The change of pelvic position results in increased flexion at the hip joints. This can cause flexion contractures if not addressed. The skin in the groin area can become warm and moist, potentially causing skin irritation. To compensate for this altered position, the lower limbs are forced underneath the body, increasing flexion at the knees, and the feet have a tendency to take the weight through the toes.

As the head repositions itself over the pelvis, the spine is forced to compromise. This results in an increased lordosis, which if left will become fixed. To compensate, the person will push their chest forwards, and the scapulae then become 'winged'.

Pelvic obliquity

This postural change is thought to be as frequent as a posterior pelvic tilt. In this position, the pelvis tilts obliquely (Figure 10.5). When palpated from an anterior position when the person is seated, the ASIS on one side will be lower than the ASIS on the other side. The person is therefore deemed to have an obliquity on the side that is lower. If an obliquity is determined, the client will require a full physical examination in a supine position, in order to ascertain whether the obliquity is fixed or flexible. An obliquity, which is found to be flexible, can be rectified by suitable seating provision. However, seating provision can only accommodate an obliquity that is found to be fixed.

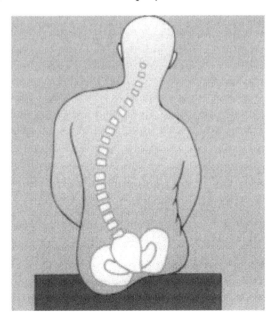

Figure 10.5 Pelvic obliquity – posterior view. With kind courtesy of Karomed Seating.

Activity 8

Sit with a pelvic obliquity for at least 10 minutes. Notice where the discomfort predominates. What position is your trunk placed in? How long could you maintain this position voluntarily?

When a pelvic obliquity occurs, the majority of the seated body weight is taken by one ischial tuberosity only. This increases the risk of pressure ulcer development under the lower ischial tuberosity, as the other supports either no or minimal body weight. Furthermore, the lower ischial tuberosity becomes able to laterally and medially rotate, lessening the person's sitting stability even more.

Once the pelvis has developed an obliquity, the upper body weight is forced over to one side, as the head realigns itself over the pelvis. The spine is forced to compromise, and a scoliosis develops. This will result in lengthening of the trunk on the side of the obliquity, and shortening of the trunk on the opposite side. If left uncorrected, the abdominal and spinal muscles will contract, and the position will become fixed.

The major cause of a pelvic obliquity is a saggy or unstable seat (Zacharkow 1984), such as a wheelchair canvas, which has stretched and bowed. However, other causative factors may initiate the development of this posture. For example, a seat that is too wide will encourage the sitter to fill the available space, in order to obtain stability. People who foot propel their wheelchairs are often forced to sit with a pelvic obliquity as they lean over to reach the floor with their feet. In addition, people who use electric wheelchairs often lean over to the side that has the control (which is why children tend to have controls that are centrally mounted, as these encourage a symmetrical posture). It is also common for people who have suffered a cerebrovascular accident (CVA) to lean heavily to one side. Frequently, they may lean heavily to the weak side; however in some instances, they lean more heavily to the side that has not been affected by the CVA. In either case, a pelvic obliquity may develop unless sitting stability is assisted.

Pelvic rotation

Rotation of the pelvis is caused by a number of reasons, such as a pelvic obliquity, foot propelling, and leg length discrepancy. In this position, the pelvis rotates forward on one side. Therefore, when palpating the ASISs, one side will be obviously further forwards than the other. The most obvious visual cue that pelvic rotation is taking place is that one leg appears longer than the other does. However, true leg length discrepancy is less common, and the only method of ascertaining whether there is a leg length discrepancy, or whether there is pelvic rotation, is by checking the position of the ASISs.

When true pelvic rotation is taking place, the upper trunk will initially be forced to follow the movement of the pelvis. However, postural accommodation soon takes place, and the trunk will re-align itself over the pelvis, which in turn will cause the spinal column to rotate, as this will facilitate function.

Advanced seating assessment

This assessment is undertaken in addition to risk assessment and interface pressure mapping. It involves assessment of the client's posture both within and outside of the seating provision, be this a wheelchair or an armchair.

Assessment of the existing seating

This assessment is undertaken with the client sitting in the existing seating provision. The assessor identifies the client's ASISs and PSISs. By palpating both the ASISs together, the assessor can determine whether the client is sitting in a neutral pelvic tilt. If this is so, then the ASISs will be level. If a pelvic obliquity is present, one ASIS will be lower than the other; if pelvic rotation is present, one ASIS will be further forwards than the other. The assessor should also palpate one ASIS and one PSIS from a lateral position. If the pelvis is in a neutral tilt, then these landmarks should be at the same height. However, if the PSIS is lower than the ASIS, then a posterior pelvic tilt is present, and if the ASIS is lower than the PSIS, then an anterior pelvic tilt is present.

In many instances, it is difficult to palpate the PSISs, as their bony prominences are subtle. However, if a posterior pelvic tilt is present, the remainder of the client's posture may give this away. For example, it may be impossible to slide one's hand under the sacrum and coccyx if the client is in a posterior pelvic tilt, as the client will be leaning on his sacrum.

If postural changes are noted in the existing seating, it is important to continue the assessment out of the chair. If no postural changes are noted, then it is likely that no postural changes have occurred.

Assessment on a firm surface

If postural changes have been determined in the client's existing seating, then it is essential to ascertain the cause of this, and whether or not the postural change can be reversed. Firstly, the client should be sat onto a firm flat surface, such as a plinth. The seat should be the correct height for the client. If necessary, the client's upper body should be supported by member of staff. The firm surface will frequently reduce the severity of the postural change, and in some instances, eliminate it altogether. This is due to the provision of the firm surface. If this is the case it can be assumed that the postural changes are caused by the seating and can be rectified by more suitable provision. Any remaining postural change can then be identified and clarified by assessment in a supine position.

Assessment in a supine position

Once a postural change has been ascertained, it is then essential to determine whether it is fixed or flexible, as this will dictate the type of seating provision that is required. This type of assessment involves examination of the movements of pelvis in all planes. It also involves examination of the movements and position of the lower limbs, and examination of the shape of the spine. In general terms, if the postural changes are deemed to be flexible, then it is possible to address them by providing suitable seating. However, if the postural changes are found to be fixed, then it is only possible to accommodate them.

This assessment must only be carried out by a suitably trained healthcare professional, as inappropriate assessment could pose a serious risk to the client. This assessment is frequently conducted at a wheelchair service or specialist seating unit.

Goals for sitting

Seating is such a complex issue, that it is difficult for clinicians to prioritize seating needs. The following list includes some suggestions, which will differ in order of priority for each client:

- Provide a stable sitting surface – this is essential in order to maximize client function.
- Promote normal pelvic and spinal alignment.
- Maintain symmetrical body alignment (Collins 2001c).
- Support the maximum surface area possible – in order to reduce interface pressures at the buttocks and thighs.
- Increase weight taken through the thighs as this will reduce the load on the bony prominences (Herbert and Kreutz 1997).
- Reduce the effects of friction and shear.
- Maintain the centre of gravity and body weight in front of the spine.
- Reduce the effects of high tone and extensor spasm.
- Provide comfort.

The sitting surface itself should also be waterproof, vapour permeable, conformable (both the cushion and the cover) and non-slip.

Cushions: construction materials and design

There are many different types of cushions on the market, and all of them have their place in providing pressure relief and pressure distribution. Few of them, however, have undergone rigorous trials in order to ascertain their efficacy in preventing the development of pressure ulcers (Lockyer-Stevens 1994), although this trend is rapidly changing. It is the responsibility of the clinician providing the seating to ensure that appropriate goals of sitting have been established for the client, and that the chosen cushion meets these principles. Clinicians need to become familiar with the different types of cushions on the market, and practised at evaluating the qualities of each cushion. It is also important for clinicians to demand suitable clinical evidence or the opportunity to evaluate products prior to purchasing them. A checklist of aspects to consider when evaluating cushions can be found in Table 10.3.

Table 10.3 Evaluating cushions

When evaluating cushions, the following questions provide a framework for deciding which cushion is the most suitable for a particular client.

- What construction materials is this cushion composed of?
- Does this cushion reduce pressure or relieve it?
- What pressure-relieving properties can this cushion offer, and how does the cushion achieve this?
- What positional properties does this cushion offer, and will this assist or hinder my client?
- What particular needs might this cushion cater for?
- Is there a client group that this cushion would be particularly suitable for?
- Is there a client group that this cushion would be unsuitable for, and why?
- What are the advantages and disadvantages of this particular cushion, for example, maintenance requirements, stabilizing properties etc?

As with all equipment for clients at risk from pressure ulcer development, cushions can either reduce overall interface pressures or relieve pressure. It is important to understand the concept of both processes.

Pressure reduction

Equipment providing pressure reduction aims to spread the weight being taken by the cushion over the maximum surface area possible, thereby reducing interface pressure (Rithalia 1996). This can be achieved in two ways: firstly, by the actual design of the equipment which conforms to the shape of the body, and secondly by the use of pressure-reducing material from which the equipment is manufactured. Cushions providing pressure reduction are known as static cushions. Due to the small area of the body taking the load in the sitting position, it is considered impossible for any cushion to reduce mean pressure below capillary pressure (Souther et al. 1974).

Pressure relief

Pressure relief occurs when the source of the pressure is completely removed (Fletcher 1996). Equipment, which provides pressure relief, includes alternating mattresses and cushions. These operate by inflation and deflation of individual cells, giving pressure relief over the fully deflated cell (Fletcher 1996). These cushions are often referred to as dynamic. Work undertaken by Kosiak (1961) confirms that pressure relief is a more superior method of preventing pressure ulcers than pressure distribution. However, these cushions offer less stable sitting posture than static pressure-reducing cushions.

Pressure-reducing cushions

Many types of materials are used to construct pressure-reducing cushions; they can be constructed from one material only, such as foam, or in combination with several other materials, such as siliconized fluid or air.

The different construction materials and design methods are discussed briefly below. However, it is for the reader to determine which ones are suitable for which client groups. Consulting the MDA (1997a) cushion comparative evaluation will assist the healthcare professional in selecting appropriate cushions for their clients. However, it should be borne in mind that a number of cushions currently on the market did not feature in this evaluation, and should not be excluded from use because of this.

Polyurethane and latex foam

Due to their versatility, these foams are commonly used in the construction of cushions. Such cushions are available in different types of density and depth. For example some cushions are as shallow as 4 cm deep, whilst others are as deep as 8 cm. The depth of foam required will depend on the size of the client, the seat interface required (i.e. wheelchair or armchair) and the pressure ulcer risk of the client. Some high-risk users manage well with foam cushions, especially if their design facilitates conformity, such as cross-cut or moulded cushions. Normally, however, foam cushions are used for clients who are low to medium risk, and those who are not continually sitting. Generally, foam only has a maximum life expectancy of one year, if in constant use. However, some foams do have a much longer life expectancy and accompanying warranties, for example, the Jay Combi, which is a moulded foam cushion. Examples of cross-cut foam cushions are the Propad and the STM cushions.

Viscoelastic foams

This type of foam gradually conforms to the shape of the user over a short period of time in response to body heat, which increases its pressure-relieving qualities, as it distributes the body weight. Cushions comprised of viscoelastic foam enhance sitting stability, due to their ability to conform. This type of foam has less 'memory' than other types of foam and so does not return to its original shape so quickly. This therefore lessens the upward pressures. These cushions tend to be used with medium- to high-risk clients. This type of material is found in the Integra range of cushions and in armchairs which have the Reflexion viscoelastic polymer incorporated into them.

Moulded foams with fluid pads

These cushions consist of an oil-based or a siliconized fluid pad on top of, or within, a foam cushion. They can be used with medium- to high-risk clients, as they generally contour well to the body and provide stability, as the fluid accommodates the pelvis. Therefore these cushions can give high levels of pressure reduction, and also optimum postural support. Examples of a moulded foam base with a separate upper cushion pad are the Jay 2 and the Flotech Solution. The foam base provides the postural support, whilst the fluid pad provides the pressure-reducing qualities. An example of a foam cushion with a fluid pad sandwiched between the foam is the Transflo. It should be noted that moulded cushions are not always suitable in instances where a large number of patients might be expected to use the same cushion, for example within hospital armchairs, because moulded cushions are size specific and should be assessed for each individual person.

Air

There are several different types of air cushion on the market. These vary from simple designs where air is pumped into a hollow cushion via a valve, to more complex cushions such as dry flotation systems, which are made from interconnecting cells of neoprene rubber. The majority of these cushions can be used with high-risk users, although it is important to ensure that such a cushion maximizes sitting stability. The designs of these cushions vary, as does the price. A simple but effective air cushion is the Repose, whilst a more complex design is the Roho. Other cushions on the market utilizing air include the Vicair range of cushions, which utilize small air filled pyramids inside the cushion base, or the Varilite range, which uses both air and foam to achieve the optimum pressure distribution.

Dynamic cushions

Dynamic cushions are designed for a very high-risk user, and are often provided at the same time as a dynamic air mattress. They are constructed of air-filled cells, which inflate and deflate at set intervals via an electric or battery operated pump. As an individual cell deflates, the area of the body in contact with it is relieved from pressure. The remaining inflated cells of the cushion support the surrounding areas of the body. Pressure-relieving cushions are indicated when a person is either at a very high risk of developing a pressure ulcer, or who has already developed pressure damage. Most pressure-relieving cushions operate by using the pump from the alternating mattress (they are generally supplied together and if not, should be). However, this does pose drawbacks. For example, if the patient has a wheelchair they are unable to move from the confined space of the bed due to the electrical supply. Some companies do supply battery-operated alternating cushions, which can allow the patient to be mobile and independent. However, their pumps can be noisy, causing some patients to reject the cushion. Examples of alternating air cushions are the Transair and the Pegasus Daycare. Such cushions can frequently be hired as well as purchased.

Conclusion

Sitting is not an easy posture to maintain for long periods of time. Prevention of pressure ulcers in the seated client will rely on an understanding of seating biomechanics, comprehensive assessment and provision of suitable seating equipment either within the armchair or wheelchair. It is unlikely that a cushion will prevent pressure ulcer development if the client is not frequently repositioned, offered bedrest, or mobilized, as the surface area to body weight ratio conspires against this. No single cushion will suit every client's needs, and so it is important that each clinical setting has a range of cushions or armchairs with integral pressure-reducing cushions available.

CHAPTER 11

Foam technology and its role in wound management and prevention

SYLVIE HAMPTON, FIONA COLLINS, KATE SPRINGETT, MATHEW PHILIP AND LEYTON STEVENS

People often need methods of helping absorb the effects of mechanical stresses, regardless of their medical or surgical state and level of activity. Someone who is bed-bound needs an appropriate mattress to help prevent pressure ulceration, whilst people who sit for prolonged periods of time without appropriate support can also develop lesions (Figure 11.1). Specialized foam can help prevent these pressure ulcers (Figure 11.2). Someone who is able to walk around, will frequently require insoles to help reduce the body loads and the potential for ulceration (Levin 1993). In each of these examples, provision of foam equipment or devices will reduce or remove the mechanical stresses implicated in pressure ulcer formation, lessen strain on intercellular structures and also reduce the blood vessel occlusion that can result in ischaemia. If tissues continue to be loaded for a prolonged period of time, they will be relatively hypoxic and consequently damaged. These traumatized tissues release inflammatory mediators (McKay and Leigh 1991; Roitt 1994), which cause an inflammatory response once blood flow is restored. The reactive hyperaemia which occurs on off-loading tissue sites is usually associated with release of oxygen free radicals (e.g. superoxides) which will result in further tissue damage (Hoekstra et al. 2002). This same mechanism is used by granulocytes in their phagocytic action against invading microorganisms and is a powerful process.

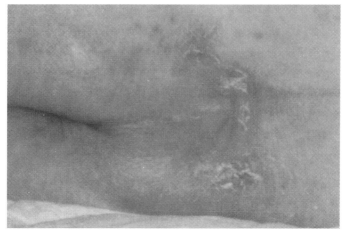

Figure 11.1 Sacral area with pressure ulcer.

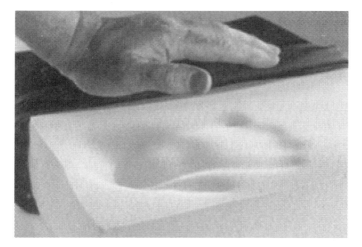

Figure 11.2 Memory foam.

The function of devices aimed at off-loading tissues or those for reducing the mechanical stresses exerted on tissues is similar. The materials used have a common theme, regardless of context. Often these devices are made of foams of one type or another and, as these different foams have different properties, they are therefore specialized and are most useful in particular circumstances. Although foams are used commonly in devices to off-load, and reduce and redistribute mechanical stresses, there is confusion over the variation in terminology used by manufacturers, mechanical engineers, clinical scientists and the different healthcare professions.

In this chapter we aim to explain the use of terms about mechanical stress, and to provide information on foams and their manufacture. A fictitious patient, Mrs Sands, is used to illustrate when and where the different foams may be used to good effect by the multidisciplinary team.

Foam technology and pressure reduction

A number of devices are used to reduce stress, and many of these are made of foams of different forms and densities, such as mattresses, seating cushions and insoles.

A key part of preventing and treating chronic wounds is to remove the cause, whenever possible, and this often involves a multidisciplinary approach. Mechanical stresses (pressure, friction, shear, torsion and tension) are frequently implicated in the cause of chronic wounds. It is often possible to remove these stresses or, if not, certainly to reduce them. Devices used for this purpose are varied but many contain foams of different types. However, it can be difficult for the different healthcare professions to identify which device or which foam should be selected for each individual patient treatment. The following information applied through the example of a patient, Mrs Sands, aims at defining some of the terms used, clarifying when and where to use the different foam products, whilst also introducing some new concepts in management of chronic wounds.

Appropriate use of foam technology is a requirement for the whole multidisciplinary team and knowledge about the manufacturing process and qualities offered by individual foams is essential, irrespective of individual clinical background.

There are a number of questions which need answering to help with selection of the most appropriate foams for Mrs Sands and to prevent further problems developing. The information in the following sections will help answer these.

Assessment

Routine multi-professional assessment procedures were undertaken, including psycho-social assessment. Relevant assessment findings are given below.

Case example

Mrs Sands, an 82-year-old lady who lives in the downstairs floor of her terraced house, suffered a L CVA which resulted in a right-sided hemiplegia. She is a full-time wheelchair user. She is unable to self-propel, and therefore uses her feet to propel herself around her accommodation. She complains of some discomfort under her right buttock.

She has had Type 2 diabetes for 30 years and has many of the complications affecting her feet and lower limbs (Figure 11.3). Peripheral sensory and motor neuropathy has resulted in marked Charcot's foot deformity (see Chapter 5). The medial longitudinal arch is raised making a very high-arched foot (*pes cavus*) and the toes have clawed making the metatarsal heads prominent. The right foot alignment, following the CVA, is such that it contacts the ground on the lateral border. This area has ulcerated in the past although she was unaware of this problem.

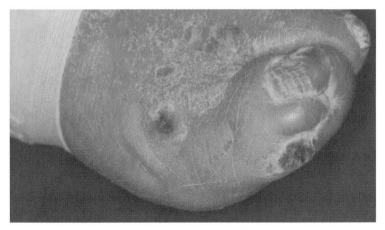

Figure 11.3 Small area of ulceration on left foot (see Plate 36).

Mrs Sands has carers three times a day, for an hour at a time, to get her up, put her on the commode at lunchtime, and also put her to bed. She has recently been admitted to hospital with diarrhoea. Within 24 hours the constant passing of faeces and continual cleaning had lead to maceration of the sacral tissues causing blistering (Figure 11.4) and leaving her very distressed.

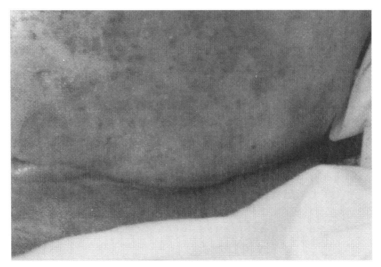

Figure 11.4 Macerated sacrum (see Plate 37).

Tissue viability assessment by the multidisciplinary team

Nursing

Mrs Sands was assessed using the Waterlow score, which placed her at the high-risk level of 24. The assessment indicated that hydration levels were low with reduced tissue turgour although nutrition was average; any problems with eating would be exacerbated by the right-sided hemiplegia as she would find managing cutlery difficult. The hemiplegia would also limit independent repositioning in bed and would also reduce mobility in general.

Doppler readings identified an ankle brachial index pressure of 0.8 (see Chapter 5), which demonstrates a reduced arterial supply of blood. This places the heels at risk when in bed or in a chair.

Maceration and excoriation were observed over the right buttock (Figure 11.4) due to faecal incontinence increasing the risk of pressure ulcer development. The medical condition of diabetes is likely to delay healing and increase potential for further skin damage.

Mrs Sands had been supplied with an air mattress on a previous admission to hospital and found it to be uncomfortable. Based on this past experience, she refuses to use an air mattress.

Occupational therapy

In the wheelchair the patient had a right pelvic obliquity and her pelvis was rotated forwards on the left. Her trunk leaned heavily to the right causing discomfort, she had a scoliosis convex to the right, there was also evidence of a posterior pelvic tilt with associated lateral rotation and abduction at the hip joints. These postural changes were associated with the way in which Mrs Sands needed to propel her wheelchair.

When supine, it was not possible to tilt the pelvis anteriorly confirming that the posterior pelvic tilt was fixed. However, the pelvic obliquity was reduced passively, as was the pelvic rotation. The scoliosis also reduced as the pelvis was adjusted in the lateral plane. There was evidence of redness of the skin under the right buttock and the likely cause for this was the pelvic obliquity in the seated position.

Podiatry

Mrs Sands has autonomic neuropathy so that although the skin feels warm, the blood flow may be through the arterio-venous anastomoses and not through the capillary plexi (Frykberg 1998). Tissue perfusion is therefore poor. There is also some evidence of macro-angiopathy through atheroma, which can occur following high blood lipids in diabetes. Ankle brachial pressure indices are 0.8 bilaterally and pulses are monophasic, but presence of atheroma may give erroneous Doppler readings (Baker and Rayman 1999). Therefore, increased attention to pressure redistribution from the heels, feet and toes is essential if pressure damage from shoes is to be prevented. Non-enzymatic glycation of soft tissue in diabetes means that skin and soft tissue biomechanics are altered and the skin is stiffer than normal (Jude and Boulton 1998; Hashmi 2000). Inspection of the skin of the foot showed a neuropathic ulcer under the second metatarsal head (Figure 11.5).

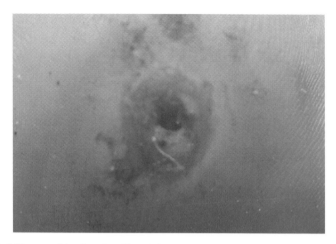

Figure 11.5 Neuropathic ulcer (see Plate 38).

Management of mechanical stress

Although normally all aspects of management would be undertaken, for the purposes of this book, only issues relating to mechanical stress (pressure, shear, etc.) will be considered.

A common, recurring theme for Mrs Sands's management involves reduction in the magnitude and duration of load. In this context load needs defining (see glossary at the end of this chapter). The load may be Mrs Sands's weight taken by a large surface area, e.g. the mattress, or the weight may be taken by a smaller surface area, e.g. the ischial tuberosity on a cushion or a metatarsal head on an insole. It is preferable for load to be redistributed over a larger surface area rather than having a high pressure on a small point such as a bony prominence i.e. point pressure. This may be achieved through use of various materials, especially foams in seating cushions, mattresses and foot orthoses (insoles).

Redistribution of pressure is a suitable method of prevention of pressure damage. This reduces load at one point and transfers it to a larger adjacent contact interface. For example, the NHS Standard Contract mattress does not allow contouring to the body shape, and so the spreading of the load from the point of pressure, that is bony prominences to a larger surface area, is not efficient. Conversely, pressure-reducing mattresses will redistribute the load over a larger surface area, as the foam conforms to the body shape. Similarly, reduction of pressure can be achieved through the use of foams, which contour to body surfaces in the foot and under the buttocks.

The length of time of loading is as important as magnitude of load. Even light loads will cause tissue ischaemia if unrelieved for long periods of time (Kosiak 1961). Therefore the site of loading needs to be changed frequently if pressure ulcer damage is to be avoided. Gebhardt and Bliss (1994) confirm this view in a study where patients were mobilized from sitting every two hours, and this reduced the incidence of pressure ulcers. Sites on the foot that take load for a long time during a stance phase have a greater chance of developing ulceration (Jude and Boulton 1998). It is important to try and change this foot function so that other areas of the foot also share the load at different times.

For Mrs Sands, an alternating air mattress and cushion would be ideal to reduce the time of loading of the tissues, thereby promoting healing. However, she has refused to use one, and so it is necessary to rely on other methods of pressure ulcer prevention such as repositioning and use of pressure-redistributing foam. Different foams for cushions, mattresses and insoles will be selected for their appropriate characteristics. Pressures can be three to five times higher on the bony prominence than more superficial tissues. For Mrs Sands, the load on her right ischial tuberosity would be immense due to the pelvic obliquity. By providing cushioning with a foam material, there is reduced shear and pressure on tissues and this will have the effect of reducing the deep bone and tissue stress.

Understanding mechanical stress and load

The term load is generally used to describe the force due to the mass of an object. For example, a patient with a mass of 60 kg will exert a force on the ground equal to this mass multiplied by the acceleration due to gravity, normally taken to have a value of 9.81 m/s^2 (see Table 11.1) Therefore the force exerted on the ground, $F = 60 \times 9.81 = 588.6$ N (see Table 11.1). It is normal to talk about the weight of the patient being 60 kg. In fact, since weight is the name given to the force exerted by an object due to the pull of gravity, the weight of a patient having a mass of 60 kg is actually 588.6 N. It is, however, more convenient to refer to mass and weight interchangeably and so it is usual to refer to the weight of the patient being 60 kg. In imperial

Table 11.1 Units of measurement

Quantity	SI Symbol	Pronunciation	Imperial symbol	Pronunciation
Length	m	metres	ft	feet
Time	s	seconds	sec	seconds
Velocity	m/s	metres per second	ft/sec	feet per second
Acceleration	m/s^2	metres per second squared	ft/sec^2	feet per square seconds
Force	N	newton	lbf	pounds force
Stress	N/m^2	Newtons per metre squared	psi	pounds per square inch

units 60 kg is equivalent to about 134 lb (pounds). The equivalent weight is simply referred to as 134 lb f (pounds force).

Acceleration

This is the rate at which the speed of an object changes with time. For example, if an object is dropped from a certain height, its velocity increases from zero the moment it is released and continues to increase until it hits the ground (see Figure 11.6).

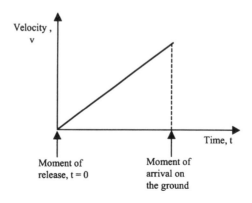

Figure 11.6 The change in speed with time for an object with constant acceleration.

The gradient of the line, which is the change in velocity over a given time divided by that time, is constant when the line is straight. This is the case with acceleration due to gravity. Note the reference to velocity rather than speed because by using the word velocity it is recognized that the quantity has both a magnitude as well as a direction. Speed is just a measure of magnitude. It is therefore usual to use the term velocity when calculations need to be carried out.

Scalars and vectors

Speed is therefore said to be a scalar quantity (having magnitude only) and velocity is a vector quantity (having magnitude and direction). Acceleration, being the rate of change of velocity, is also a vector quantity.

A force is the result of a mass being accelerated (force = mass × acceleration). The weight of a person remains the same although the person is hardly ever seen to accelerate except when falling! This is because, the weight of the person is balanced by the force of the ground wherever he or she is standing, reacting against the weight. This reaction force is said to have the same magnitude as the weight and acts in exactly the opposite direction to the weight as can be seen in Figure 11.7. If forces are acting but there is no motion, then we can say that the forces are in equilibrium.

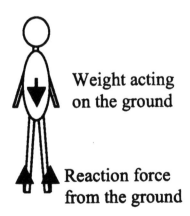

Figure 11.7 Example of forces in equilibrium.

Uniaxial load

When the load or force acts along one direction, we refer to it as uniaxial loading. If the person in Figure 11.7 is standing on top of a cylindrical column as shown in Figure 11.8, the result would be a uniaxial compressive force acting along the length of the cylinder or its main axis.

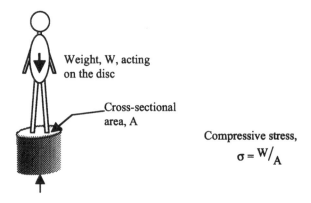

Figure 11.8 Stress within a body due to an applied external force.

This force is shared by the area that supports it. The effect of the force on the material that supports it is called stress. This is defined as the force divided by the area at right angles to the force, supporting it. This is usually referred to as the cross-sectional area. The resulting stress will be compressive and acts along the axis of the disc. This would be referred to as a *uniaxial compressive stress*.

Compressive and tensile stresses are vector quantities as they have both a magnitude and direction.

The stress in the object is not dependent on the material making up the object, providing the material has the same properties in all directions. As a result of this stress, the object deforms and the amount of deformation is however dependent on the material properties. For example, in Figure 11.8, a column of rubber with a Young's Modulus of $0.01\ GN/m^2$ (this is 0.01 giga newton per metre squared and is the same as $10\ N/mm^2$) would deform by about 20 000 times as much as a steel column of the same cross-section and height. This is because, the Young's Modulus of steel is approximately equal to $200\ GN/m^2$ (which is the same as $200\ 000\ N/mm^2$). This deformation is defined by the term, strain, which is the change in dimension along the stress axis divided by the original length along that axis. Therefore, if a person with a mass of 80 kg stands on a column of height, h = 300 mm and the cross-sectional area is 30 000 mm² (this is approximately 195 mm in diameter), then:

- force applied by the person on the disc = 80 kg × 9.81 m/s² = 784.8 N
- stress in the disc = 784.8 N/30 000 mm² = 0.0262 N/mm² = 26.2 kN/m²
- This stress acts along the direction of the applied load and is compressive.
- Strain is given by, stress divided by Young's Modulus, E.
- Therefore strain in the rubber disc = 0.0262/10 = 0.00262
- In the steel disc, strain = 0.0262/200 000 = 0.00000013

Strain values are usually very small and can be expressed as a percentage of the height by simply multiplying by 100. Since strain is the change in dimension divided by the original length, we can see that the rubber column would deform by about 0.8 mm whereas the steel column would deform by only 0.00004 mm!

Pressure

This is the term generally used when the force is acting uniformly in all directions such as the pressure due to air or a fluid. For example atmospheric pressure of 1000 mbars (millibars) is the same as 0.101 N/mm² (newton per millimetre squared). Therefore the air exerts a force of 0.101 N on every square millimetre of surface. This is the same as the weight due to a 10.1 g mass. Within a solid, the term, stress distribution is used instead of pressure.

In another example, when someone sits on a cushion, their weight causes a pressure within the cushion (Figures 11.9a, b, c and d). The cushion reacts so that the person feels a reaction force. This reaction force is distributed over the part of the person's body in contact with the cushion, causing a stress over that part of the body. When a thicker, softer cushion is used so that the person can 'sink into' the cushion more, more of the body surface is in contact with the cushion and so the stress on the body is reduced although the force is still the same. Hence the cushion will feel more comfortable.

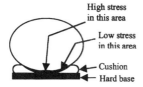

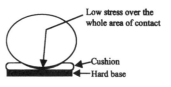

(a) - Body on a thin soft cushion: the weight is transferred to the hard base and so the seat feels uncomfortable.

(b) - Body on a thin relatively hard cushion: the weight is supported by the cushion and so the seat feels more comfortable than in (a).

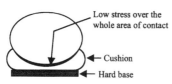

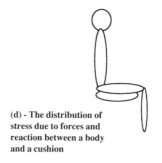

(c) - Body on a thick soft cushion: the cushion deforms around the body and so the weight is supported by an even larger area than (b) and so the seat feels even more comfortable than in case (b).

(d) - The distribution of stress due to forces and reaction between a body and a cushion

Figure 11.9 The distribution of stress due to forces and reaction between a body and a cushion.

Stresses are likely to be high when either one or both of the surfaces in contact with each other has a high rigidity or stiffness. When measured precisely, this is called the Young's Modulus, E (also called Elastic Modulus), of the material. It is a measure of the amount of deformation that results from a given applied load – the greater the deformation, the smaller the value of E.

A person wearing stiletto-heeled shoes will damage a floor more easily than a person of equal weight wearing 'flat' shoes although the weight or force applied on the floor is the same in each case. In the former case, the weight is transferred to the floor across a smaller area and so the stress (or force per unit area) is greater. This is referred to as the contact stress.

Atmospheric pressure can be expressed in many different units. It is often measured in terms of a column of mercury and so the standard atmospheric pressure, which is said to be equal to 1 bar, is also equal to 760 mm Hg (mm of mercury). The other possible ways of describing the same quantity are:

1 bar = 1000 mbar (millibars) = 101 kPa (kilopascals) = 0.101 MPa (megapascals) = 0.101 N/mm² (newton per millimetre squared) = 0.101 MN/m² (mega newton per metre squared)

Shear force and shear stress

Shear stress is the stress resulting when one body, attempting to slide past another, encounters resistance. The force could be a force of resistance due to friction. The effect of this shear force can be seen with a pack of cards. Squash the pack between two hands so that the palms are in contact with the external faces of the outer cards. Then apply a sliding force with one hand. The pack should deform as the cards, if new and smooth, slide past each other. Whereas under a pulling or pushing force, an object would change its volume, under a sliding force, the volume is unaffected. This can be seen with the cards since no card has deformed after sliding although they have moved relative to each other.

Consider what happens when a person is walking and the sole of the shoe comes into contact with the ground. As the heel strikes the ground, there is both a downwards force and a backward force. I am sure we have all experienced the effect of trying to take a normal step on an icy surface and finding that there is no grip there! This 'grip' is the resistance we need to project ourselves forward when walking. This grip is a shear force. This is different from the direct forces considered so far in that it acts parallel to the surface it is acting on. This is illustrated in Figure 11.10.

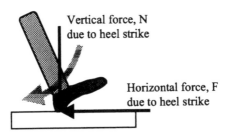

Figure 11.10 Shear force and direct force during walking.

If the area over which the heel makes contact with the ground is A, then the direct stress acting downwards would be N/A and the shear stress over the same area would be F/A. Notice that the direct and shear stresses are different by nature. The maximum shear force that can be applied on the surface without causing sliding depends on the nature of the surface and is defined by its coefficient of friction, μ (pronounced mu). This is the ratio of the friction force acting along the surface divided by the downward (or normal) force acting on the surface; that is,

$$\mu = F / N$$

We can rewrite this to give the maximum frictional force,

$$F = \mu N$$

When the heel strikes the ground, it is held in place while the leg rotates because the forces acting are in balance (or equilibrium). The downward force of the leg is balanced by an equal reaction force acting in the opposite (upward) direction. Similarly, the horizontal force applied by the heel is balanced by the frictional reaction force of the ground acting in the opposite direction. Note that, although vertical and horizontal forces are discussed in this example, it is equally true on an inclined surface. It is important to remember that in any situation, we identify the force acting at right angles to the surface as the normal force and the force acting parallel to the surface as shear force.

Now consider the cube of material in Figure 11.11a. The symbols for the forces and the area have been kept the same as in Figure 11.10. If the forces applied are on the top surface, then to maintain equilibrium, there has to be corresponding reactions of the same magnitude but in the opposite direction on the bottom surface.

Here there is a new problem. Although the forces are in equilibrium, the cube will still rotate clockwise because the forces F are separated by the height of the cube. It may not be obvious here but imagine that the forces were being generated by a circus artist standing on a sphere. As she slides her foot across the top of the sphere, there will be an equal frictional reaction generated on the ground in the opposite direction to compensate. However, the effect of the two forces would be to cause the sphere to rotate. This is precisely her intention since she is aiming to roll the sphere as she stands on it. In the same way, the cube could rotate because of the two horizontal forces.

Turning forces, moments and couples

To be precise, there are two equal and opposite forces where their lines of action are different. This action of a pair of equal and opposite forces with different, parallel lines of action, is called a couple (Figure 11.11b). The couple has a value equal to the

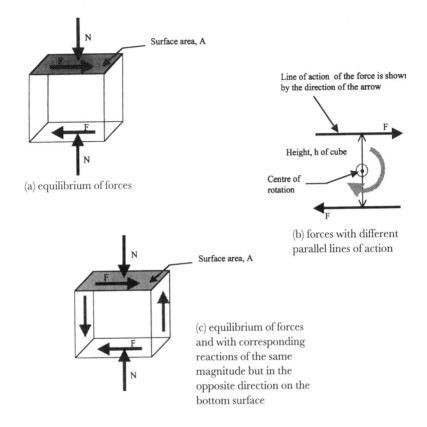

(a) equilibrium of forces

Line of action of the force is shown by the direction of the arrow

Height, h of cube

Centre of rotation

(b) forces with different parallel lines of action

Surface area, A

(c) equilibrium of forces and with corresponding reactions of the same magnitude but in the opposite direction on the bottom surface

Figure 11.11 Forces and moments in equilibrium.

magnitude of the force, F multiplied by the perpendicular distance between their lines of action, which in the example given above is the height of the cube. To prevent this rotation, a couple of equal magnitude and acting in the opposite direction, has to be applied. The easiest way to do this is to apply two forces each of magnitude, F on the other sides of the cube as indicated in Fig 11.11c.

The force in this case is a turning force since it has a tendency to cause rotation. The value of this turning force is called its moment. The moment is defined as the magnitude of the force multiplied by the perpendicular distance from the line of action of the force to the centre of rotation.

Torsion, torque

Whereas a couple acts in a plane, a lot of damage can be done during twisting along an axis. This is the result of actions such as a couple acting across planes. Imagine a man standing upright with arms outstretched (Figure 11.12). If he twists his body by rotating about his shoulders whilst maintaining his feet in one position, he has effectively applied a torque to his body. The value of the torque is the same as the moment of the force about his centre. At his feet, there will be an equal torque but in the opposite sense, due to the reaction of the ground.

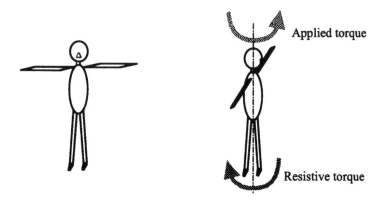

Figure 11.12 The effect of twisting force on a person.

Impact energy

When discussing the cushioning effect of a load, reference is often made to the sudden application of a load. For example, a falling person may suffer little injury if the fall is cushioned by a soft object. Let us call this a cushion again. A good cushion must satisfy four criteria:

1 In the same way as the cushion distributed the stress in Figure 11.9c, the stress must be distributed so that no part of the body feels a particularly high stress.
2 At the point of impact, the cushion must deform to allow the energy of the object to be transferred to the cushion.
3 The object that is moving, must also be brought to rest within the cushion; that is to say, the speed of the object must be allowed to decrease from its value at impact to zero before the object passes through the cushion.

4 The energy carried by the object must be absorbed by the cushion. Otherwise, the object will bounce back off the cushion. This is the impact energy.

The impact energy is equal to the difference in kinetic energy of the object and the cushion. If the cushion is stationary, it does not have any kinetic energy. The kinetic energy, W of the object is then given by,

$$W = \tfrac{1}{2}\, mv^2 \text{ (see Table 11.1)}$$

where m is the mass of the object and v is its velocity.
Examples:

1 If a glass jar is to fall onto a hard surface from a height of a metre for example, the energy carried by the jar is mostly reflected back into the jar (Figure 11.13). Just as a wave reaching the sea shore can be reflected back out, at the point of impact, a shock wave (or pressure wave) is sent out into the hard surface. Another wave is returned into the glass itself. Each of these can further reflect within each body. If the maximum stress resulting in the jar is greater than the failure stress for the glass, then the jar will shatter.

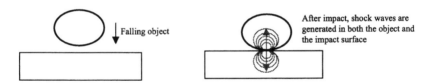

Figure 11.13 The generation of shock waves during impact.

2 If the glass jar is to fall onto a rubber or foamed polymer surface, a significant amount of the energy is absorbed as the latter deforms and so the stress developed in the glass will be reduced. The surface is said to be shock absorbent.
3 If a person is to fall over onto a concrete floor, most of the energy at impact will have to be absorbed by the person. Hence it is important that the stress is distributed over as large an area as possible. Therefore it is no surprise that a fit person, reaching out with their wrist to stop the fall is more likely break a bone than a drunken person falling uncontrollably.

When there is a sudden impact, shock waves are generated. This is a dynamic situation where the stress is changing with time. Consider another example, when the heel of a person strikes the ground during walking. The shock waves give rise to very high stresses for a short time (Figure 11.14a and b). If the person comes to a halt, the stress will decrease to a fixed value based on the weight of the person and the area of the feet supporting the weight (Figure 11.14c). This is a static load.

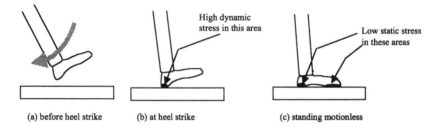

(a) before heel strike   (b) at heel strike   (c) standing motionless

Figure 11.14 Changing stress on the foot during walking.

Materials in the sole of a shoe, for example, are designed to cope with both the rapidly changing stresses during walking and the static stresses when standing still. Similarly, foams used for cushioning are also designed to distribute stress and absorb energy. When someone sits on a cushion, their weight causes a pressure within the cushion. The cushion reacts and causes a pressure over the ischial tuberosity.

The best way to absorb the energy may be by exploiting the properties of several materials. Layers of material may be put together forming either a coating or the bulk of the cushion, mattress or insole. For example, the fabric cover on a mattress is composed of a number of layers (waterproofing, knitted fabric, etc.) or the mattress may be formed from a number of layers of different materials, similarly for cushions and insoles. These layers may be referred to as laminations.

Viscoelastic or thermoelastic foams

Polymeric materials of the type used for the manufacture of foams may be viscoelastic. This means that they have a combination of characteristics that allow them to behave as partly viscous and partly elastic materials. They react differently according to the rate at which load is applied. For example, when falling onto a cushion, the rate of loading is high whereas when normally sitting, the rate is low. At the higher rate of loading, the material will give a greater resistance to deformation than at the lower rate encountered when sitting normally. In this way, viscoelastic foams are able to damp dynamic oscillations and give better stability to the user.

Resilience

Rubbers and foams also have resilience. This property measures the amount of elastic energy absorbed by the material. This energy is stored by the material and then returned when the load is removed. For example, the person sitting on a resilient cushion will gain a 'helping hand' in getting off the cushion as the cushion returns this energy. On the other hand, a very viscous material would absorb all the energy permanently when the load is applied and more effort has to be applied to get off such a cushion. They have a different role.

Foams made from predominantly viscous materials have low memory and do not instantly try to regain their original shape. They are often referred to as 'squidgy' foams and have little resilience. Such foams respond to body heat and form a 'well' around bony prominences. Because the foam does not struggle to regain shape, only doing so once pressure is removed, there is very little pressure placed under the patient.

The above definitions of mechanical load and shear can be used by the multidisciplinary team to establish the different foam requirements of individual patients. It is important that the selected foam can help to reduce both load and shear by redistributing the load and supporting the patient. For instance, the foam supporting feet would generally take 100 per cent of the body weight or load. The ischial tuberosities would take 75 per cent of the body weight. The bony prominences of a prone patient would take equally distributed loads along the length of the mattress. These differences must be taken into account when purchasing foams.

Nevertheless, selection of appropriate foam for each requirement is difficult. The most expensive of these requirements can be the mattress and cushion.

The following questions must be asked prior to purchase of any foam:

1 How can the aetiological mechanical stresses of pressure, friction and shear stress be reduced by the use of foam?
2 How can comfort be improved or maintained with the use of foam?
3 Is there a life-span for the foam equipment and devices?
4 What are the mechanical stresses that need to be considered in ulcer management?
5 What mechanical stresses will affect the lifespan of the material?
6 What factors need to be considered when purchasing a foam product?
7 What are the characteristics of foam products?
8 Why has Mrs Sands developed chronic wounds at the sites described?
9 What are the different clinical requirements that Mrs Sands has from the different foam products?

Static mattresses and cushions: making an informed choice

At some point every patient uses a foam mattress or cushion so purchasing the right internal foam and cover is a critically important decision if pressure ulcer prevention is to be achieved and cross-infection is to be avoided. Each manufacturer claims to provide the best product on the market, yet prices vary considerably and faced with vast amounts of technical and commercial information it is easy to suffer from an information overload. So how do you ensure that the decision you make is the right one?

A start is by clearly defining key criteria for what is required. This requires an informed decision-making process to identify the suitability of a particular mattress. It also requires careful examination of the evidence that manufacturers provide on their product. It is the responsibility of the manufacturer to provide evidence validating their claims. The section below explains some of the key criteria which may be helpful in the decision-making process as to which mattress to choose.

It doesn't matter what criteria selection is made, the question and answer must always the same, *yes*!

Yes. It's waterproof.
Yes. It will last for the length of the guarantee.
Yes. It's fire retardant. And so on . . .

There are two words for the purchaser to use when in discussion with the supplier: prove it.

CE marking is mandatory and it is a criminal offence to offer for sale products not meeting the essential requirements. Medical Device Directive 93/42/EEC covering medical devices has been mandatory since June 1998. Under CE marking regulations a manufacturer has a clear duty of care to see that medical devices are suitable, which means that they shall be safe and perform as stated by the manufacturer. In other words they must be able to prove the claims they make.

But foam is foam, or is it?

What sorts of foam are there?

Foam manufacture is a chemical process; the chemicals used to form the foam react and expand rather like a loaf of home-made bread. Chemicals including isocyanate and polyol are whipped by a large mixer and placed onto a moving conveyor and within a few minutes they form a foam loaf, which is then cut into usable lengths. They are cured for around 24 hours before they can be cut to shape.

The two principle properties, which vary, are density and hardness. Density means the weight of material within a stated volume and hardness refers to the amount of force required to compress the foam. Varying the amount of water and isocyanate within the process can control both density and hardness. Both these characteristics are verified using British Standard BS4443 parts 1 and 2, and these should be available for each batch produced.

Foams are manufactured for a multitude of purposes ranging from sponges for washing the car to high-quality contract mattresses. A sponge that is fine for washing the car would not be suitable for a mattress (i.e. 'fit for purpose'), as they have different properties. This variation can be just as pronounced within different mattresses and to help recognize the difference, look for the following:

1 Fatigue test: The foam is pounded for 16 hours with a 12 stone weight and retested for hardness and thickness in order to simulate 'in use' deterioration. It is then allocated a rating: L, A, S or V, L being suitable for padding, etc., A for general-purpose seating and S for standard NHS contract mattresses. If you want the mattress to last, settle for nothing less than V, that is Very severe use and again ask for the proof. Proof should be available in the

form of a certificate and contain the reference to BS4443 Part 5.

2 Compression test and wet compression test: Here samples are placed between two plates, compressed and then placed in differing environments, for example at an incline of 70° for 22 hours, this artificially ages the foam and the tests are repeated to gauge their performance after a long period of use. Comparing independent results is an excellent tool.

Most covers are made of polyurethane, but what are the different types of covers? All hospital healthcare workers are aware that beds move between wards and units. Therefore, in hospital, quality, pressure-reducing/relieving mattresses are needed throughout the whole of the care unit. In contrast, in nursing homes and the community, the choice of mattress and cover type can be individualized to the patient.

Most covers are manufactured using the Transfer coating method rather than the Direct coating method, so how is this done? Transfer coated fabrics allow a waterproof fabric to be produced which maintains its stretch and drape. Also, unlike direct coated fabrics, in a transfer coating process a uniform layer of the polyurethane is produced prior to its adhesion to the fabric ensuring that the polyurethane layer is of even thickness across the fabric.

A measured amount of polyurethane is first applied to paper on a conveyor system. Once cooled a second or intercoat is applied in the same manner, this is designed to protect against any fibre penetration and any possible defects in the topcoat. At the third stage a polyurethane adhesive is applied before the fabric is finally introduced and the paper removed.

Here are some of the desirable features that a good cover should have:

1 Two-way or multi-stretch properties balanced to the end use, so as not to modify the properties of the support system being covered.
2 Resistance to abrasion damage: the material is tested to BS5690. It is particularly important is to find out how the fabric performed after the abrasion test.
3 Water vapour permeability: how can you keep water out of the mattress foam inner, but let moisture escape from the skin's surface? This is achieved via one of two methods, in essence by having holes that are big enough to let vapour through but not

water or by introducing a hydrophilic material, which attracts moisture but is a barrier to liquid.

4   There are two methods of test for vapour permeability: the Paynes cup method and BS7209. Ask to see the results.
5   Water penetration: the cover material should tested under high water pressure, in excess of 120 kPa without letting in water. The test certificate should clarify how waterproof it is, preferably to BS5455, for the life expectancy of the cover.
6   Resistance to microbiological attack: the polyurethane should contain some form of anti-biological element.

So what criteria can be applied? The list is endless but there are a few identified key points that narrow the choice without compromising the quality. In no particular order of importance, they are:

• Longevity: You need to know the mattress is going to last, so what do you look for? First simplicity and clarity in a warranty and a guarantee that both foam *and* cover will last at least three years. You need then to establish confidence that it's likely to last beyond that and the very best indicator is a proven track record. Beyond that, ask for certification regarding the British Standards.
• Maximum contour capabilities: Contouring the foam reduces tissue compression, reduces surface tension and ultimately the ability of the foam to push back against the bony prominence. The cells operate individually to respond to shearing forces, effectively reducing pressure and mechanical stress.
• Pressure mapping results: Pressure mapping is a method of measuring interface pressure using a computer, and may be considered to be more sophisticated in its approach than ordinary pressure monitors. Clients are positioned over a sheet of sensors, allowing measurement of a wide surface area. In addition to pressure, readings such as peak pressures can be determined in addition to force versus time and other similar measurements. No pressure measuring tool will be entirely accurate, as they cannot conform exactly to the skin (Clark 1994). Also, as it is estimated that the majority of the pressure experienced is concentrated deep within the tissues (McClemont 1984), it must be accepted that pressure measuring devices can only provide an estimate of the pressures being exerted on the tissues. Pressure mapping devices do not necessarily indicate

the client's degree of risk, as some clients can withstand higher pressures without tissue breakdown, whilst others can sustain tissue damage (Medical Devices Agency 1997a).

Care should be taken because with manipulation of the sensitivity scale it is very easy to create a poster, photograph or any other marketing literature demonstrating the 'ours against theirs' with bias to the manufacturer. This bias can be assessed as most manufacturers should be able to demonstrate in person the capabilities of individual mattresses. A good manufacturer, if asked to do so, will demonstrate on site and with independent models. Remember that pressure mapping is an indication only, it is a prelude to the real evidence of clinical trials.

- Fire retardancy: An absolute minefield, it needn't be so confusing. Here are a few simple guidelines to follow:

1 A mattress should be tested to BS7177:1996.
2 Importantly the mattress should be tested on the top *and* the bottom to at least crib 5.
3 If it says it is tested to BS6807:1996, then that's fine as long it is top and bottom.
4 The supplier should supply the certificate proving the test.
5 The test should be carried out by an independent test house, ideally UKAS accredited.
6 There are no guidelines as to the time between tests. However, common sense must prevail, remembering the duty of care. The exact requirements for compliance are set by each care unit, for example, a psychiatric unit might insist that the mattresses comply with a crib 7 test.

- Strike-through: Ask the following questions:

1 Has possible leakage through the zip been designed out? In other words, is there a flap over the zip and is the zip welded?
2 Has possible leakage through the seams been designed out; that is, have the seams been welded?
3 Has the manufacturer incorporated methods to reduce damage by bed cradles?
4 Has the manufacturer designed out the need to allow a mattress to dry before turning over?

5   Does the manufacturer follow the guidelines recommended by the NHS concerning 'white backed cover' for the easy identification of stains? Some covers are black inside and this masks any strike-through that may occur.
6   Has the manual handling issue been addressed to reduce the requirement to flip the mattress?

Using the above information can ensure that the right choice is made when deciding which mattress to buy. Remember to collate the evidence, let the supplier do the work for you, let them validate the claims they make and let them address the issues that are important to you and your patient.

'Value for money' is quality you can quantify!

Rationale for selection of the various foam devices for Mrs Sands

Nursing

As Mrs Sands refuses an alternating air mattress it is essential to select an appropriate pressure-reducing or redistributing foam mattress. It is also important to reposition Mrs Sands at regular intervals to avoid overloading tissues and inhibit ischaemic changes. The load needs to be evenly redistributed to minimize the high pressures found on bony prominences. Mrs Sands will need to be repositioned according to the clinical needs identified through assessment. Blanching erythema and leg oedema over the feet influence repositioning requirements, although the 30° tilt would be appropriate generally (see Chapter 9). This is particularly important following CVA as incorrect positioning and incorrectly placed limbs can lead to tissue damage through shearing and friction. Assessment findings will dictate the type of mattress and cushion she requires, however, a more detailed discussion on assessment and mattress selection is given below. Mrs Sands's nutritional levels do not cause particular concern, although she requires rehydration. Diabetes is a concern, however, as unstable glucose levels can lead to poor clinical outcomes and increase potential of clinical infection.

An air mattress would offer pressure relief over a set period, whereas a foam mattress offers pressure reduction. Pressure relief is achieved by alternating inflation and deflation of the cells in the air mattress. On deflation of a cell, the contact area is given a relief of pressure for 6–10 minutes. The inflated cells then deflate and the next small area of tissue is left without load. The area of tissue with reduced load will be the size of the individual cells, which vary with mattress type. Constant low pressure has been shown to cause marked tissue damage in rats, therefore static redistribution of load is not fully effective without regular repositioning. During the experiments undertaken by Kosiak 1961, the rats with least tissue damage had been exposed to alternating pressure. Pressure reduction is where the load is constant and is generally measured against a NHS Kings Fund contract mattress. However, the NHS mattress is known to generate loads of up to 130-150 mmHg (Medical Devices Directorate 1993), whereas modern pressure-reducing foams generally offer an average reduction in load of 40 per cent. When a patient is prone, the load is taken over a larger surface area and therefore a foam mattress, with a plan of regular repositioning, would meet Mrs Sands's needs, particularly as she refuses to use an air mattress. Nevertheless, when reclining in bed, the tissues of her heels, sacrum and ischial tuberosities are at increased risk of tissue damage from pressure, friction and shear stresses. The tissue maceration following faecal incontinence will add to this risk.

The composition of the covering material could affect the characteristics of the foam mattress and therefore needs to be selected to assist with redistributing the load. For example, the NHS Kings Fund contract mattress has a polyurethane vinyl cover, which is deliberately smaller than the foam core, so that once in place it forms a firm protective cover for the mattress and prevents bony prominences from sinking into the foam, preventing redistribution of load. The cover then functions almost like a drum where objects contacting its surface bounce off. This covering material also does not allow evaporation of perspiration, thereby increasing moisture at the contact surface. This increases the risk of pressure sore development through an increase in friction and shear stresses (Torrance 1983), and provides a good pathogen culture medium. Conversely, modern material covers for mattresses are vapour permeable and have multidirectional stretch. The multidirectional stretch allows bony prominences to sink into the soft foam below, which redistributes the load onto adjacent tissues. These modern materials are also vapour permeable and permit perspiration evaporation, thus maintaining the skin surface microenvironment at 'normal' levels. To maintain its flexibility and pliability, skin needs about 10–20 per cent water content in the stratum corneum (Potts et al. 1985), so it is inappropriate to dry the skin totally.

Mrs Sands needs a soft but supportive foam for her mattress to redistribute load away from her sacrum, trochanter, heels, shoulders, knees and ankles when lying down. However, when sitting in bed then pressure will need redistribution from ischial tuberosities and heels. To provide the support and softness required, mattresses are often produced in layers of different density foams. The edge of the mattress needs to be fairly firm to prevent Mrs Sands rolling out of bed and to allow her to easily lever herself to a standing position from a sitting position. If the selection of foam is appropriate for her requirements, and repositioning and continued assessment is part of the nursing plan, it is unlikely that tissue damage would occur.

Occupational therapy

The qualities of foam in a cushion will be somewhat dependent on the supporting surface provided by the armchair or wheelchair. For example, a wheelchair canvas will easily hammock, causing cushions to become rounded in shape and reducing the ability of the both ischial tuberosities to be supported at the same time, thus overloading one site and increasing risk of pressure sore development. Overloading of one ischial tuberosity is referred to as a pelvic obliquity. If this position is not redressed, a resultant scoliosis will occur, which may increase the need for bespoke seating. An armchair with rubber webbing that has deteriorated (sagged, or snapped) will cause a similar problem. Therefore, cushions used in wheelchairs normally require a rigid base. The rigidity can be provided by the use of plywood, however, it has been documented that wood will significantly increase interface pressures on the cushion (Medical Devices Agency 1997a).

As Mrs Sands has a posterior pelvic tilt it is likely that a large portion of her thighs will no longer be supported, increasing interface pressures under the ischial tuberosities and inappropriately loading the sacrum. Furthermore it is likely that a pressure ulcer will develop under the right buttock due to the existing pelvic obliquity, although, as it has been determined flexible, this can be addressed.

She will require a cushion that will be firm enough to support her posture in the most symmetrical way possible, which can realign her ischial tuberosities but which is soft enough to provide pressure reduction. It is unlikely that the use of foam alone will meet Mrs Sands's needs. Mrs Sands required a specialized cushion, which accommodated the pelvis in a fixed posterior pelvic tilt whilst providing the sacrum with pressure reduction and redistribution of load. It also needed to reduce the pelvic obliquity on the right side, thus inhibiting pelvic rotation on the left side, and allowing realignment of the legs. Reduction of the pelvic obliquity will also assist with correcting the scoliosis to some extent, but a specialized foam backrest was also required to provide postural support and correct the scoliosis.

In a sitting position a smaller surface area of the body contacts the supporting surface in comparison to lying down, and this will result in much higher interface pressures as the load is not shared elsewhere. Seventy-five per cent of the body weight must be supported by the thighs and ischial tuberosities and so it is essential that any cushion provision is the correct size (Collins 2001a). The cushion must be large enough to accommodate the length and width of the buttocks and thighs. A gap is needed behind the back of the knees of 2 cm in order to prevent compression of the popliteal fossa. This is important to blood flow, to prevent damage to the popliteal nerve, and to allow the knees to rest at 90° angle. This angle is necessary to prevent stretching of the hamstrings, to allow a more even loading of the buttocks and thighs to minimize point loading and potential heel ulcer formation, and will allow the feet to rest flat on the floor. If the feet are flat on the floor, they will take some of the body weight whilst sitting, which will not occur if there is asymmetry in the seated position, or if the body has slid down in the chair. The feet in the correct position will take 19 per cent of the body weight, reducing the load on the ischial tuberosities.

Ongoing assessment, utilizing Mrs Sands's comments, is necessary to ensure her comfort. It is crucial that Mrs Sands's posture is improved to increase symmetry and thereby to redistribute the load. It would also improve the cosmetic appearance of her position. At the same time, the cushion must provide adequate stability in order to enhance her function. Most importantly it must be comfortable. People frequently need to try several cushions before they identify the most suitable and comfortable one for them, and this is always negotiated with the therapist. Different materials can be used in the cushion to achieve different functions. The level of pressure ulcer risk will determine whether a rigid base foam is used in combination with a softer body contact foam as in the case of a patient with low risk. Mrs Sands, however, requires a contoured cushion, which provides her with stability and positioning. Therefore a more rigid, closed-cell foam was a more suitable base foam for this need. However, due to her complex physical condition, she will require maximum pressure redistribution and it is unlikely that this can be offered by foam, particularly when placed on top of a rigid, closed-cell foam base. Therefore a cushion that had a rigid, closed-cell base with a corresponding pressure-reducing fluid pad was selected, in order to reduce interface pressures at the body's contact surface.

The cushion cover will require the same properties as that for a mattress (see above), but with two exceptions. Firstly the cushion base needs to inhibit movement of the cushion on top of the seat surface. This can be achieved either by a non-slip surface or by the use of velcro or ties. Secondly, at this present time, it is not possible to obtain a chair upholstery material, which is vapour permeable, multi- or two-way stretch, waterproof and which can withstand continuous day-to-day use. (Mattresses do withstand the use as a sheet is always placed between the patient and the mattress cover.) In a cushion, the main problem with a vinyl covering is the moisture build-up at the contact interface and sliding causing friction and shear stresses, which predispose to pressure ulcer development.

Podiatry

Complications in diabetes can lead to amputation (Edmonds and Foster 2000). Risk of amputation can be lessened by reducing load over the stress points at the foot or ground interface and maintaining tissues in a viable state (e.g. minimize callus formation, inhibit skin maceration, use of appropriate topical preparations). It may be appropriate for an insole to be manufactured to off-load and cushion the ulcer site, and to provide shock absorption (see glossary at the end of this chapter) and thermal insulation. During locomotion, other mechanical stresses affect the foot and it may be necessary to select insole materials capable of reducing these (i.e. pressure (force/area), torsion, shear, friction and tension). The style and fit of footwear (socks, shoes, slippers) need checking for materials used and space available for orthoses (insoles).

It is necessary to keep Mrs Sands independent within the confines of wheelchair use. She will need to be ambulant moving from her wheelchair for daily activities. Non-enzymatic glycation of tissues can occur in diabetes (Jude and Boulton 1998, Hashmi 2000), making tissues stiffer, so it is worthwhile considering selection of materials and footwear to compensate for tissue changes in the foot. The aim of this form of management is to spread load from a point source to share this over a larger surface area, and to reduce magnitude and duration of impact against the ground. A foam material will be needed to compensate for reduced shock absorption in the soft tissues in the early phase of contact with the ground. This foam will also need to be firm enough to provide a fairly resistant surface to push off against at toe-off, otherwise it becomes very tiring to walk. Any abnormal bony/soft tissue projections will need to be accommodated by the insole to redistribute load away from that one small site and to share the load with adjacent tissues. This can be achieved by cutting a shape into the foam material around the site of increased load. Sometimes use of layers of different density foams (see glossary) can achieve a similar effect. Alternatively, a button of a low/light density foam can be inserted into the cut out shape. All of these methods allow change in the rate of loading of the foot tissues and increase the area of contact, thus minimizing the potential for ulcer development. However, at the sites of high loading the foam material can bottom-out quickly (see glossary).

Mrs Sands will need insoles for both feet, but it is essential to check she has sufficient room in her footwear, otherwise the additional bulk of material will cause ischaemic changes. The aim of insoles for Mrs Sands is to accommodate her foot shape thereby providing increased comfort and preventing further damage, but not to change structure or function. Although Mrs Sands will perceive little change in comfort because she has peripheral sensory neuropathy, the insoles will reduce the risk of neuropathic ulceration. She will need insoles made of layers of foams that have different properties, which will allow some shock absorption on contact, redistribution of load during stance, and sufficient rigidity to allow efficient toe-off. The firmer foam will need a shape cut or moulded into it to accommodate the prominent second metatarsal head to redistribute load away from this area and share this with adjacent structures. The most superficial layer may be constructed from a low/light density thermoplastic foam material, which will provide some insulation from extremes of temperature. Body weight, and body heat will cause compression of this thermoplastic foam at sites of increased mechanical stress under the bony and soft tissue prominences, the material will conform to all contacting surfaces, thus ensuring a more uniform loading of the foot.

The covering material must allow multidirectional stretch and be robust enough to withstand friction and shear without changing the properties of the foams underneath and needs to be washable. It is likely that Mrs Sands has only been supplied with one pair of insoles, so they have to be robust enough to be transferred from shoe to shoe, providing that they fit each footwear type. Because there is often a point load on the insole material, the life expectancy of the foam is often short. After issue and a follow-up assessment, the insoles need to be checked at least every six weeks for bottoming out, and to ascertain if they are causing increased loading on other sites. Ideally Mrs Sands or her carer should check her feet frequently (daily) for signs of abnormality, and she will need to attend for regular checks (Hutchinson et al. 2000).

Glossary

This glossary explains a number of terms introduced in the above example.

Load
Force applied by an object on another object (e.g. weight of the patient on a mattress, cushion, insole).

Force is mass × acceleration (Newton's second law). For example, a person standing on the floor applies a force on the floor that is equal to the mass of the patient × acceleration due to gravity. In this case there is no actual movement because the floor applies an equal and opposite force.

Any mass under an applied force will accelerate unless acted on by an equal and opposite force (called reaction).

Pressure or stress
This is the effect of a load on a given area (surface area). Pressure = force / area supporting the force.

Pressure is used when applied over a volume. For example, when someone sits on a cushion their weight (load) causes a pressure on the cushion. The cushion reacts and causes a pressure over the ischial tuberosity. The tissue of the ischial tuberosity is considered under stress.

With use of a thick cushion, the pressure of the body is lower as force acts over a larger area (the cushion reaction is over a larger area). The body tissues respond.

A measurement of pressure is mm Hg. It cannot be applied directly to load as load is usually measured in N pressure × area. Pascals are a better measure as this measures stress or pressure (force/area). For example, air pressure is 760 mmHg = 1 bar = 1.01 kPa (kilo pascals).

Lamination
This is where layers are put together; they may form a coating or the bulk of the cushion, mattress or insole. In other words, the fabric cover on a mattress is composed of a number of layers (waterproofing, knitted fabric, etc.) or the mattress may be formed from a number of layers of different materials, similarly for cushions and insoles.

Acceleration
This is the gradual change of speed of an object. The rate of change of speed, e.g. if a person was to slip and fall, they suddenly feel the effect of acceleration due to gravity, their speed increases from zero to a higher speed. The speed always changes as they fall.

Most foams are viscoelastic
Different foams deform at different rates with different relaxation times for each foam type. Viscoelastic foam damps oscillations following full loading.

Cushioning
A cushioning material is one which very quickly deforms to match the surface contours of the object forced onto it. Thus the contact surface is high and the energy of the object is transferred to the cushion and absorbed.

Shock absorption
This is the amount of shock waves that the surface can absorb. For instance, a soft, dense foam will absorb and dissipate shock whereas a hard surface will not. A person falling hard onto foam may not feel it as the shock dissipates into the foam. However, a person falling onto the hard ground will absorb the shock into their own body. This term is the technical equivalent of cushioning.

Stress distribution
This refers to the showing of stress due to an applied load. By having a material that conforms to the contact surface, the load is shared over a larger area, thus reducing stress.

Shear
Pure shear stress is where the deformation takes place at right angles to the direction of application of the load, as opposed to direct stress where the deformation occurs in the direction of the applied load. Shear stress acts within a plane.

Resilience
This is the ability to absorb elastic energy, energy that is returned when the load is removed.

Viscoelastic or thermoelastic foams
These foams have low memory and do not instantly try to regain their original shape. They are often referred to as 'squidgy' foams. They also respond to body heat and form a 'well' around bony prominences. Because the foam does not struggle to regain shape, there is very little pressure placed under the patient.

Conclusion

The use of foam is an important part of overall care for patients whose tissues are at risk of developing of chronic wounds. The mechanical stresses of pressure, shear and friction are implicated in the development of pressure ulcers. Foam materials are useful for reducing these stresses and for cushioning, shock absorption (depending on thickness of the material and area of coverage) and thermal insulation, but they need to be selected as 'horses for courses' or fitness for purpose. The covering material also needs to be considered as this will affect the contact surface microenvironment and may affect the characteristics of the foams. Different professions, not only clinically, but also engineering and manufacturing, have a common need for knowledge of these materials and terms used. The case example of Mrs Sands highlights the importance of multi-professional involvement, working with the patient and the need for understanding the terminology.

CHAPTER 12

The process of audit and research in tissue viability

The concept of evidence-based practice has a basic rational and sensible grounding. The concept is one of uniformity of practice with each professional aware of good practice and with a commitment to fulfilling and supporting standards, offering the best quality care to all patients and the elimination of variations in practice (Humphries 1998). In order to provide a pathway toward evidence-based practice the Government has introduced a process of clinical governance (discussed later in this chapter) and has set two groups the task of monitoring practice. The two groups are the National Institute for Clinical Excellence (NICE) and the Commission for Health Improvement (CHI). To enable audit of standards, first the standards must be decided and this is achieved through a process known as benchmarking.

Benchmarking in tissue viability

Benchmarking is a method of identifying the best nursing provisions within a ward department, measured along a qualitative continuum (Bland 2000). However, to enable benchmarking to become a way of life for all healthcare professionals, there needs to be a consensus on practice issues and, at present, there is no consensus. Purvis (1996) carried out an audit which identified that, out of 331 patients with leg ulcers, 278 treatment variations were used.

Following the audit, Purvis recommended that a standardized approach should be adopted as, without a standardized approach, variations in practice could lead to poor practice with clinically ineffectual and costly care.

Kop (2000) suggested there are two main reasons for practice variations; there is no agreed standard of best practice, which leaves practitioners to choose what they believe to be the most appropriate treatment; and best practice has been agreed, but practitioners may not be aware of it.

To address the problems associated with practice variations, the Government introduced a new initiative, the Essence of Care: Patient-focused Benchmarking for Healthcare Practitioners, which sets out a tool to advance the clinical governance agenda and to improve the eight fundamentals of care. These eight fundamentals involve personal and oral hygiene, nutrition and continence (Casteldine 2001). The chief nurse's office produced a benchmarking 'toolkit', which (among other issues) aims to provide practitioners with guidance in treatment, management and prevention of wounds.

There are seven phases of benchmarking:

1 Agree area of practice: sharing evidence-based good practice with others.
2 Establish a comparison group with consumer representation: membership would consist of those in clinical practice or with the power to affect patient care. This group will enable adequate resources to be planned for.
3 Agreeing best practice: discuss and agree what evidence of practice provides a basis for advising care.
4 Scoring and rescoring: practioners score the benchmark and offer rationale for the score. This score is based on evidence of good practice.
5 Compare and share: each member compares her own scores and offers rationale for where the development effort should be placed
6 Action: the group action plan is built into the ward development plan. This is ongoing – assessed and redeveloped at regular periods
7 Dissemination: the progress in the ward development would be shared/disseminated with colleagues

Most guideline development process involves a 'consensus panel' (Grimshaw 1995) and the process of benchmarking relies on just such a consensus group. The above phases require that one person becomes 'leader' of the benchmark process, organizing meetings of the consensus panel and driving forward the process of identifying areas of best practice and distributing the information to others. The discussion in the group provides information and expertise and offers 'ownership' in the process of standardizing practice. The group responsible for developing the benchmark process, would require expert support through structured and critical literature reviews.

Benchmarking is considered the way forward for healthcare professionals but is time consuming and this makes the process difficult. However, benchmarking will safeguard high standards, creating a clinical environment where excellent clinical care can flourish (Bland 2000).

Once the benchmark is set, audit is the natural process that follows.

Research and audit

Research and audit are closely linked and it is often difficult to decide whether it is a research project or an audit that is being undertaken. However, the two are distinctly different in many ways with research asking how practice can be changed or 'what would happen if'? Research will 'take chances' providing it is ethically acceptable; audit, however, will not as it investigates present clinical practice and asks the question 'is this best clinical practice?' Whereas research will direct the practitioner to new and better methods of care – audit will direct the practitioner into providing better methods of care based on the present methods. Barton and Thompson (1992) define this as follows: 'Research practice asks "what should be done" or "what is best clinical practice" whereas audit asks "has it been done?" and "has best clinical practice been achieved locally?"'

Research must be conducted within the framework of specific aims and objectives (Bader 1998). Bader writes, 'As in any research, it is important to progress in directions of potential promise and be willing to rethink areas and working hypotheses which are not proving useful. At all times, the clinical problem must be kept in mind'. An experienced researcher may easily achieve this but when research is undertaken by the inexperienced professional, it is more difficult to deviate from the original research proposal. Time constraints and fear of making mistakes can compel the researcher to continue, even when it is obvious that the data are not providing the required answers.

Technology is advancing human existence and people, who would not have survived their illness 10 years ago, are now living longer due to the provision of life-saving/extending resources and drugs. Three points arise from this:

1 Increasing amounts of people are attending hospital to utilize the resources or to be given the drugs.
2 Increasing amounts of people are living longer and are more likely to use hospital facilities.
3 Higher numbers of patients with acute and increasingly complex illnesses can lead to escalating incidences of pressure ulcers.

The first two issues lead to increasing numbers of people passing through the hospital system and this has an impact on bed management. Patients with hospital-acquired pressure ulcers remain in acute wards five days longer than those without development of pressure ulcers (Collins 1998b) and this has a high implication for acute bed management and reduces quality care by causing pain and distress for the patient. Hibbs (1987) made a claim that pressure ulcers are 95 per cent preventable. If that is an accurate statement then the question must be posed, why are pressure ulcers costing the National Health Service £1000 million per year (Bader 1990a) and why are pressure ulcers still occurring? The only way to answer this question is through the use of audit.

Audit

Audit can be amazingly simple to perform and yet can make immense changes to clinical practice or even give reassurance that quality care is of a high standard. There are many frameworks that can be used in setting standards and forming audits although this chapter does not attempt to explain the processes involved or to introduce the tools that promote audit. The aim of this section is to assist the practitioner in developing audit in a simple and easily applied way. The audit mechanism can be used to develop pressure ulcer prevention in hospital or community and will support the Tissue Viability Nurse Specialist with large audit or the nurse on a ward with local audit. The audit tool follows a design developed within the Eastbourne Trust and has been assessed and evaluated for its use in changing practice and developing education needs within the trust.

Pressure ulcer formation can be an excellent indicator of quality care within a hospital or community. High incidence or prevalence of pressure ulcers demonstrates that prevention is not high priority within that area. Nevertheless, high incidence does not indicate (necessarily) that nursing care is of low standard. Nurses have traditionally taken the blame for the formation of pressure ulcers; many years ago, this may have been true when nursing was a popular career and there were few staff shortages. At that time, the ratio of nurses to patients was sufficiently high to allow time for the repositioning of patients (when required) and, in addition, the nurses were not tied to the mass of technology that is faced now in clinical practice. Today we are more aware of how pressure ulcers may be prevented and we understand that 'two-hourly-turns' can never be enough for those moribund patients who would develop pressure ulcers even if turned hourly. Two hours was always too short a time for those patients in pain or distress and who required to be left in peace. Excellent provision of resources will prevent pressure ulcers and will offer the patient increased comfort. How do we know that this is so? Through audit!

Clinical governance

Clinical governance is to offer national regulation of practice and will be supported through the National Institute for Clinical Excellence (NICE). The Royal College of Nursing (1998) defined clinical governance as 'A framework which helps all clinicians, including nurses, to improve quality care and safeguard standards of care continuously'.

NICE is an academic institute set up to identify the best clinical evidence and to develop recommendations for its use (McClarey 2000). The Commission for Health Improvement (CHI) was introduced at the same time as NICE and both bodies are part of clinical governance. Their role is to promote or guide by the following means:

* dissemination of information;
* overseeing risk management;

- reviewing research findings;
- auditing methodology;
- ensuring audit is undertaken in the clinical area;
- listening to patients' views;
- encouraging development of pathways of care;
- clinical supervision;
- overseeing continuing education;
- monitoring current practice;
- team building;
- disseminating guidelines;
- ensuring safe standards are achieved;
- supporting health professionals in delivering clinical governance.

Clinical governance is a framework, which can be used to build improved standards of care within the NHS and will affect all aspects of care by ensuring personal responsibility and accountability from all clinicians and managers. The process will also ensure that clinicians of all grades will be free to air concerns and will have opportunities to make decisions and enable them to present their views.

Audit is an essential part of the process as NICE and CHI will use the results of audit to produce baselines and provide comparisons between different trusts. This will ensure that each NHS employee will be working toward achieving the highest standard possible. Professionals will be made to answer for their methods of treatment as all treatments become standardized. The aim of clinical governance is to standardize in order to promote good practice. The doctor or nurse who uses outmoded and unproven methods will be made to answer for their actions. If they are unable to offer satisfactory explanations, they will be expected to adapt to proven researched methods used in other areas.

The process of audit

Pressure ulcers will develop on patients who are nursed on mattresses that are inappropriate for the risk of pressure ulcers and when pressure is unrelieved for long periods of time. Nurses generally strive to place patients on an appropriate mattress, one that relieves or reduces pressure but access to this equipment relies on whims of the management, whether they see pressure ulcer prevention as a priority and provide money for purchase and hire, or whether they give it low priority. Without the audit process, complaining about lack of resources would be a meaningless exercise, with managers refusing to purchase required equipment without the proof of clinical effectiveness. Therefore, the first consideration in any pressure ulcer audit is a baseline with an appreciation of the overall problem of:

- how many pressure ulcers are within the hospital, nursing home or community?
- are pressure ulcers hospital-acquired or non-hospital-acquired?
- what are the grades of pressure ulcers?
- which speciality has the highest incidence of pressure ulcers?
- what is unique about that particular speciality that produces the highest incidence?
- what can be done, generally, to prevent pressure ulcer occurrence?
- what type of mattress is the 'at risk' patient nursed on and is it appropriate?
- what types of mattresses are there within the trust?
- are those mattresses in good condition or wearing out?
- what type of chair and/or cushion does the patient sit on during the day?
- how many air mattresses are owned by the trust and does that match with the high risk scores of patients. i.e. are there 100 patients with a risk score that is high but only 50 air mattresses (that may indicate the need to purchase 50 more air mattresses)?

At the same time, a baseline of nurses' educational needs in pressure ulcer prevention can be useful.

The following work will demonstrate how an audit tool can be developed. The suggested audit tool (Figures 12.1 and 12.2) is specifically for a hospital setting but could be adapted for nursing homes or community settings.

The audit tool will be developed using five stages. Each stage will develop the audit and refine it until the results offer a pathway of progress to the auditor. Each audit will indicate where problems may be found and the auditor can decide on how to overcome those problems. The second audit (3–6 months later) would demonstrate whether the measures (applied following audit one and used to overcome the identified problems) have achieved success in reducing the pressure ulcer incidence. By using this action research or problem solving approach, there will be a rolling strategy for reducing incidence of pressure ulcers.

Hospital		Patient information label	

Pressure sore audit form for the individual patient

WARD		INVESTIGATOR		BED IDENTIFICATION	

SITE OF SORE (Code listed below)				
Sore present on admission (Y/N)				

If sore not present on admission, when was it first noted.				
1–4 days				
5–6 days				
< 7days				
Not known				

How long established?				
< 7days				
< 28 days				
2–3 months				
3–12 months				
< 12 months				

Grade of sore				

Sore coding							
Sacrum	01		Natal cleft	02		Ischial tuberosity	03
Trochanter	04		Heel	05		Elbow	06
Ankle	07		Other	08			09

Figure 12.1 Hospital audit tool.

Name of nursing home . . . . Room . . . . Investigator . . . . Date							
BED IDENTIFIER							
BED OCCUPIED (Y/N)							
PATIENT AGE							
GENDER (M/F)							
DATE ADMITTED							
RISK ASSESSMENT SCORE							
MATTRESS TYPE (1/2/3/4)							
CONDITION OF MATTRESS							
REPLACEMENT DATE IF BO							
ADDITIONAL SUPPORT							
CUSHION TYPE (A/B/C)							
CHAIR TYPE (A/B/C)							
NUMBER PRESSURE ULCERS							
GRADE OF ULCER							

Please give the date or "N" if the mattress has 'bottomed-out' (BO) but not replaced on date of audit.

Figure 12.2 Nursing home audit tool.

Stage 1: Lead-nurses

Nurse education is the most important component of the problem solving process. However, there is difficulty in hospitals with teaching the entire workforce. Hospitals are a mobile workforce with agency nurses and staff changes ensuring that teaching is a bottomless pit. The most sensible way of developing nurse education is by dissemination or the 'cascade' system where one nurse from each ward is taught a subject and that nurse passes that knowledge to all other nurses on her or his ward. This system of lead-nurses, is effective providing the nurse is happy to pass on the knowledge.

The system of lead-nurses is particularly effective in audit. Each lead-nurse is educated in the audit requirements and in identification of pressure ulcers and mattress types. This nurse is then totally responsible for completing the audit on the appointed day and for the identification of pressure ulcers.

Stage 2: Introducing clinical audit

Undertaking an audit can be a lonely business. An important element of any audit, and one that can remove the isolation of the audit process, is the involvement of the Clinical Audit Team (CAT). These teams are expert at producing audits and know the process. They can:

- assist in educating the lead-nurses;
- produce the data collecting forms required for the audit;
- advise the auditor on how to organize the audit;
- assist with analyzing the data;
- assist with writing the final report;
- advise on the development of the next audit.

Therefore, forming a partnership with CAT is beneficial and reassuring and will promote the audit process.

Stage 3: Baseline

The first audit will be difficult and will consume an enormous amount of time and commitment from all those taking part in developing the audit tool. The organizer of the audit could approach all concerned managers to ask for support, particularly with free time for lead-nurses who should be supernumerary on the day of the audit. Every ward would be advised of the date of the audit and who will be completing the audit on that particular ward.

The audit will cover a 12-hour period over one day and would include all hospital in-patients present between 12 midnight on day one and 12 midnight on day two. The supernumerary nurse will begin at bed one and will check every patient's pressure areas for redness or breaks in the skin and will record the findings on the data form (Figure 12.1). The primary data collector will be informed and they will check the pressure areas for grades of ulcer, etc. Only one or two nurses should be allowed to identify grades to ensure accuracy of grading identification as the greater the number of nurses involved, the greater the potential for diluting the grading results (identification may differ between the nurses).

The mattress will be checked for condition as follows:

- Is there a brown patch in the centre? If yes, then there is an indication that the cover has delaminated allowing the entry of body fluids into the foam. The mattress must be opened and the foam checked. Any staining of the foam and the mattress must be condemned.
- Join the hands together into a fist and press into the mattress where the patient sits. If the metal bed-base can be felt then the mattress must be condemned.
- Any tears or cuts in the cover means the mattress must be condemned. A torch shone through the cover from inside will show pin-prick holes. Any staining of the foam also informs the examiner that there is a hole in the cover and it must be condemned.

Doctors often have the habit of pushing syringe needles into the cover as a safety precaution. They are generally unaware that this immediately opens the mattress to a risk of cross-infection.

Stage 4: Analysis

Following the day of audit, the results should be analysed. Statistics that arise from the results would indicate where further education is required or which department requires an increase of pressure ulcer prevention resources.

Audit will clearly demonstrate where patients are being nursed on inappropriate mattresses for their risk score and where patients with grade 0 and 1 (EPUAP) pressure ulcers are not being nursed on an appropriate mattress. It will also indicate whether patients are developing pressure ulcers because they spend too long in chairs with inappropriate chair cushions.

Subsequent audits would follow the data collection format of the baseline. There may be additional data required for future audit and this will be determined by the results of the previous audits.

Research

Research is difficult to undertake and to understand. Pure research is unlikely to be applied without a total application to the subject and that requires an expert professional dedicated to the particular subject. Nevertheless, this should not prevent inexperienced nurses and doctors from working with the research process and learning valuable lessons from it. Without the inexperienced professional experimenting with research, pure research would be unlikely to occur, particularly as the inexperienced professional is giving the care and is aware of research requirements.

Disraeli said there were 'Lies, damned lies and statistics' meaning that statistics can be used to prove whatever the research wishes to prove. Leaving out some findings and including others can 'massage' the actual true findings of a study. Professionals are being increasingly taught how to critically analyze research papers so that poor methodology and 'massaging' of findings can be identified. This is not to intimate that all researchers are trying to present biased findings. Most are honestly and openly trying to identify potential improvements in the world of tissue viability.

Nevertheless, many studies are often so small in sample size that the findings cannot been seen as significant, even though the researcher has, mistakenly, presented it as such.

Randomized controlled trials (RCTs) are now (correctly) seen as the 'gold standard' of all studies in tissue viability (Fogg and Gross 2000) and the NHS Executive recommend RCTs as the most reliable evidence for the efficacy of interventions. The RCT is an experimental method used when two or more treatment procedures are to be compared. This ensures that a control is in place and that the research has a valuable contribution to make. Randomized trials are generally considered the most rigorous way of determining whether a cause and effect relationship exists between intervention/treatment and outcome, and for assessing the effectiveness, including cost-effectiveness, of an intervention or treatment (Getliffe 1998). Nevertheless, there are those who find controlled trials do not 'fit' into the holistic approach prevalent in contemporary nursing practice; it is too reductionist in approach to serve the needs of the patient as a whole being or nursing as a caring profession (Black 1998). RCTs can take many months or perhaps even many years as a very large number of subjects are required in the studies to relieve all of the variables that will always come with ill health. Nurses generally need answers quickly such as whether a mattress will offer clinical efficacy and cost effectiveness. This rapid answer cannot be obtained from RCTs. These results come from clinical experience and evaluations.

Research is promoting evidence-based nursing and this is vital to the future credibility of nursing as a profession. Nevertheless, dogmatically refusing to listen to experience also has huge implications on standards of care. All professionals are aware that clinical effectiveness is important and each product or treatment should be individually judged. The experience of many professionals is scorned when there is little actual proven evidence to support their experience. One such experience could be potassium permanganate. Dermatologists recommended the use of this substance for many years, claiming that it 'dries out' wet eczema and reduces bacterial contamination. This theory was scorned because there has been no research trials carried out on its use and other professionals doubted that the mild antiseptic action could have any effect on wound healing (Wound Care Journal 1995). The problem here is not the fact that the experience is not believed but that the dermatologists not only did not undertake to show, and write up, the effectiveness of the treatment but also appeared to continue using it as a 'blanket' therapy on many unnecessary wounds. This lowered the effective ratio and led to disbelief as a therapy. The treatment obviously has some benefit or the very experienced dermatologists would not continue using it. The outcome of this is that a substance that may benefit patients, is falling into disuse among professionals who demand proof and, until it is provided, will not listen to the voice of experience. Nurses are being increasingly highly educated and this process will assist them with critiquing research. Without education and the ability to understand the jargon of research, many papers will be taken at face value and used as 'evidence' when implementing new methods of care. Nevertheless, there is often a lack of research evidence in practice with nurses (Hunt 1996):

- not understanding research findings;
- not knowing about research findings;
- not believing the research findings;
- not knowing how to apply the research findings;
- not being allowed to use the research findings.

Research findings can also be misleading. One paper in question could be a paper by Gould et al. (1998) Gould et al. compared a long-stretch bandage (Setopress) with a short-stretch bandage (Elastocrepe) over a 16-week period. The study was a randomized, observer-blind, parallel group study of 39 patients of whom seven had bi-lateral leg ulcers. Results of the study showed that the long-stretch bandage had a higher healing rate (58 per cent) than the short-stretch bandage (35 per cent) with median healing times of 12 weeks for long-stretch and 23 weeks for short-stretch (statistically significant at $P = 0.04$). However, the study used Elastocrepe bandages for the study and this is not a recognized short-stretch bandage. The researchers were able to call it 'short-stretch' because the bandage stretched a 'short way'. However, nurses using Elastocrepe would know that it does not hold its extensibility and would, therefore, never use it as a compression bandage and would only use it as a retention bandage. The results of this study were accurate as a comparison between Elastocrepe and multilayer bandages but the misnomer was very misleading and uneccessarily damaging for short-stretch compression therapy.

Another misleading research project was the Landis (1930) work where healthy, young subjects' nail beds were used to identify at what pressure capillary closure occurs. The result was an average of 16–32 mmHg of pressure. This result does not, even in the simplest terms, relate to ill, moribund, immobile and elderly patients. However, companies who wish to sell their product constantly quote mmHg pressure that they relate to their mattresses. Even worse, those who are purchasing the mattress unquestioningly, accepting the results and applying them to suit their own situation. Accepting results and not critiquing the research methodology could be considered a dangerous practice.

Nevertheless, the process of research is extremely important to the future of the health service. Nurses are becoming increasingly adept at undertaking research and doctors traditionally are expected to undertake research. Studies in wound care, however, are difficult to undertake. Patient compliance, patient retention in the study, ethical considerations, time and cost all combine to prevent good studies being completed. Many healthcare professionals are overcoming these difficulties, however, and useful and interesting results are being formulated.

Conclusion

The future of research and audit has become almost compulsory and the future of wound care and pressure ulcer prevention is almost assured. Nevertheless, improvements will not be made to practice until all of the process of benchmarking, audit and research are given high priority by the staff who apply the care.

Activity

Using the audit tool in Figure 12.1 or 12.2:

- decide how this tool could be effective within your area of practice;
- develop your own audit tool using these figures as a guide.

CHAPTER 13

Ethics, the law and accountability in wound care

The law and tissue viability

Ignorantia Juris Nemineum Excusat (ignorance is no excuse). In the eyes of the law, it is important for the professional to be aware of any law relating to their profession. If they are unaware of the law when they commit an error, their ignorance will not be taken into consideration and they will be found guilty.

The Law of Tort is a judge-made law, which defines duties of care in all aspects of life. Law of Tort applies to a professional who is paid money to perform a service for people that others are unable to perform. This imposes a duty of care on the professional to take responsible steps at a particular level when performing that duty (Johnson 1994).

In contrast, the issue of ordinary care, the law requires the nurse/doctor to undertake those tasks within their level of competence. If this is observed, the person will be judged according to level of experience that they could reasonably be expected to have reached. However, if the person (nurse or doctor) undertook tasks beyond the level of competence, without checking with a more experienced superior, he or she would be judged on the level of the superior. For example, a nurse taking on the doctor's role will be judged by the standard of a reasonable doctor. Nevertheless, a judge would use the Bolam case (*Bolam* v *Friern Hospital Management Committee* 1957) to assess whether a reasonable level of care had been given. An expert witness would determine for the court, not what the expert would be expected to do in such a case, but what a nurse of the same level could be expected to have done in similar circumstances. If a reasonable level of care was given for the expected level of the nurse, the ruling would be in the favour of the nurse. However, if the judge considers that the nurse did not reach the standard expected of his or her level, the ruling would be against the nurse.

Each professional must abide by the code of 'a duty of care' and each professional owes the patient a duty to act with all reasonable skill and care. A mere failure to act or omission is not necessarily tantamount to negligence and a litigant must prove there was a breach in the duty of care and that the breach was the cause of the damage (Hine 1993). The most important case, against which all other similar cases are judged, is the *Bolam* v *Friern Hospital Management Committee* (1957), which led to the declaration: 'The test is the standard of the ordinary skilled man exercising and professing to have that special skill. It is sufficient that he performs within his competence and, if this is observed, the person will be judged according to level of experience that they could reasonably be expected to have reached.'

Therefore, the nurse should work within the guidelines of the United Kingdom Central Council (UKCC) (1992) in exercising professional accountability, and should only undertake those tasks in which he or she has received education and can be judged as competent. However, it would not be considered enough to merely receive education, as, in the exercise of accountability, the nurse must be expected to achieve and maintain high standards.

Johnson (1994) states 'A doctor is not negligent if he acts in the practice accepted at that time by a body of competent professional/ medical opinion even though other doctors adopt a different practice'. This can be applicable to the use of Edinburg Solution of Lime (EUSOL) (see Chapter 3). There are professionals who strongly believe that EUSOL is harmful, whereas, other professionals believe just as strongly that EUSOL is not harmful. Therefore, a doctor who is sued for use of a harmful substance is likely to prove that EUSOL is not harmful and will have a body of professional people and evidence to prove that it debrides and cleanses wounds.

The work that began the debate on EUSOL was undertaken on a rabbit's ear chamber on a healing wound when it was found that the microcirculation was damaged through the use of EUSOL (Leaper and Simpson 1986; Brennan and Leaper 1987). However, traditionally, EUSOL was used on very sloughy or infected wounds where healing was not an issue. Nurses decided that EUSOL should never be used even though the researchers themselves had said it should only be used with caution. This led to many debates between doctors and nurses and (sometimes) a refusal to use the product.

Case scenario: using EUSOL

A consultant prescribes EUSOL for a sloughy pressure ulcer. The nurse refuses to use it as she or he believes it to be harmful to the patient. The pressure ulcer deteriorates and becomes infected. The patient dies as a result of septicaemia and the family sues the hospital. Where does the nurse stand in this situation? We know that the wound would have deteriorated anyway and the death of the patient was not related to the nurse's refusal to use EUSOL. However, the consultant points the finger in the nurse's direction and he has proof that EUSOL will always clean the wound. His proof comes in the form of written papers (there are many) showing EUSOL to be effective and he has the support of many other consultants that EUSOL is effective.

This scenario is not meant to encourage nurses to use EUSOL, there are many other, less painful and less harmful dressings that will provide better care. It is to show that the law is not as clear-cut as supposed and that the nurse requires stronger evidence than just research papers. If faced with this situation, the nurse should always use the TVN or a manager for support.

Litigation for negligence is increasing with damages against doctors showing the largest upward trend. Most cases of medical negligence are settled out of court and, therefore, there are only a few cases that reach the public domain. Nurses are becoming increasingly accountable for their actions and, although a nurse has not yet been sued as an individual, the day is approaching when vicarious liability does not offer protection as it did.

Vicarious liability and tissue viability

Vicarious liability means that the employer is responsible for the actions of employees. This means that the individual employee is unlikely to be sued although their employing body may well be sued because of the professional's breach of duty of care. If a patient develops a pressure sore because adequate care was not provided and equipment was not made available to the patient when required, the trust may be sued. Nevertheless, it would be the nurse responsible for the ward or the patient's care that would be called to court to answer the allegations. It is worth noting at this point that if the care has not been documented, in the eyes of the law, it has not been provided. Tingle (1997) identified poor communication, insufficient documentation and non-reflective practice as areas of concern in law.

However, the nurse is also responsible for his or her actions. For example, consider the scenario where a sister in a nursing home is ordered by the owner to remove a resident from an air mattress. The sister tries to persuade the owner to change their mind but the decision was made and the resident is duly removed from the air mattress and placed on a foam mattress. The resident develops a pressure ulcer and the next of kin complains, leading to the sister being struck off of the nursing register. How could this occur when the sister had fought for the air mattress to remain *in situ*? If the sister obeyed orders to remove the resident from the mattress but had not initiated any other preventative methods, including not recommending nor instigating repositioning, then she would be clearly guilty of negligence.

Ethics in tissue viability

Wound care is becoming an increasingly scientific discipline in its own right and is being taken up, almost exclusively, by the nursing profession who are seeking to establish its own independent and distinct body of knowledge (Hampton 1997f). However, wound care has traditionally been taught subjectively, using anecdotal evidence (Flanagan 1994) and personal preferences for selection of dressings without the objective, research-based evidence to support the choice of wound treatment. Flanagan (1992b) found that nurses were reluctant to make decisions about the type of dressing to use and suggested that this reluctance was due to a lack of confidence and resistance from colleagues.

Selection of an inappropriate wound cleansing agent or dressing may have serious consequences (Wood 1976; Brennan et al. 1985). The UKCC (1992) for nursing dictates that nurses must be competent in any area that requires them to give treatment or care to patients. Moore (1992) writes, 'there is still a body of opinion that favours the use of inappropriate wound cleansing agents'. If this is coupled with Flanagan's discovery of nurse reluctance to make decisions, it could mean that some patients may be receiving poor quality, even potentially dangerous, wound care.

Nursing is moving rapidly toward autonomy and nurse prescribing. The UKCC directive that competence is a prerequisite to giving care, means that nurses are required to have knowledge of wound care before making decisions on dressings. However, due to poor staffing levels and cost of study days, nurses are finding increasing difficulty in acquiring that knowledge.

This section asks whether it is ethical for nurses to prescribe wound care if they are not educated or knowledgeable in wound healing and treatment and reviews ethical principles in relation to the care of the patient with a wound.

Ethical principles related to wound care

Benjamin and Curtis (1992) write, 'Ethics is an attempt to formulate and justify systematic responses to what ought to be done in a given situation'. This statement reflects the ethical problem with prescribing wound treatment. Wound care is only a small part of nurse/doctor training and it is then the responsibility of the individual professional to educate themselves in this area. If the employing body does not offer the education it would be difficult for the nurse to receive the required knowledge and to gain competency in making decisions. Nevertheless, the patient with a wound requires appropriate wound care and if both doctor and nurse have received little education in the principles of wound treatment, the decisions on wound care may have to be based on ritualistic practices and not on research-based evidence. If that is the case, then the practitioner may be ignoring the directive from the UKCC.

Patient advocacy

Patient advocacy can be an emotive subject. Nurses may not wish the responsibility of the role of advocate (Culley 1997) whereas some nurses may become antagonistic within the role, determined to defy doctors when they believe their patient is in danger of poor practice. However, the role of advocate is not one of refusal to give prescribed care, but is one of patient support. The UKCC (1996) code of professional conduct offers the core functions of patient advocacy as 'informing, supporting and protecting the patient'. Concern about aspects of the patient's care must be reported and this is the primary act of patient advocacy. Failure to report acts or words that are negligent is a failure of the nurse to safeguard the patient and the nurse must then share the blame for any harm resulting from the negligence (Young 1991).

The patient is entitled to be given a clear, concise and understandable explanation of their condition, disease, the planned treatment or investigations, any alternative procedures available, any significant after effects and the chances of success or serious side effects (Culley 1997). It is the role of the nurse to ensure that the patient has had the opportunity to discuss the issues arising from this and that there is clear understanding of all side effects.

Ethical theories

Teleological theories

Teleological theories are based on good or bad actions and the consequence of those actions. Good consequences come from 'right' actions; bad consequences come from 'wrong' actions. There are, however, difficulties in defining what is 'good' and what is 'bad' and several ideas emerge to rationalize the theory.

Utilitarianism

Utilitarian principles stem from maximizing the overall good to the highest number of people and, as such, offers a simple solution to every problem (Benjamin and Curtis 1992). The theory dictates that acts can be useful or not useful and that useful acts produce good effects, whereas, acts that are not useful cause harm and that any act should supply the greatest happiness for the greatest number of people. Bentham (cited by Curtin and Flaherty 1982) argued that people should act to maximize pleasure and minimize pain but also that pleasure should be measured in terms of quality and quantity.

To examine theories of utilitarianism as applied to wound care, one would need to define 'good' or 'happiness'. Patients may be given the greatest 'happiness' knowing that their wounds are cared for by a professional, particularly if the patient is unaware that the professional lacks knowledge in wound care. Perhaps 'bad' or 'not useful' acts could be those of professionals giving wound care that delay healing, even though the recipients of the treatment are unaware that harm is being done and are happy with the care. Nevertheless, Bentham's argument of 'maximizing pleasure and minimizing pain' would indicate that the 'pain' of delayed healing is wrong and the 'pleasure' of having a wound healed is right particularly as healing rates can be measured in both quality and quantity.

Nevertheless, the basis of utilitarian principles is that of consequences arising from acts or decisions that have been carried out and whether those consequences are 'good' for the larger group or 'bad'. 'Good' outcomes, for the largest number of people, are the aim, regardless of the consequences to the individual.

Rowson (1993) writes 'From the utilitarian perspective, the right kind of professional-patient relationship is one in which the professionals use their expertise to decide what is in the best interests of the patient with the patient's own role that of compliance' (otherwise known as justified paternalism).

Justified paternalism

Justified paternalism lends itself to the culture of nursing. It is easy to make decisions in isolation of the patient because the nurse makes similar decisions daily with the patient accepting the nurse in the parental role. However, if the nurse embraces the UKCC (1989) directive that 'the practitioner should explain the procedure to the patient without bias and as in as much detail of possible reactions, complications and side effects as the patient requires', thereby allowing the patient to give informed consent, the paternalistic-based decision is unacceptable as the consequences may cause harm (delayed healing, infection, etc.) of which the patient would be unaware. Informed consent automatically removes paternalism to some degree as 'informed' means that the patient will be aware of the procedure and the possible consequences and can refuse to give consent if they wish to do so. To apply the term 'paternalism' here would be a contradiction of terms. The UKCC (1989) stands firm on this by stating: 'The practitioner must be sure that it is the interests of the patient that are being promoted rather than the patient being used as a vehicle for the promotion of personal or sectional professional interests'. This stand gives the nurse complete responsibility as the patient's advocate and utilitarian views become 'toothless tigers'.

Applying the principles of utilitarianism to wound care is obviously difficult and conflicting and generally does not permit the individual patient to make a choice. Rowson (1993) argues that involving patients in decision making can increase their motivation to get well, whilst this involvement may make decision making difficult for the professionals. A paternalistic decision would allow the practitioner to treat a wound without interference, particularly as a patient may wish to change a decision when they have full information on the action of the dressing and this could make treatment difficult for the practitioner.

The professional also has a right to respect and autonomy and Rowson offers an example of a patient who demands a skin graft for an ulcer. The nurse believes it would be more beneficial for the wound to heal slowly but, as it is the patient's wish, the surgeon must carry out the procedure. In this case, the professional's expertise and judgement has been ignored – eliminating their own individual rights. The utilitarian view would be that the happiness of the largest group (patients) does not justify maintaining the individual's (the nurse's) rights or autonomy.

Respect for autonomy

Seedhouse (1993) argues that autonomy is central to healthcare and that the person's chosen direction should be respected, whether or not the health worker approves of that direction. The utilitarian might say that, in wound care, offering the highest good to the most people would be to allow nurses (whatever their knowledge base) to prescribe care for the patient; the consequence of this would be that the patient will have their wounds dressed when required, nurses and doctors will be satisfied that they have given excellence in care and managers will not be forced into supplying expensive study leave that they can ill afford.

However, this solution is not as simple as first thought as lack of knowledge could lead to the patient receiving wound care that will delay healing and may cause systemic side effects. Nurses are accountable for the care that they give and lack of knowledge is not an excuse for giving poor quality care and, therefore the study leave is justified. There is also a potential that delayed healing may have a cost implication as the patient's discharge could be delayed because a wound is not healing.

The act-utilitarian theme, as described by Steele and Harmon (1983), 'may have some actions emerge that cause both happiness and unhappiness necessitating the choice of an alternative – one that results in the greatest good for the greatest number of people'. It could be argued that the patient body represents the greatest number and that their happiness or good is the issue. As inappropriate wound care may cause harm, nurses should be educated in wound care with management being responsible for the cost of that education. Nevertheless, any increased cost to the financially compromised community and hospital trusts will ultimately reflect on patient care and may cause reduction in the money available for other treatments. There is also difficulty in providing nurses to replace those who are taking time off to study and this may result in reduced numbers of qualified nurses caring for patients on the wards.

With wound care, it may be difficult to predict the consequences accurately or to prove responsibility for poor outcomes, and therefore utilitarian principles are difficult to apply. Nevertheless, nurses are accountable for their actions and have a duty to care. They may be faced with a moral dilemma – the possible poor outcome of actions they are pressured into, or the duty to act for the complete benefit of the patient who requires care – even if that care is of a poor standard.

Deontology

Seedhouse (1993) describes deontology (the duty to care) as 'not [being] the result that matters but that the person acted according to a perceived duty and intended that some good should come out of it'. Seedhouse also writes that a central feature in deontology is integrity, relying on honesty not based on expedient calculation. Applied to wound care, this would mean that the patient would be well informed of decisions and the consequences of treatment and that the nurse would have a responsibility to obtain knowledge in wound care. The Kantian theory is based on a moral issue. Providing the reasons for an action are pure, then the nurse's decisions in wound care would be morally justified.

However, this theory is also difficult to apply as it is rigid and supports only the one person – the patient with the wound. It does not take into account the consequences of the nurses' education with escalating costs and reduced levels of qualified staff, which affects the care of the many other patients. Nevertheless, delayed discharge from hospital, through poor wound healing, also has a consequence, that of blocked beds and postponed elective surgery with an increased waiting list and possible penalties for the trust concerned.

Kant (cited by Seedhouse 1993) strongly believed that respect for individuals is the primary test of one's duties and that people should not be exploited for any reason. This is the principle of 'universalizability', that each person should act as another would do in a similar situation and means that every decision to act should be based on whether it would be a generally accepted (or normal behaviour) to act that way. This theory puts heavy reliance on the individual to behave in a 'normal' manner and frowns on any act that promotes self-interest, which would not be done by others in a similar situation.

Wound care is often a ritualistic practice and regularly offered to patients by nurses and doctors with little education in wound healing principles. According to Kantian theories, lack of education is not a problem as it is common practice for wounds to be treated by practitioners with little wound healing education. However, this theory may mean that patients are receiving inappropriate care for their wounds and that healing is delayed and this is not how practitioners with wound healing knowledge would treat wounds. Nevertheless, the practitioners with wound healing knowledge are in the minority and (according to Kant's theory) they could be considered abnormal and wrong to practise wound care as they do. Marks-Maran (1993) states that nurses are both accountable and responsible. Applied to wound care, this would mean that nurses are responsible for taking care of the patient's wound – dressing it when required. However, as an accountable practitioner, the nurse should be able to explain why that dressing was applied, justifying the action and understanding the rationale and the consequences of selecting that particular dressing in that circumstance.

Seedhouse (1993) writes, 'For Kant, moral issues are not complex or insoluble – ethics are not a frustrating form of cerebral perpetual motion – rather it is possible to be moral and moral in exactly the same way as all others by the use of reason'. According to Seedhouse, it would not be enough to give wound care simply because it is part of the nurse's job and if care is given under instruction or pressure from hospital managers then the nurse would have no moral defence for his or her actions.

Rowson (1993) writes that 'An accountable person examines a situation, explores various options, demonstrates a knowledgeable understanding of the possible consequences and makes a decision which can be justified from a knowledgeable base'. This reflects the ideology of the UKCC 'Scope of Professional Practice' and does not agree with Kant's theory of right.

The Rawlinson theory

Rawls's (1973) theory of justice is loosely based on Kant's theory of a duty to care mixed with some utilitarian ideology and suggests that those in a disadvantaged position should not be hurt, thereby respecting individual rights, but that consequences of actions should also be considered. Seedhouse (1993) writes on Rawls's theory that the basis of it is that each person would have an equal right to all others with any inequalities arranged so that it would work to everyone's advantage.

This theory could dictate that each person would receive research-based wound care with nurses acquiring the same knowledge base; this care would increase the speed of patient discharge and the consequence would be that more people would be given the operations they require. If this is not possible, then the introduction of wound care specialist nurses (to advise on wound care), or early discharge to the district nurses' care, could perhaps speed up the process. This could lead to each person with a wound receiving equal care without disrupting the common good by blocking beds.

However, forming a place for specialist nurses may well be against the Rawlinson principle as that could be considered an inequality with a nurse receiving education that is denied to the wider group of nurses. Rawls believes there should be an equal distribution of resources (Seedhouse 1993) and offering higher education to a limited group is possibly unjust. It is also possible that patients in one district will receive expert advice on wound care and another patient, in a district without a specialist nurse in wound care, will receive advice that is not from an expert.

Non-normative theories

Ethical emotivism

The theory is that the right and wrong of a situation relies on the emotional response of the person dealing with the situation and how that person can raise a similar response in others. Therefore, a manager can believe that it is wrong to take nurses away from the ward for education as this reduces the care given to a greater number of patients. If the manager can persuade the nurse to reflect those thoughts, then treating wounds without knowledge of how to treat them would not be seen as wrong.

Curtin and Flaherty (1982) write, 'The emotivists' claim that ethical judgements have no basis in reality strains credibility'. This would reflect on wound care particularly as the wound exists and can lead to morbidity and even death. No amount of persuasion could detract from the fact that, although some patients may receive less attention, this patient may die without appropriate wound care and that must be ethically wrong.

Ethical scepticism

The sceptic claims that people do not know right from wrong (Curtin and Flaherty 1982) as people often disagree and two opinions cannot both be correct. Nevertheless, as a judgement must be made on wound care and the results of that decision has the potential for disastrous consequences, it would be desirable to accept the solution that causes the least harm and this must be based on ethical principles.

Ethical relativism

Relativism is a theory that relates right or wrong to the individual circumstance or situation and the choice of action would be right if the individual believed it to be right. This supports the saying 'ignorance is bliss!' as, if the individual believes the wound care they give is adequate then that is good enough as they acted according to their own values. This theory does not recognize the limitations of experience in wound management and certainly is not supported by the UKCC Scope of Professional Practice (1992), which states that the nurse must 'Honestly acknowledge any limits of personal knowledge and skill and take steps to remedy any relevant deficits in order effectively and appropriately to meet the needs of patients'.

Curtin and Flaherty (1982) state that 'although non-normative theories increase understanding and tolerance, both of which are important in decision making, they are not enough to determine right and wrong'.

Conclusion

Ethical principles are complex and in wound care it would be difficult to adopt one ethical theory over another as each theory lends itself to a 'catch 22' situation where the nurse is both wrong and right when making decisions. If the health service was such that each nurse was given the necessary training in wound treatment, then the ethical question would not arise. Nevertheless, in the modern climate of insufficient trust funding, it is unrealistic to expect nurses to acquire necessary knowledge. This leads to the dilemma of whether the nurse should refuse to give treatment without the knowledge and competence to back up the decisions – possibly leaving the patient completely without treatment – or whether the nurse should give treatment knowing that the UKCC directs that procedures should only be carried out when the nurse is competent, with delayed wound healing as a distinct possibility.

Kant's theory of duty is possibly the only theory that can be adjusted to 'fit' the ethics of wound care as Kant sees nurses as morally responsible for the care they give and, providing the motives for the actions are pure, then the decisions would be moral.

The health service is extremely low in funds and this is not likely to improve in the near future. Nurses are being made accountable for gaining competence in all areas within their scope, but time and funds are not realistically available to them.

Inferior wound care is not acceptable and, according to all of the theories, unethical. However, it is difficult to point a finger at the area of responsible as each group has its own difficulties; the nurse is not given the means to obtain the required knowledge, the hospital management is unable to accommodate education requirements and the Government does not supply the necessary funding.

One thing is certain, no matter what the academics agree in ethics, the nurse has a duty to the patient that is dictated by the governing body (the UKCC). This is inescapable and competency must be the nurse's first consideration when giving wound care. It is the nurse's own responsibility to gain that competence and to ensure that the individual patient's needs in wound care are addressed. This does not allow discussions of ethics and how they may be applied to nursing the patient with a wound. Nor does it allow any degree of paternalism as each patient must be informed and public trust and confidence must be justified according to UKCC dictats.

Nevertheless, there is an answer that may satisfy ethical principles. One nurse on each ward could be given the education and training required to support excellence in wound management and this nurse could then be responsible for cascading the information down to colleagues and ensuring that prescriptions for wound care are based on good practice. This would reduce the cost of education with only one nurse on each ward being given study time and, as fewer nurses leave the ward for tissue viability education, there would be reduced numbers of bank nurses required to replace them. Kantian theories of duty-based care could then be applied, the patient would receive excellence in wound care, the other patients would not be denied the attention of nurses otherwise struggling to receive education and the cost of education would be lower for the trust.

It could be said that this solution also fits with Rawls's theories as inequalities would be arranged so that it works to everyone's advantage with everyone receiving equal rights. Any solution that is reached to the satisfaction of all parties must also satisfy the utilitarian view as the greatest happiness will be given to the greatest number of people.

It is important that practitioners have a clear understanding of the law and how it applies to each particular field. In tissue viability, the law is for the practitioner if they have worked within their own competencies, have behaved ethically and have confirmation that reflective practice and evidence-based rationale has been used to form decisions.

CHAPTER 14

The specialist nurse in wound management

One of the most significant developments in the United Kingdom is the emergence of the clinical nurse specialist (Bale 1995). Specialist nurses have appeared on two levels of equal importance as:

- the nurse who has a specialist knowledge and fully uses that knowledge in the day-to-day practice of her or his duties (the clinical nurse specialist);
- the nurse who has a specialist interest in a subject and uses that knowledge as part of the daily discharge of duties (the link-nurse or lead-nurse within a ward, community setting or nursing home).

The first level practitioner, the clinical nurse specialist, requires an in-depth knowledge of tissue viability and a high level of skill in wound management and pressure ulcer prevention. The idealistic vision of a specialist nurse would be one who acts in the capacity of advisor to nurses or doctors who, for whatever reason, were unable to make a rational decision on a wound in their care. The role of the specialist nurse would be to discuss the wound, to use the situation to teach and to give options of care so that the practitioner could reach their own, informed decisions on wound care. However, in reality, it is more likely that the responsibility for decisions will be passed to the specialist nurse with the nurse/doctor allowing that responsibility to be passed on. The reasons for this are complex but the following may give some explanation:

- the nurse or doctor with responsibility for the patient, is under pressure from other duties;

- the nurse or doctor has little interest in tissue viability;
- the nurse or doctor has never received education in wound care;
- dressing selection is difficult due to the vast range of dressings and the amount of new dressings being introduced to the market;
- the nurse or doctor has an erroneous idea of the clinical nurse specialist role and believes the role to be one of 'wound care nurse' rather than advisor and educator.

For the sake of public safety, the UKCC wishes all those practitioners calling themselves 'specialists' to undergo courses leading to a recordable qualification of specialist practitioner (Humphries and Masterson 1998) and there are several universities where this qualification may be obtained. However, at present it is not compulsory for nurses to undertake a specialist practitioner course before calling themselves 'specialist' (Humphries and Masterson 1998).

Role development

The role requirements may be variable depending on the philosophy of each individual employing trust. Nevertheless, the role can be definable independently of the variables within each trust. In developing the role, the specialist will need many physical and theoretical skills including:

1 diagnostic skills
2 counselling skills for patients with intractable wounds or social problems
3 prescribing and monitoring care
4 change management
5 organizational competencies
    - maintaining a clinical caseload of more complex cases;
    - dexterity, required to manage difficult-to-dress wounds;
    - the ability to manage rapidly changing situations;
    - the ability to gain the confidence of the patient;
    - educational.

The role will constantly develop and change and will require the ability to think laterally and to not feel threatened by change.

Without this ability the role of the specialist will never be 'special'. Wound care is particularly liable to change as developments show treatments or products, once frowned on, as now being extremely useful (maggots therapy, iodine, sugar paste, etc.). Hence, the specialist must be able to move from a stance of not recommending a treatment to recommending it; a difficult situation for anyone.

In the United States, Masters degree level is the minimum standard for the specialist nurse and that will soon be expected in the UK. However, Flanagan (1997) found that 39 per cent of tissue viability nurses (TVNs) in the UK had no academic qualifications. It is beholden on the TVN to gain academic education and clinical expertise through practice and this is often difficult in the current climate of cost cutting in the health service.

Education

The tissue viability specialist nurses are responsible for increasing their own education in wound care so that the knowledge can be adapted for educating students, nurses, doctors, physiotherapists, occupational therapists, patients and carers. However, the education is not necessarily the primary source of knowledge for the TVN. Knowledge can be vital when acquired through 'hands on' experience. Knowing and applying results of research in the clinical setting, depends on the type of patient on whom the research was carried out. If the subjects were healthy individuals – as in the Landis research (1930) (see Chapter 9) then results in practice will not be the same as those identified through research. The TVN will know from experience that research results still have to be taken in the context of interventions and use of equipment being successful for those patients with differing variables (Hill 1995). Failure to listen to the 'voice of experience' could lead to a loss of valuable knowledge in pressure ulcer prevention and the value of many dressings in the wound healing process.

Education of all those involved in tissue viability is a vital part of the TVN role. Without the ability to teach and to pass on information and knowledge, tissue viability will not progress with pressure ulcer prevalence suffering as a consequence.

Practitioner

The TVN is generally autonomous, prescribing and/or recommending care and, as such, is a role model for general nurses. It is important that the TVN maintains a clinical caseload with, usually, more complex cases. The availability of the TVN for referrals, often at short notice, of clients for whom first line policy has failed or is not appropriate is invaluable (James 1994). The TVN will produce and promote standards, be responsible for written protocols in wound care and will develop assessment tools for use by the generalist nurse. The TVN will also undertake audit in tissue viability and will use the results of the audit to develop standards and to establish education requirements.

Researcher

The TVN must be responsible for developing wound care and pressure ulcer prevention within their own area and, on a larger scale, with their peers throughout the UK. This involves small- and large-scale studies and research projects and may involve multicentred trials. The findings of these studies must then be implemented, and disseminated, through written papers and through practice example within the workplace. This involves the TVN as a change agent, acting as a catalyst for change within the organization (Bale 1995).

The importance of the tissue viability nurse role is evident. The generalist nurse is expected to hold a vast amount of knowledge and skills and can be a 'jack of all trades'. When the limit of knowledge has been reached in areas such as mobilizing the patient, the nurse could be expected to liaise with a colleague who may have a greater and more specialized knowledge in that area, for instance a physiotherapist. It would be difficult for the nurse to give the level of mobilization required whilst siting cannulas, physically caring for acutely ill patients, preventing pressure ulcers and giving wound care – along with all the vast amount of tasks expected from the ordinary nurse on the ward or in the community. Add to this the thought that nurses cannot be expected to know how to treat more complex, specialist cases and it is evident that there is a place for the clinical expert in any field. This will ensure that patients are supplied with the highest quality care possible through supplying information and education to those working in the field.

Nevertheless, there is a potential for the specialist nurse to deskill the generalist nurse, particularly if the specialist undertakes the role of decision making and wound dressings in isolation. Therefore, the most important role of the specialist is as educator and advisor – leading or being consulted for their level of knowledge and expertise.

There may be an argument against specialism if specialist nurses are reluctant to share knowledge in order to retain power. 'Knowledge is power' (Emerson cited by Frazer 1991) and individuals may be tempted to keep their knowledge and skills to themselves as this would ensure their role. The specialist nurse may be given power through consultants who recognize that the knowledge level is high whilst the generalist nurse may have comparatively low knowledge in wound care. This may demonstrate that the specialist nurse is not acting as educationalist, which should be a vital and important part of the role.

New products would not be reviewed successfully without the specialist nurse to co-ordinate the evaluations and to disseminate the findings. Large-scale clinical trials could not be successfully undertaken without the co-operation and co-ordination of the specialist nurse.

Decisions on mattress purchase could be fragmented and expensive without the specialist to review and trial different types of mattress on the market. These decisions also rely on a multidisciplinary involvement with physiotherapists deciding on mobility potential from mattresses, resuscitation officers reviewing resuscitation potential on mattresses (are they too soft to support resuscitation) and electrical engineers reviewing the strength of the mattress and the quality of the compressor that inflates the mattress. The Infection Control specialist nurses would review the potential for bacterial growth within the mattress. The TVN would be expected to co-ordinate the involvement of the team and would review all required evidence. The tissue viability nurse will also undertake clinical evaluations particularly in relation to the potential for pressure ulcer prevention with the mattress.

The specialist nurse is involved in ensuring cost savings, so the savings that are made negate the argument that specialist nurses are expensive. However, the specialist nurse in tissue viability is likely to request more expensive, higher quality mattresses and this may be seen as an unnecessary expense by managers with little knowledge in the life-threatening horror that may be associated with pressure ulcer development. Collier (1995) found that it can cost £40 000 for one patient with a pressure ulcer. However, unscrupulous managers may balance that cost against the cost of admitting a patient for surgery in the place of a patient who was discharged home, sooner, without an ulcer.

Review of market developments and liaison with company representatives, reading specialist journals and attendance at conferences and product exhibitions keeps the TVN aware of new products and developments in wound care (James 1994) in a way that the general nurse is possibly unable to do. Expertise, understanding and teaching wound healing and developing tissue viability within the workplace, offers credibility and respect to the TVN role.

One area that is important is audit of pressure ulcers and wounds such as leg ulcers. Without audit it is impossible to evaluate whether care is successful. The generalist nurse would be unable to co-ordinate audits throughout the hospital or community trust without the support of the specialist.

The tissue viability nurse as a change agent

Wound care has traditionally been taught by word of mouth for doctors and for nurses with each professional continuing the practice of their predecessors and mentors. It is the role of the TVN to look at those practices and either support them or act as a change agent in promoting improved practices. This requires distinct interpersonal skills, particularly as other professionals may feel threatened or bruised when told that their own standards may not be achieving the required level of best practice.

The TVN has the responsibility of offering seamless care to the patient and liaison between community and hospital is an important aspect of that care. Often there are political problems between two separate areas with each area believing they have superior knowledge and skills to the other area. It is the role of the TVN to work with that political agenda, using change management skills with the aim of achieving seamless patient care.

Each TVN will promote quality care in an individual way. Changing inferior practice in wound care may be difficult as many nurses and doctors have been undertaking wound care in their own way for many years and may resent being told their practice was poor. However, it would be wrong for one professional to hold up another professional to scorn by challenging them in front of others. The TVN requires an opportunity to show the benefits of changing practice through providing evidence-based care that produces excellent results, such as demonstrating high healing rates. Being challenged will not alter a medical consultant who insists on using a product, such as hydrogen peroxide or EUSOL. However, should the TVN or generalist nurse have evidence of another, improved practice, they can show, through example and through written evidence, that the new method achieves better healing rates.

The author's (Hampton) personal style is to await an opportunity to demonstrate how a different product can improve on healing rates and, although this has taken time, it has greatly changed practice within the trust and has earned respect from consultants and senior nurses. The opportunity may not always present itself openly but change management may sometimes be subliminal. For instance, any education, given to junior nurses and students, will develop their practice, giving them opportunities to demonstrate, both by example and through their questioning of those whose practice is under observation.

Bureaucracy and local politics may also be immense obstacles for the TVN to overcome and this requires skills of negotiation. Managers may be defensive of budgets and may see the role of the TVN as one that places demands on that budget; this is difficult to overcome. However, with the appearance of clinical governance and the input of CHI (Commission for Health Improvement) to monitor good practice, there will be a change of climate. Budgets will assume less importance than quality of care, delivered within budgetary constraints. The budget will still be considered when giving care but the quality of the care will become increasingly important, leading to better equipment and reduced pressure ulcer incidence with increased wound healing rates.

To achieve these changes in practice, the TVN must have excellent communication and change management skills that often require the background education found in a degree programme. Therefore, it is imperative that the TVN is part of higher education.

Change management

Strong hierarchical structures in the NHS, particularly in the nursing profession, with communication often highly formalized, can lead to a lack of co-operation (Broome 1990). This is particularly seen in specialist nurse roles when innovation is directly in conflict with managerial financial constraints or as a threat to the nurses directly caring for patients. Broome identified that an individual must be ready to change and must feel secure in change through 'ownership' of the change. However, it is not easy to introduce the same culture to managers who are often cost driven. Nevertheless, a problem-solving approach assists with this problem (Figure 14.1) and if managers do not respond to the first request for change, then it is re-evaluated, a new problem/solution identified and introduced. This process will be supported by a new job description.

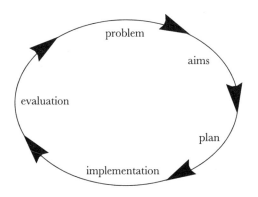

The problem-solving approach removed personal frustration as if one method does not achieve the desired results, another method will be considered, implemented, evaluated and the process continued until the goals are achieved

Figure 14.1 The problem-solving approach.

Advanced practice

It may be argued that many TVNs have been working at advanced practice level for some years, without the recognition of higher pay or without a title to recognize the position. Many TVNs are already at first and/or second degree level, autonomously prescribe wound care, work independently without support, develop and promote standards, guide and advise other professionals, manage a caseload of patients and manage budgets. They also develop relationships with other professionals for the advancement of tissue viability and make cost savings in resources without compromising quality. All of which would be required of an advanced practitioner.

The title 'Advanced Practitioner' is likely to offer very little to the role of the TVN and this is also likely to be taken into consideration by a clever government when considering who should receive the accolade of 'consultant nurse'. If the TVN is already practising at that higher level, it is unlikely that they will receive a different pay structure. Nevertheless, all nurses should be working toward advanced practice (whichever field they are in) so that patients can be offered the highest achievable quality care.

Clinical practice

Each TVN will have a different job description, with some responsible for hands-on patient care and others in an advisory role. Without a 'hands-on' role it is very difficult to develop wound care linked with experience. How will the TVN know that the advice they have provided is sound without seeing the results. However, if the TVN takes over the care of each patient with a wound, the general nurse will quickly become reliant and will become deskilled in wound care. The role, therefore, should be a fine balance of guidance, advice, education and actual hands-on care.

The TVN must ensure accurate diagnosis by liaising with all other professionals such as vascular consultants, diabetes specialist nurses, pain specialist nurses, etc. The role then becomes one of support, ensuring that the care plan is appropriate and complete and that follow-up visits show that the care is being followed. On discharge, the TVN must liaise with any carer or community nurse to ensure that care is continued at home.

The tissue viability nurse as a purchaser

One of the most important roles among the many that the TVN must undertake, is that of purchaser. High expenditure on a few high grade mattresses leaves the path open for pressure ulcer prevalence to increase. The concentration of resources on expensive mattresses may mean that basic foam mattress requirements are ignored and this ignores the utilitarian principles of the greatest good for the greatest number of people. If the greatest expenditure is on the lower grade mattresses with emphasis on quality and proven efficacy, then the requirement for higher grade mattresses may be null and void as pressure ulcer prevalence reduces.

The TVN is responsible for purchasing the highest quality resources at the lowest possible cost. Quality must never be compromised but, at the same time, the TVN must promote healing and maintain prevention in as many people as possible. It is therefore important that the money is used wisely.

At the time of writing the process of tender is requested for products that will cost over £10 000 per year; it is the only way to reduce overall cost of products and can be long and drawn out. The process involves the production of a specification – identified and important elements required of the equipment or dressing. This could be the type of foam used in mattresses (see Chapter 11), the cover design, research results on the product among many other specifications that are required. The TVN presents the specifications to the Supplies department and that department asks at least three companies to present the dressing or equipment that can match the specification.

The system of tender can be manipulated to suit the person producing the specification. If a certain mattress or dressing is required, the specification could be made to include that product and exclude others. This is probably never used in practice but is an option in theory. The safest form of tendering is generally through the NHS Supplies department, where the department is responsible for setting tender and purchasing. As they purchase in bulk, their purchase price can be very low. They then resell to the NHS hospitals and community at a mark-up to them but a reduced price for the purchaser. The purchaser prefers this system because the tendering work has been completed for them, supplies are guaranteed and they do not require storage facilities as NHS Supplies will deliver what is required when it is required. A simple and cost-effective method of purchase. The TVN is then responsible for selection of the required products from those within the NHS Supplies department catalogue. The problem that is then posed is how the TVN can extract the required and valid information from studies that may not relate to moribund or poorly patients.

Factors influencing the delineation of the TVN's role

'The appointment section of nursing journals illustrate why there is widespread confusion about nursing jobs titles. Advertisements include jobs for E-grade nurse practitioners' (MacClaine 1998). MacClaine also writes that 'the Clinical Nurse Specialist (TVN) must be willing to relinquish the protection offered by the medical delegation of tasks to embrace a philosophy of autonomous practice in which they are happy to take full responsibility for their actions and decisions'. This would place the role of TVN beyond the scope of an E-grade position and within the scope of H- or I-grade. Clinical nurse specialists (TVNs) have proved their effectiveness and realized the sense of job satisfaction that comes with greater responsibilities (Davis 1992; Kaufman 1996). However, the lack of agreement between trusts on the role of the TVN can leave nurses with a lower grade open to abuse from employers. They may be expected to work at a higher level – particularly when it is seen that other TVNs can make high quality and high cost-saving decisions in an autonomous manner. To protect the patient, there must be some consensus between trusts and employing aspects of a universal TVN job description.

The role of the tissue viability specialist is as educator, researcher, practitioner and consultant. However, other aspects must also be considered and aspects that can be identified within a SWOT (strengths, weaknesses, opportunities and threats) analysis would be motivation, economic considerations and change management, with audit supporting all of the factors. The identified factors can be examined and balanced against the advanced practice and professionalism required for an improved job description in tissue viability.

SWOT analysis of the tissue viability nurse role

The SWOT analysis (Table 14.1) shows interesting bias with strengths of the role being mainly educational opportunities; weaknesses mainly economic; opportunities mainly social and threats mainly economic or political. In developing a job description for the TVN, it is important to establish the future aim for the role and to look at how the negative areas of a SWOT analysis can be overcome through the development of new objectives and through the use of a problem-solving approach.

Table 14.1 The SWOT analysis

Strengths
Offers education in tissue viability to ward nurses
Focuses on new developments
Undertakes large-scale clinical trials
Audits tissue viability and uses the audit to develop problem areas
Rationalizes resources and saves the trust money to spend on patient services
Reduces pressure ulcer prevalence and, therefore, reduces patient discomfort, complaints and saves the trust from 'bed blocking'
Excellent support in all areas from the nurses on the wards

Weaknesses
Can fragmentize nurses' knowledge
Lack of financial support
Lack of possible recognition (from hospital mangers) for quality improvements and initiatives
Politics among departments can make it difficult to change practice
Low grade of pay for the TVN does not match the high responsibilities
No opportunities for promotion

Opportunities
Facilitates large changes in practice in tissue viability
Offers seamless care for the patient as the TVN can work closely with community care
Education opportunities are immense as tissue viability courses and conferences are continuous throughout the year.
Invited to travel the world to give lectures in tissue viability
Freedom to develop the role without interference

Threats
Could be isolated
Lack of finance may lead managers to see the role as potentially expensive if money for resources are requested
Specialist nurses are easily removed with redundancy when a trust is in negative equity
The role may become 'stagnant' and stop developing leading to a threat of conclusion of the job

---

The tissue viability nurse as an educator

Effective learning is a two-way process with good teachers constantly acquiring new knowledge during the process of imparting their own (Schurr and Turner 1982). However, this concept implies that the educator has an open mind and is willing to accept their knowledge limitations. Within tissue viability, it is unlikely that one could ever be described as an 'expert' in that field because wound treatments change rapidly and what is true today will almost certainly not apply tomorrow. Therefore, although education must be an important part of the job description, professional development should lead the way along with a willingness to learn from others. Those specialists who keep knowledge to themselves will lose the opportunities gained by learning from others.

Learning involves three stages, personal experience, reflection and transformation of knowledge and meaning (Butterworth and Faugier 1992). This implies that learning is best accomplished by 'doing' rather than through classroom lectures. This style of education has been demonstrated as successful in Eastbourne (Hampton 1997d). Therefore, the new job description should facilitate principles of best practice with nurses encouraged to discuss care for their patients as a learning opportunity, instead of 'handing over' the problem to the TVN. Teachers serve many functions in the teaching process; they stimulate enthusiasm, arouse curiosity and cultivate the crucial will to learn whilst acting as role models for their students (Williams 1992). As a role model and ward-based educator, the TVN can 'capture' those nurses who would not wish to attend a formal study day, thereby promoting the ideals in tissue viability.

Flanagan (1992a) believes that education is an integral part of the TVN's role with identification of training needs, implementation and development of educational programmes for nurses, other staff and patients.

At present, nursing care is failing the patient because the care is driven by tradition rather being than patient-driven (Walsh and Ford 1992) and it is not acceptable that poor practice is based on 'we have always done it this way!' (Williams 1992). It is, therefore, important for any education to be firmly supported by research-based evidence that the prescribed care is founded on sound rationale.

The tissue viability nurse as a researcher and auditor

Christensen et al. (1994: 311) wrote on nursing research as 'A spirit of enquiry that helps to guide the systematic exploration of accumulated nursing knowledge as well as nursing practice issues and problems'. Nursing is a research-based profession (DHSS 1972) but, today's information is based on yesterday's research and there is uncertainty whether it is relevant for tomorrow (Rees 1992). Therefore, the most acceptable research is action research – ongoing research that develops and changes with the outcomes of evaluation (Gibbings 1993).

Although randomized controlled trials are now accepted as the gold standard in research (Fogg and Gross 2000), the philosophy of action research is possibly better suited to evaluation and audit. As this process has been successful (Hampton 1997a, 1997b, 1997c) it would be valuable for any TVN job description to support a similar formula.

The tissue viability nurse as advanced practitioner and consultant

Flanagan (1992a) stated that a 'clinical nurse specialist does not practice nursing in the traditional manner; experience and education, together with freedom from daily patient care, allows the specialist to make an objective assessment of wound management problems and offer innovative solutions'.

The advanced practitioner practises within a framework of theoretically based knowledge, combines that knowledge with expertise and is essential in influencing quality care. Studies have shown the improvements of quality care that can be achieved through the introduction of specialist nurses in patient care (Wright 1991). A multi-professional group including community GP and district nurse, hospital nurse, hospital consultant and nursing homes will consult the experienced TVN, which advances the opportunity for education. Any job description should reflect this.

Economics

Although current trends in healthcare reform result from economic constraints, they nonetheless present opportunities for nursing to develop further in the advanced practice role (Deane 1993). The TVN can use the outcome of research and audit to demonstrate savings for the hospital trust if essential financial responsibility (for purchasing resources) is fulfilled. There is an opportunity for the TVN to reorganize dressing supplies, limiting choice for normal dressing regimes but widening choice on an ad hoc basis for dressing difficult wounds. Combined with education, this can offer effective care and cost savings in any healthcare setting. There is also an opportunity to develop pressure ulcer prevention through proactive actions rather than being reactive to an established ulcer. Purchasing good foam basic mattresses will reduce the need for expensive air mattresses and purchasing several (cheaper) air overlays instead of the expensive dynamic air replacement mattresses has far-reaching consequences. Seven air overlays can prevent ulcers in seven patients at a time whereas, for the same cost, the expensive replacements can treat only one patient. Although this is a utilitarian view, it can be argued that if the ulcers are prevented, there is less need for the replacement mattresses. A TVN can apply knowledge and experience in decision making in wound care and pressure ulcer prevention and should be allowed to make, and answer for, those decisions.

Motivation

Motivation may depend on the expectations of those around and a lack of motivation may derive from the feeling that the TVN is unable to influence the course of events (Hinchcliffe 1995). The TVN must have the freedom to make decisions and the means to purchase requirements. However, it would be unwise for the TVN to arrive at the decision without consulting colleagues, as they will require 'ownership' of any change if they are to apply and support the consequence of the change. Motivation and driving force can be the ability to measure and identify the benefits brought about by changes and also seeing the transformation and motivation of colleagues, achieved through change management.

Job description for the role of tissue viability nurse specialist

The following job description is loosely based on the generic framework of competencies devised by the National Association of Tissue Viability Nurse Specialists. It is not the definitive answer to the role of the tissue viability, but it will enable qualified nurses, wishing to enter the field of tissue viability, to base their future educational requirements on the obligations of the job description.

Job title:	**Tissue Viability Nurse Specialist**

Qualifications:	RN Educated to 1st and/or 2nd degree level Portfolio of relevant experience and achievements Knowledge of developing standards Demonstrable knowledge of research and audit Demonstrable knowledge of wound healing principles and dressing application
Skills:	Proven managerial skills Proven ability to think analytically Excellent written and verbal presentation skills Excellent interpersonal skills
Grade:	H/I
Accountable to:	(Appropriate department dictated by the trust. i.e. Quality Assurance)
Department:	
Role:	To provide a resource of specialist nursing for patients with compromised tissue viability by providing advice and clinical support combined with clinical decision making and the ability to monitor and improve standards of care.
Job purpose:	The tissue viability nurse is responsible for providing a strategic approach to the prevention and management of pressure injuries and treatment of chronic wounds. The post holder will be responsible for implementation and evaluation of the strategy and will offer education in pressure damage prevention to underpin the successful implementation of the strategy.

Clinical practice:
1 Will act as a specialist nursing resource for individualized patient care based on sound clinical evidence.
2 Will act as a role model to students and colleagues through professional and knowledgeable leadership.

3 Will be responsible for ensuring a strategic approach to the prevention and management of pressure injuries and treatment of chronic wounds.
4 Will act as patient advocate applying knowledge, skills and clinical evidence as a sound basis for ethical care.
5 Will undertake audit of all services provided through tissue viability ensuring the development of quality care.
6 Will undertake change management in areas identified through audit or through development of knowledge.
7 Will consult with relevant professionals and departments to develop a cost-effective formulary in wound management.

Key responsibilities
1 Provision of clinical evidence and advice in the purchase of new resources.
2 To provide staff with the means to obtain appropriate pressure-reducing equipment when required.
3 To ensure that all staff, involved in patient care, are aware of methods of prevention of pressure ulcers.
4 To co-ordinate a programme of audit in pressure ulcer prevention.
5 To develop standards and audit in relation to management and treatment of chronic wounds.
6 To act as a specialist resource for the management of patients with compromised tissue viability.
7 To establish a professional relationships with all relevant professionals and departments.
8 To identify educational needs of staff, patients and carers in relation to tissue viability and to implement and evaluate educational initiatives.
9 To conduct investigations and to develop research appreciation and critical awareness of staff whilst demonstrating the application of evidence-based practice.
10 To identify where cost savings can be made without compromising quality of patient care.
11 To maintain up-to-date knowledge of chronic wound practices and in reduction of pressure injuries and to contribute to advances of knowledge in this field.
12 To implement, and collaborate with, research in promoting quality and high standards in tissue viability.
13 Dissemination of research findings to all.

Working relationships
1   To work with the Audit Department to improve and/or maintain excellent standards of care in tissue viability.
2   To support Quality Assurance in ensuring standards are achieved and maintained in tissue viability.
3   To work with Infection Control to ensure cost-effective and high standards are maintained in prevention of cross-infection.
4   To work with the Wound Care Group in reviewing the efficacy and cost-effectiveness of wound dressings.
5   To work with medical staff to consult, advise and to act as a resource in the treatment and management of difficult wounds.
6   To work with nursing staff to advise on wound care, pressure ulcer prevention and to assist in producing audit leading to cost-effective and high standards of patient care.
7   To work collaboratively with the Community Trust and local nursing homes in all aspects related to tissue viability.

Summary

The tissue viability nurse specialist will be responsible for the development of knowledge within the specialist area, the dissemination of information and promotion of standards.

Conclusion

Professionalism and development of skills of the specialist nurse role requires that proficiency, advanced practice and education is promoted by the job description. However, there is not a formal route to exploit when attempting to change managerial viewpoints. It must be the intention of any job description, to open this route – to allow pursuit of the ideal goal in achieving the highest care possible in tissue viability.

Nevertheless, the TVN will practise within a framework of theoretically-based knowledge, combining knowledge and expertise and supported by a partnership with other departments within the trust and in alliance with other professionals such as community practitioners, hospital nurses, occupational therapists, physiotherapists and doctors.

The TVN role is an important part of providing quality patient care. Without the guidance of a specialist, tissue viability could become expensive and patients could receive care that is not based on research with good clinical evidence. Education of those caring for wounds would be lacking; the future of tissue viability could be bleak. Trusts that employ a TVN should offer support to ensure that research, audit and educational development is undertaken and cost-effective care is provided.

Whilst the TVN is an essential person in influencing quality care in the traditional practice settings, there are now opportunities with clientele and practice settings which have expanded beyond the conventional boundaries (Sparacino 1992).

Appendix

Some recognized dressings

COTTON WOOL AND GAUZE

Dressing pads Gamgee Gauze	Highly absorbent and used as secondary dressings for highly exuding wounds.
	Cotton wool and cotton gauze were traditionally used to clean wounds or as a primary dressing. Gamgee or dressing pads can be useful in containing large amounts of exudate. Use of cotton wool can cause trauma to tissues (Flanagan 1997) and can shed fibres in the wound giving a focus for infection (Wood 1976). This greatly limits the use of cotton wool for cleaning or cotton gauze as primary dressings, although the use of dressing pads or wadding (e.g. Gamgee, Surgipad, multidress) still has a place as a secondary dressing. Cotton gauze is still used in some countries for 'wet to dry' debridement where gauze is soaked in saline and then placed in the wound and allowed to dry. It is then ripped out and is a successful debriding method. Not used in the UK because of the probability of pain for the patient.
Rationale for use	Exudate management as secondary dressing. Can offer protection for vulnerable wounds.

ALGINATES

Algosteril Algisite* M Curasorb Kaltogel, Kaltostat, Melgisorb Tegagen, Seasorb Sorbsan Sorbalgon Algisite	For medium to high exudate and cavity wounds. Produced from seaweed with high calcium content. All alginates transform to gel in the presence of exudate, are hydrophilic and are useful in highly exuding wounds but are best avoided in low exudate wounds (Miller and Dyson 1996). Some alginates contain mannuronic acid, which breaks down quickly in the presence of sodium and rinses quickly away. Others contain guluronic acid, which maintains its structure making removal, in one piece, easy. Highly absorbent. Keeps the wound bed moist, is easily removed and can reduce pain as exposed nerve endings are protected (Flanagan 1997). However, the osmotic pressure caused by the alginate's hydrophilic nature can possibly increase pain in a wound that is dry. Requires a secondary dressing to:

- support the alginate *in situ*
- maintain a moist environment.

	Some alginates also have proven haemostatic properties and are therefore useful in wounds prone to bleeding. To reduce bleeding, an alginate should be placed in the wound for 10 minutes and then removed and replaced with another alginate sheet. Alginates high in guluronic acid (e.g. Kaltostat) will retain shape within the wound bed. Mannuronic alginates (e.g. Sorbsan) (Dealey 1994a) lose the shape and are easily washed away from the wound with
Alginate Ribbon Kaltostat Sorbsan Melgisorb	saline. Alginates require a secondary dressing to maintain a moist environment, particularly when used as a haemostat.

Rationale for use	Maintain a moist environment. Management of exudate in medium exudate wounds. Non-traumatic removal. Useful as haemostat.
Combiderm	Used for moderate exudate. The dressing is self-adhesive and has a central island of super absorbent cellulose granules which wicks exudate. Retains fluid, keeps the wound bed moist but not wet and will not adhere to the wound. Differing sizes of dressing and a sacral shaped dressing.
Combiderm N	Same as above but non-adhesive.
Rationale for use	Management of exudate in medium to high exudate wounds.
Transorb	A, hydrocellular, self-adhesive wound dressing with a highly absorbent core. Transorb combines the film, a foam, and a hydrogel, to form an absorbent wound dressing. Transorb provides a moist wound environment.
Rationale for use	Management of exudate in medium to high exudate wounds. Useful in reduction of overgranulation (see Chapter 2).
Allevyn Cavity	A foam pad of differing sizes and shapes covered with a non-adherent surface designed as a cavity dressing and for high exudate. Will not adhere to the wound bed and the hydrophilic foam centre absorbs exudate whilst the hydrophobic outer cover keeps wound moist but not wet. Does not debride necrotic or sloughy wounds and requires secondary dressing.
Cutinova Cavity	Cutinova Cavity is a sterile wound dressing

made of a polyurethane matrix with embedded absorbent particles.

Rationale for use   Maintain moist environment.
Manage medium exudate wounds.
Protect vulnerable areas.

Cavicare   Foam dressing designed for medium to high exudate. The dressing is prepared by the practitioner by mixing two elements, one of polymer and the other a catalyst that is easily reconstituted if kept in the fridge prior to use. The cold slows the process as the mixture vulcanizes at room temperature (Williams 1995). Because the practitioner reconstitutes it, it fits the shape of the cavity wound perfectly. Can be washed and soaked in chlorhexidine (10 minutes), rinsed in sterile saline and replaced in the wound. Changes in the wound size can be judged by the need to reduce the size of the foam. Prevents premature wound closure (Williams 1995). Requires secondary dressing and does not debride necrotic or sloughy wounds. The dressing can 'set' very quickly, therefore, speed of reconstitution and application is necessary.

Rationale for use   Cosmetically acceptable in face wounds.
Useful for medium exudate.
Conforms to even difficult wounds.

HYDROCOLLOIDS

Replicare Cutinova hydro Comfeel Easyderm Granuflex Hydrocoll Tegasorb	Especially suitable for chronic wounds such as pressure sores, leg ulcers, superficial wounds and low exudate. Particularly suitable for wounds that require desloughing and for providing a moist environment to promote healing. Consist of a mixture of pectins, gelatines, sodium carboxymethyl cellulose and elastomers.

Hydrocolloids are available in a number of forms, as wafers, extra absorbent wafers, extra thin wafers, granules, powders, gels and pastes. On contact with wound exudate, the hydrocolloid material dissolves into a gel. This gel provides many of the favourable conditions of moist wound healing. But, as it mixes with exudate, it has a particular 'yellow' appearance and can exude a characteristic odour. Although this is normal and to be expected with these products, those handling the dressing, and also the patient being treated, need to be aware (Flanagan 1997). Care should be taken to ensure that the correct size of dressing is applied, that is one large enough to cover the wound with an overlap of at least 5 cm. Hydrocolloids can reduce dressing change interval to around five days. The hydrocolloid pastes are easily used and

Bordered Duoderm extra thin

are effective desloughing agents. Excellent for small cavity wounds. Can reduce pain through moistening the nerve endings (Flanagan 1997).

Granuflex paste

Provides optimum wound-healing environment (Flanagan 1997) and can be left *in situ* for five or six days. (remove if 'strike-through' is apparent). Hydrocolloids also provide a hypoxic environment, which promotes angiogenesis in the first stage of healing. The patient is able to bath/shower without removing the dressing.

NB: Easyderm does not provide a hypoxic environment but is a 'breathable' dressing. Peri-wound areas can become macerated, particularly when used in conjunction with a hydrogel. Not suitable for highly exuding wounds.

Rationale for use

Occlusive, can reduce bacterial contamination.

Provides a hypoxic environment for the wound and increases potential for angiogenesis.

Absorption of exudate enables the dressing to conform to the wound.

Provides a moist environment.
Does not require a secondary dressing.
Cosmetically acceptable.
Non-traumatic removal.

HYDROCOLLOID AND HYDROFIBRE

Versiva	Versiva is a hydrocolloid base that maintains a moist interface with the wound whilst a hydrofibre centre and foam third layer will absorb fluid.
HYDROFIBRE Aquacel Aquacel ribbon	A hydrofibre dressing is also a hydrocolloid. Particularly useful in cavities and highly exuding wounds. It is a foam pad of differing sizes and shapes covered with a non-adherent surface, which will not adhere to the wound bed. The hydrophilic foam centre absorbs exudate and the hydrophobic outer cover keeps wound moist but not wet. Requires secondary dressing and does not debride necrotic or sloughy wounds although the moisture from the exudate in the hydrocolloid will support autolysis. Available on drug tariff.
Rationale for use	Maintains a moist environment. Management of medium to high exudate. Potential reduction in bacterial colonization. Non -traumatic removal.

FOAM

Allevyn Cutinova Cutinova Thin Flexipore Lyofoam Tielle Spyrosorb Trufoam Mepilex	Foam dressings are for moderate exudate and superficial wounds. They are not interactive and will not reduce bacterial colonization or deslough wounds. May be useful for reducing overgranulation. Some sheets may have a non-adherent surface and an occlusive surface. Foam sheets are hydrophilic and absorb quantities of exudate. All sheets have a non-adherent surface

and can be used as a second dressing with a desloughing agent next to the wound. However, care must be taken as maceration can occur when hydrogels are used in conjunction with some foam sheets. All sheets are easily applied and highly absorbent. Cutinova Foam is a sterile wound dressing consisting of a polyurethane matrix and a polyurethane top film. Cutinova Thin is designed for the care of granulating, moderately exuding superficial wounds such as leg ulcers, secondary treatment of abrasions and skin graft donor sites, stage I–II pressure ulcers, partial thickness burns, post-surgical hypertrophic scars and secondary treatment of wounds after hand and plastic surgery.

Mepilex is a silicone dressing with Safetac. Safetac provides an adhesive backing that adheres to good skin but not to broken skin.

Rationale for use	Absorption of exudate. Maintains a moist environment.

DISPERSION THERAPY

Vacutex	A hydrocellular, non-woven, three-layer dressing which comprises of 100 per cent polyester outer layer, 80 per cent polyester inner layer and 20 per cent cotton fibres. The perforated layer prevents the micro fibres from shedding into the wound. The non-woven outer layers are able to transport, lift and hold exudate by capillary action. The woven inner layer prevents 'strike-through' by allowing exudate to move across and through the fabric (dispersion technique) and not to pass directly to the surface of the fabric. The inner and outer layer combine to draw the exudate away from the wound surface. This action may remove pathogenic bacteria and

potentially lower the bacterial count in the wound bed. The material is used to line ski jackets because of the warmth that is generated. This may also be a reason for rapid healing rates as the dressing would provide increased warmth to the wound.

Rationale for use   Absorption of medium to high exudate.

Tenderwet   A multilayer wound dressing pad with a core of super-absorbent polyacrylate. The superabsorbent compound is activated before use with Ringers or Hartmanns solution. The absorbent layer has an affinity for protein solutions and less of an affinity for isotonic solutions. The absorbent pad takes up exudate in preference to the Hartmanns/Ringers solution and releases the isotonic solution into the wound bed. The dressing continues to release solution into the wound, keeping the wound moist and absorbing microorganisms, thereby, cleansing the wound bed. The dressing is changed after 12 hours. Reduces exudate in a wound, and is suitable for all wounds.

HYDROGELS

Aquaform
Geliperm
Granugel
Intrasite
Purilon
Nugel
Sterigel

Hydrogels are high in water content and are useful in rehydration of hard eschar and promotion of autolysis. Used for sloughy, necrotic wounds (Bale and Harding 1990) and are ideal for cavities, leg ulcers and pressure sores. The hydrogels are suitable for cavities and are effective for desloughing and debriding wounds (Bale and Harding 1990). They can macerate peri-wound areas in highly exuding wounds that are occluded. Hydrogels are available in sheets or gel. The sheets are made up of gelable polysaccharide agarose, cross-linked with polyacrylamide. This material provides a moist environment for healing in flat wounds such as burns, fungating lesions, skin graft donor sites or dry to slightly exuding wounds. Novogel contains glycerine, which may reduce bacterial colonization. Gels may reduce pain as the moistness of the dressing 'bathes' exposed nerve endings.

HYDROGEL SHEETS

Novogel Second skin Hydrosorb Cica C Silgel	Some gel sheets containing silicon are used for reducing hypertrophic scarring. Cica C and Silgel are marketed particularly for this reason.
Intrasite conformable	This is a new dressing that has the appearance of paraffin gauze but contains hydrogel instead of paraffin. This does not stick and conforms well the wound. Should be placed on the wound in layers, i.e. the dressing could be folded. Care should be taken to ensure that peri-wound maceration does not occur.

ENZYME

Varidase	Streptokinase and streptodornase (Varidase) are two enzymes traditionally used to promote debridement of necrotic wounds. Streptokinase is thrombolytic and acts directly on a substrate of fibrin by activating a fibrinolytic enzyme in human serum breaking up thrombi (Martin 1996). Streptodornase liquefies the viscous nucleoprotein of dead cells or pus. The joint action of the two enzymes rehydrates the hard necrotic material in a wound and allows the secondary dressing and/or irrigation to remove the liquefied material. Useful, therefore, for hard eschar and black/green necrotic tissue. The

recommendation of the *British National Formulary* is that it should be applied as a wet dressing and changed one to two times daily, although it can be left for longer periods when mixed with hydrogel and placed under a hydrocolloid. Can be useful as a cavity dressing but is difficult to apply to the wound unless mixed with hydrogel. There is some doubt as to efficacy (Martin 1996) and the cost of Varidase (particularly if used twice daily as recommended) is prohibitive. Changing dressings twice daily is difficult to achieve and Varidase is often soaked into gauze and placed on the eschar. Although this may help the gauze, it is unlikely to benefit the wound. Flanagan (1997) writes 'it is not successful on dehydrated and hard eschar'.

Mepital
Omiderm
Tegasorb

Used for superficial wounds, burns, leg ulcers and donor sites. Useful in moderate to high exudate (used with secondary dressing) and can be left *in situ* with the secondary dressing changed PRN. Mepital contains Safetac, which will only adhere to dry skin and therefore will not cause pain on removal. These are hydrophobic dressings, which allow the exudate to pass through into the secondary dressing. Non-adherent and easily applied.

MULTIDRESS

Multidress
  compress
Multidress
  ribbon
Multidress WCL
Multidress
  standard
Multidress Extra

Designed for moderate exudate, the dressings contain gelling fibres which retain fluid and keeps the wound bed moist but not wet.
The dressings will not adhere to the wound. The dressing range provides similar characteristics to other conventional dressings but the addition of gelling fibres gives enhanced performance including lower adherence and superior performance.

Exu-dry   Designed as a one-piece wound dressing made
                   up of multilayers. Exu-dry's speciality upper
                   extremities dressings are designed to conform
                   readily and comfortably to the contours of the
                   upper extremities.

Primapore   Primapore dressings combine an absorbent pad
                   with a soft and conformable fixative layer for the
                   simple and effective management of sutured
                   wounds.

Melolin   An absorbent pad bonded to a wound contact
                   polyester perforated film, which is useful for
                   superficial wounds. Easily applied and easily
                   obtained with some absorbent properties.
                   Claimed to be non-adherent although it has been
                   known to adhere to wounds (Hampton 1997f).
                   This dressing has limited absorbency and is most
                   suitable for lightly exuding wounds (Bale 1991a).
                   A layer of viscose rayon covered with non-woven
                   material and bonded to a polyethylene film.
Release   Absorbent dressing with perforated film backing.
Skintac
Telfa   A layer of cotton enclosed in a perforated film
                   (Bale 1991a), which is useful for superficial
                   wounds. Easily applied and easily obtained with
                   some absorbent properties.

NA DRESSINGS

                   NAs (non-adherent) are a single layer of knitted
                   viscose, which requires secondary dressing to
                   absorb exudate.
Cicaplaie   Cicaplaie is a sterile adhesive wound dressing
Tricotex   that is designed for post-operative use, for cuts,
                   lacerations and sutured wounds.

NA Ultra   NA Ultra contains silicone, which improves the
Paratex   non-adherence of the dressing.

TULLE DRESSINGS

Jelonet
(impregnated with
paraffin)

Tulle dressings are sheets of gauze impregnated with various amounts or loading of paraffin. Antiseptics and other agents can also be added. They have the advantage of being cheap and when correctly applied (i.e. in sufficient thickness) can be of low adherence to the wound surface.

Suitable only for superficial wounds and can adhere to wounds and cause trauma on removal. If painful on removal, the tulle should not be applied a second time unless used in sufficient thickness to prevent adherence. Useful when applied to peri-wound areas that are macerating or with several layers (up to five) on low exudate wounds. Paraffin gauze requires frequent dressing change to prevent adherence particularly as paraffin is hydrophobic and cannot be freed by irrigation once attached to a wound bed. A useful tip for removal of tulle that is stuck is to apply a hydrogel and massage it through the dressing. Always requires secondary dressing.

Bactigras
(impregnated with
chlorhexidine)

Bactigras is an antiseptic (chlorhexidine) dressing. (Refer to Chlorhexidine Chapter 3.)

Fucidin
Sofra-Tulle
(impregnated
with antibiotics)

Fucidin and Sofra-Tulle are antibiotic impregnated tulle dressings, which can lead to antibiotic-resistant infections and sensitivity (Hampton 1997d). With leg ulcer patients, additives frequently cause allergic reaction and antiseptics have been shown to delay healing (Leaper 1987). Clinically infected wounds are always best treated systemically.

NON-MEDICATED FILM

Bioclusive Cutifilm EpiView Opsite Tegaderm Transite Smartfilm 1000 Hydrofilm Mefilm	These films are made up of a clear polyurethane type film and are coated with an adhesive. Wounds can be viewed without dressing removal. Due to their highly elastomeric and extensible properties, these dressings are conformable and resistant to shear and tear. They are semi-permeable and as a second dressing, can help to provide an optimum wound-healing environment. Will not absorb exudate and may require aspiration of exudate to avoid premature leaking. (This can be done by use of a small needle and syringe and a new patch of film to cover the puncture site.)

MEDICATED FILM

Arglaes	Contains silver as an antimicrobial agent and delivers a controlled antibacterial effect in the wound. Silver has been used for centuries as an antibacterial agent. Useful in infected superficial wounds and is resistant to shearing forces. The dressing is semi-permeable and the wound may be viewed without dressing removal. Will not absorb exudate. May require aspiration of exudate to avoid premature leaking (as above).

LIQUID FILM

Cavilon SuperSkin	Liquid film is useful for macerated/excoriated tissues over peri-wound areas or around stomas. Protects tissues from urine, faeces and dribbled saliva and is also useful for nappy rash. Both films are painless on application although SuperSkin *may* feel warm when applied to wet tissues. Can protect tissues for up to 72 hours and are useful as protection for surgical wounds. SuperSkin is rough to the touch which may increase adherence. Cavilon is easily applied with a 'lollypop

stick' applicator. Both films are also useful to increase adherence of other, difficult to apply dressings such as faecal collectors or hydrocolloids.

CARBON

Carbonet
Actisorb Silver 220
Clinisorb
Carboflex
Lyofoam C
Carbopad VC

Designed for malodorous wounds, as charcoal dressings filter and deodorize. Actisorb contains silver as an antibacterial agent but should be used as primary dressing. Carboflex has a unique five layer construction, comprising a Kaltostat, and Aquacel wound contact layer, activated charcoal cloth, absorbent padding, with an EMA film cover. Lyofoam is absorbent with an activated carbon centre. It is thought that carbon looses its ability to absorb odour when wet.

SUGAR PASTE

Thick paste
Thin paste

Useful for malodorous wounds and colonized wounds as sugar has an osmotic effect on bacteria and 'pulls' fluid out of the cell so the bacteria cannot survive. Once the bacteria is removed the odour is reduced. Anecdotally appears to promote autolysis and is inexpensive but messy. Some sugar pastes contain iodine, whilst others contain hydrogen peroxide. However, sugar paste is sometimes difficult to obtain and is largely unresearched.

ANTIBACTERIAL

Iodoflex
Iodosorb

Iodine is slowly released from the powder base and 'bathes' the wound in iodine over a 72-hour period. Useful for malodorous and colonized wounds. Promotes autolysis/desloughs and absorbs large quantities of exudate. Can be applied under a film dressing to allow viewing of the wound. When the dressing appears white, the iodine is depleted and must be changed. Cannot apply more than 50 gms for each application or greater than 150 gms per week. Duration of treatment should be no longer than three months but when the wound appears to be granulating, the iodine cadexomer should be discontinued. Hyperphillic dressings can often be painful because of the 'pull' of the dry dressing on the fluid within the cells.

Inadine
Poviderm

A povidone-iodine based dressing can be traumatic when applied to an open wound and has been thought to be damaging to wound healing (Rodheaver 1989). Nevertheless, it is an antiseptic that is undergoing a revival and iodine is now considered to promote wound healing in chronic wounds (Gilchrist 1997). Used for colonized and superficial wounds iodine has been shown to be useful in MRSA infection (Hampton 1997a). However, pus quickly deactivates the iodine and therefore its use in heavily colonized wounds is wasteful. The dressing is easily applied and non-adherent and is useful in wounds that are superficial but at risk of infection.

Acticoat (with
Nanocry-
stalline Silver)
Acticoat 7

Silver interferes with electron transportation and binds to DNA of bacteria. It induces cell membrane interactions causing structural damage.
Acticoat dressing is an effective antimicrobial barrier dressing. The nanocrystalline coating of silver rapidly kills a broad spectrum of bacteria in as little as 30 minutes. The dressing consists of three layers: an absorbent inner core sandwiched between outer layers of silver coated, low adherent polyethylene net. Nanocrystalline silver protects the wound site from bacterial contamination whilst the inner core helps maintain the

moist environment optimal for wound healing. The nanocrystalline coating of silver rapidly kills a broad spectrum of bacteria in as little as 30 minutes and is effective for up to seven days.

Acticoat 7 dressing consists of five layers: two layers of an absorbent inner core sandwiched between three layers of silver coated, low adherent polyethylene net. Nanocrystalline silver protects the wound site from bacterial contamination whilst the inner core helps maintain the moist environment optimal for wound healing.

Acticoat
Avance
Silver sulphadi-azine (Flamazine)
Arglaes
Actisorb silver 220

All of these dressings contain silver to reduce bacterial colonization and to reduce potential for clinical infection.

Bactigras

Chlorhexidine has a low toxicity to living tissues and is effective against a wide range of Gram-negative and Gram-positive organisms (Morrison 1989).

IMPREGNATED BANDAGES

Calaband
Icthopaste
Steripaste

The bandages (apart from Zipzoc) are generally 'pleated' on the leg to prevent constriction when they dry. If the pleating is performed by winding the bandage backward and forward over the leg, the bandage is then easily removed. The bandage treats the whole leg rather than just the wound and applies wound healing principles by keeping the wound warm, moist and occluded. Can be cooling to irritated legs. May contain parabens or lanolin, both of which are causes of skin sensitivities. The bandages are easy to apply, can be left for up to one week and are inexpensive.

Visco paste	Types of bandages include: zinc impregnated,
Zipzoc	coaltar impregnated, calamine impregnated,
Quiniband	zinc mixed with 50/50 (Zipzoc) (50 per cent
	paraffin 50 per cent petroleum jelly).

LARVAE THERAPY

Maggots are not a new component in wound care, they have been found in wounds over centuries and have possibly been responsible for saving lives on many battlefields (Morgan 1997b). Green bottle larvae are known to digest devitalized tissue only and do not normally harm healthy tissue. Patients may dislike the idea although those patients with malodorous and long-standing wounds often welcome this treatment to speed up the healing. The action of the larvae is thought to stimulate wound healing and the maggots eliminate all but one type of bacteria from the wound, which eliminates malodour. Treatment with maggots can be cost effective as debridement is rapid although nurses may find it distasteful to apply. The maggots produce powerful proteolytic enzymes that degrade and liquefy necrotic tissue and can, therefore, be successful in debriding wounds.

LEECHES

Leeches have been used as therapy for centuries. They are particularly useful following surgery and for haematomas. They inject an analgesic substance into the tissues along with an anticoagulant and once introduced to the skin, they attach themselves in the form of a C and feed for 20 minutes. The action of the feeding stimulates blood supply to the tissues and the anticoagulant prevents clotting and the wound will continue to bleed for up to 24 hours. The action of sucking draws blood supply into damaged tissues and the anticoagulant they introduce helps to reduce haematoma. At £9 per leech, they can be expensive and nurses may find them distasteful to apply. Patients may also dislike the idea. See Figures 3.6, 3.7a and 3.7b, which show the difference leeches can make to a badly bruised area.

NEGATIVE PRESSURE

(Vacuum-assisted closure or VAC)
The VAC is a fairly new concept. It is a machine that can introduce intermittent or continuous vacuum therapy to a wound. The suction stimulates the blood supply to the wound bed and removes exudate and so it is possible that the VAC can reduce the incidence of infection or colonization as bacteria may be removed from the wound by the suction. Removes exudate and stimulates blood flow. Creates a hypoxic environment encouraging granulation tissue across the wound bed. The patient needs to be near to an electrical supply and so it limits movement. However, a new ambulatory machine has been produced which can be used in the community. Therapy is expensive and, with dressings, can cost as much as £40 per day at the time of writing.

WARM-UP

Warm-up is a new concept in wound healing. It is a clear plastic film dressing positioned on an adherent foam ring and is free from contact with the wound. A plate is placed into a pocket in the clear film dressing and is connected to a battery pack. The temperature of the wound is elevated above normal and remains at that temperature for one hour, three times a day. When the plate is removed the wound bed can be seen clearly through the film cover. Exudate is collected in the foam ring that supports the film. The warmth from the dressing causes vasodilation and encourages blood supply into the wound bed and increases tensile strength in the healed wound (Stadelmann et al. 1998). Price et al. (2000) found that subjects receiving radiant heat to their wounds experienced a statistically significantly faster rate of healing.

GROWTH FACTORS AND NATURAL DRESSINGS

Vivoderm Dermagraft Apligraft	Suitable for wounds that require skin grafting. Vivoderm (hyaluronic acid) is developed from the patient's own skin and Dermagraft is developed from human skin. Both products can be used to treat large areas of tissue loss. (Hyaluronic acid is intrinsically involved in the process of wound repair and enhances neo-angiogenesis and cell migration.) It is a natural product that is easily applied. Dermagraft is largely used to treat diabetic foot ulcers and Vivoderm has been used to treat burns. Both treatments are initially expensive but can be cost-effective if wounds heal faster through treatment.
Oasis Promogran	Oasis and Promogran are a new stage in natural dressings. Oasis is made from porcine small intestinal submucosa, a naturally occurring extracellular matrix and Promoran containing 55 per cent collagen.

LASER

Suitable for most wounds but there is little evidence that it stimulates wounds to faster healing. However, the author uses it when the wound bed is filled with granulation tissue because, at this point, the laser appears to give tensile strength to the wound. However, it requires expert handling and so this limits its use.

INFRARED

An old concept that has a renewed application. Utilizes the natural production of nitrous oxide in the body to cause vasodilation.

Not yet on the market at time of writing. Practitioners should ensure that any infrared device used in wound care has received clinical evaluations and studies prior to purchase and use.

For non-healing intractable wounds.

HAEMOSTAT

Surgicel
Traumacel

Surgicel is a haemostatic mesh, which is used to control bleeding, generally post surgery.

Traumacel is copolymer of anhydroglucuronic acid and anhydroglucose. Used for controlling capillary bleeding in wounded tissue. Available as a gauze, powder or spray.

SKIN ADHESIVE

Dermabond
Histoacryl blue

A topical skin adhesive that is used to approximate the edges of traumatic wounds on the face, trunk and limbs. Removes the pain of suturing and stitch removal.

Bibliography

Abatangelo G (1998) Background to tissue engineering. Presentation at Eighth Annual Meeting of the European Tissue Repair Society, Copenhagen.

Adam K, Oswald I (1983) Protein synthesis, bodily renewal and the sleep-wake cycle. Clinical Scientist. **65**: 561–567.

Agate J (1972) Geriatrics for Nurses and Social Workers. London: Heinemann.

Akasaka Y, Fujita K, Ishikawa Y, Asuwa N, Inuzuka K, Ishihara M, Ito M, Masuda T, Akishima Y, Zhang L, Ito K, Ishii T. (2001) Detection of apoptosis in keloids and a comparative study on apoptosis between keloids, hypertrophic scars, normal healed flat scars and dermatofibroma. Wound Repair and Regeneration **November-December**: 501–505.

Alberman K (1992) Is there any connection between laundering and the development of pressure sores? Journal of Tissue Viability 2(2): 5–6.

Alexander NM, Nishimoto M (1981) Protein-linked idiotyrosines in serum after topical application of povidone-iodine. Journal of Endocrinal and Metabolism **53**: 105–108.

Alhady SM, Siavanatharajah K (1961) Keloids in various races: a review of 17 cases. Plastic Reconstructive Surgery 27: 335–338.

Allen S (1988) Ulcers: treating the cause. Nursing Times **84(51)**: 62–63.

Allman RM (1989) Epidemiology of pressure sores in different populations. Decubitous **2(2)**: 30–34.

Andrews AM, Thomas S, Wilson M (1998) The effect of hydrogels on maggot growth. Presentation at Eighth Annual Meeting of the European Tissue Repair Society, Copenhagen.

Angle N, Bergan JJ (1997) Chronic venous ulcer. British Medical Journal **314**: 7086 1019–1023.

Apwlqvist J (1998) Improvements in the prophylactic and conservative treatment approach. Presentation at Eighth Annual Meeting of the European Tissue Repair Society, Copenhagen.

Arao H, Shimada T, Hagisawa S (2001) Morphological architecture and distribution of blood capillaries and elastic fibres in the human skin. Journal of Tissue Viability **11(1)**: 39.

Archer HG, Barnett S, Irving S et al. (1990) Controlled model of moist wound healing: comparison between semi-permeable film, antiseptics and sugar paste. Journal of Experimental Pathology **71**: 155–170.

445

Arthur J (2000) When is reduced–compression bandaging safe and effective? Journal of Wound Care **9(10)**: 469–471.

Arturson G (1993) Management of burns. Journal of Wound Care **2(2)**: 107–112.

Asatekin M (1975) Postural and Physiological Criteria for Seating – A Review. Journal of the Faculty of Architecture **Spring**: 55–83.

Ashurst PJ (1975) Granulation in chronic leg ulcers: a trial with a new material. Practitioner **215**: 353–358.

Atherton P (1998) Aloe vera: magic or medicine? Nursing Standard **12(41)**: 49–54.

Backhouse CM, Blair SD, Savage AP, Walton J, McCollum CN (1987) Controlled trial of occlusive dressings in healing venous ulcers. British Journal of Surgery **74(7)**: 626–627.

Bader D (ed.) (1990a) Pressure Sores: Clinical Practice and Scientific Approach. London: Macmillan.

Bader DL (1990b) The recovery characteristics of soft tissues following repeated loading. Journal of Rehabilitation and Research Development **27**: 115–126.

Bader DL (1998) The role of the researcher in tissue viability - a personal view from a biomedical engineer. Journal of Tissue Viability **8(2)**: 19–23.

Baker N, Rayman G (1999) Clinical evaluation of doppler signals. The Diabetic Foot **2 (1) (Suppl)**: 22–25.

Bale S (1991a) Wound dressings. Wound Care Society Educational Leaflet. No 5. Huntingdon: Wound Care Society.

Bale S (1991b) A holistic approach and the ideal dressing. Cavity wound management in the 1990s. Professional Nurse **6(6)**: 316.

Bale S (1992) Pressure sore management in a patient with complex problems. Journal of Wound Care **1(3)**: 12–13.

Bale S (1995) The role of the clinical nurse specialist within the health-care team. Journal of Wound Care **4(2)**: 86–87.

Bale S (1997) A guide to wound debridement. Journal of Wound Care **6(4)**: 179–182.

Bale S, Harding KG (1990) Using modern dressings to effect debridement. Professional Nurse **5(5)**: 244–245.

Bale S, Crook H, Lloyd-Jones R, Banks V, Hagelstein S, Rees-Mathews S, Harding KG (1998) Interim results of a randomized controlled trial of two pressure-relieving systems in the prevention of pressure sores in patients with fractured neck of femur. Presentation at the Seventh European Conference on Advances in Wound Management, London

Banks S, Bridel J (1995) A descriptive evaluation of pressure reducing cushions. British Journal of Nursing **4(13)**: 736, 738, 740 passim

Banks V (1998) Nutrition and pressure area management. Journal of Wound Care **7(6)**: 318–319.

Banwell PE, Holten IW, Martin DL (1998) Negative pressure therapy: clinical applications and experience with 200 cases. Presentation at Eighth Annual Meeting of the European Tissue Repair Society, Copenhagen.

Baragwanath P (1994) The management of a patient with a factitious wound. Journal of Wound Care **3(6)**: 286–287.

Barbenel J, Jordan M, Nicol S, Clark M (1977) Incidence of pressure sores in the Greater Glasgow Health Board area. Lancet **11**: 548–550.

Barbul A (1997) Wound healing in sepsis and trauma. Shock **8(6)**: 391–401.

Barbul A, Lazarau SA (1990) Arginine enhances wound healing and lymphocyte immune responses in humans. Surgery **108**: 331–337.

Barbul A, Lazarou SA, Effron DT, Wasserkrug HL, Efron G (1990) Arginine enhances wound healing and lymphocyte response in humans. Surgey **108**: 331–336.

Barnett A (1992) Prevention and treatment of the diabetic foot ulcer. British Journal of Nursing **2(1)**: 7–10.

Barr JE (1995) Principles of wound cleansing. Ostomy and Wound Management **41(7a suppl)**: 15–21.

Barrett E (1987) Putting risk calculators in their place. Nursing Times **83(6)**: 65–70.

Barton AA (1983) Pressure sores. In Barbenel JC, Forbes CD, Lowe GO (eds) Pressure Sores. London: Macmillan, pp 53–57.

Barton A, Barton M (1981) The Management and Prevention of Pressure Sores. London: Faber & Faber.

Barton AG, Thompson RG (1992) Is audit bad research? Audit Trends **1(2)**: 1–3.

Bassan M, Shalev O, Dudai M (1982) Near fatal systemic oxygen embolism due to irrigation with hydrogen peroxide. Postgraduate Medical Journal **58**: 448–450.

Beck U, Brezinova V, Hunter WM, Oswald I (1979) Plasma growth hormone and slow wave increase after interruption of sleep. Journal of Clinical Endocrinal Metabolism **40**: 812–815.

Beedle D (1993) Beating the bug. Nursing Times **89(45 suppl)**: 2–4.

Bell M (1994) Nurses' knowledge of the healing process in venous leg ulceration. Journal of Wound Care **3(3)**: 145–150.

Bendy RH, Nuccio P, Wolfe E (1964) Relationship of quantitative wound bacterial counts to healing of decubiti: effect of topical gentimicin. Antimicrobial Agents Chemotherapy **4**: 147–155.

Benjamin M, Curtis J (1992) Ethics in Nursing. Oxford: Oxford University Press.

Bennett G, Moody M (1995) Wound Care for Health Professionals. London: Chapman and Hall.

Bentley JP (1967) Rate of chlondroitin sulphate formation in wound healing. Annals of Surgery **165**: 186–191.

Bergstrom N, Demuth P, Braden B (1987) A clinical trial of the Braden Scale for predicting pressure sore risk. Nurse Clinician NA **22**: 417–428.

Bernabei R, Landi F, Bonini S, Ondor G, Lambiase A, Pola R, Aloe L (1999) Effect of topical application of nerve-growth factor on pressure ulcers. Lancet **354**: 307.

Berry DP (1992) Pilonidal sinus disease. Journal of Wound Care **1(3)**: 29–32.

Bessman AN, Sapico FL (1992) Infections in the diabetic patient; the role of immune dysfunction and the pathogen virulence factors. Cited by: Reiber GE, Lipsky BA, Gibbons GW (1998) The burden of diabetic foot ulcers. The American Journal of Surgery **17(2A)**: 5S–10S.

Bibbings J (1986) The History of Wound Dressings. London: Balliere Tindal, p 169.

Birchall L (1993) Making sense of pressure sore prediction calculators. Nursing Times **89(18)**: 34–37.

Black S (1998) Editorial. Nursing Researcher **6(1)**: 3–4.

Blair D, Wright D, Backhouse C, Riddle E, McCollum C (1988) Sustained compression and healing of chronic venous ulcers. British Medical Journal **297**: 1159–1161.

Blakeslee S (1993) The most important hours of your life. Daily Mail, 6 August, p9.

Bland M (2000) Producing clinical benchmarks for practice. Professional Nurse **15(12)**: 767–769.

Bliss M (1993) Aetiology of pressure sores. Reviews in Clinical Gerontology **3**: 379–397.

Bliss MR (1998) Hyperaemia. Journal of Tissue Viability **8(4)**: 4-13. Cites Lewis T, Grant R (1935) Observations upon reactive hyperaemia in man. Heart 1925–6 **XII**: 75–120.

Bliss MR (1998) Hyperaemia. Journal of Tissue Viability **8(4)**: 4–13. Cites Michel CC, Gilmott H (1990) Microvascular mechanisms in statis and ischaemia In Bader DL (ed.) Pressure Sores. Clinical Practice and Scientific Approach. Basingstoke: Macmillan Press, pp 153–156.

Bliss MR, Silver JR (1988) Pressure sores. In Monk BE, Graham Brown RC, Sarkany I (eds) Skin Disorders in the Elderly. Oxford: Blackwell, pp 97–112.

Bloomfield SF (1985) Eusol BPC and other hypochlorite formulations used in hospital. Pharmacology Journal **253**: 153–157.

Bolam v Friern Hospital Management Committee [1957] 2 All ER.

Boon H, Freemand L, Unsworth J (1996) Larvae help debridement. Nursing Times **92(46)**: 76–80.

Bowler PG, Jones SA, Davies BJ, Coyle E (1999) Infection control properties of some wound dressings. Journal of Wound Care **8(10)**: 499–502.

Bowler PG, Duerden BI, Armstrong DG (2001) Wound microbiology and associated approaches to wound management. Clinical Microbiology Reviews **14(2)**: 244–269.

Braden BJ, Bergstrom N (1988) Clinical utility of the Braden scale for predicting pressure sore risk. Decubitus **2(3)**: 34–38.

Bradley L (2001) Pretibial lacerations in older patients: the treatment options. Journal of Wound Care **10(1)**: 521–523.

Brand PW (1978) Pathomechanics of diabetic (neutrophic) ulcer and its conservative management. Cited by Laing P (1998) The development and complications of diabetic foot ulcers. The Journal of American Surgery **176**: 11s–19s.

Brennan S, Leaper D (1987) The effects of antiseptics on the healing wound: a study using the rabbit ear chamber. British Journal of Surgery **72**: 780–782.

Brennan SS, Foster ME, Leaper DJ (1985) Antiseptic toxicity in wounds healing by secondary intention. Journal of Hospital Infection **8**: 263–267.

Bridel J (1992) Pressure sore development and intra-operative risk. Nursing Standard **7(5)**: 28–30.

Bridel J (1993a) Assessing the risk of pressure sores. Nursing Standard **7(25)**: 32–35.

Bridel J (1993b) The aetiology of pressure sores. Journal of Wound Care **2(4)**: 230–238.

Brienza D, Karg PE, Brubaker CE (1996) Seat cushion design for elderly wheelchair users based on minimization of soft tissue deformation using stiffness and pressure measurements. IEEE Transactions on Rehabilitation Engineering **4(4)**: 320–7.

Briggs M (1996) Surgical wound pain: a trial of two treatments. Journal of Wound Care **5(1)**: 456–460.

Briggs M (1997) Principles of closed surgical wound care. Journal of Wound Care **6(6)**: 288–292.

Broome A (1990) Managing Change. London: Macmillan.

Brunner L, Suddarth D (1975) Textbook of Medical-Surgical Nursing. 3rd edn. Oxford: Blackwell Scientific, p 242.

Bryan C, Drew C, Reynolds D (1983) Bacteraemia associated with decubitus ulcers. Archives in Internal Medicine **143**: 2093.

Bryant R (1992) Acute and Chronic Wounds: Nursing Management. St Louis, MO: Mosby.

Bull J (1930) John Bull – family doctor. Journal of Tissue Viability **6(3)**: 120.

Burman PMS, O'Dea K (1994) Measuring pressure. Journal of Wound Care **3(2)**: 83–86.

Burr S (1999) Emollients for managing dry skin conditions. Professional Nurse **1(1)**: 43–48.

Burton P (1995) Prevention is better than cure. Journal of Community Nursing July: 18–20.

Butterworth C, Faugier J (1992) Clinical Supervision and Mentorship in Nursing. London: Chapman & Hall.

Bux M, Baig MK, Rodrigues E, Amstrong D, Brown A (1997) Antibody response to topical streptokinase. Journal of Wound Care **6(2)**: 70–73.

Cabak V, Dickerson J, Widdowson E (1963) Response of young rats to deprivation of protein or of calories. British Journal of Nutrition **17**: 601–616.

Callum MJ (1987) Hazards of compression treatment of the leg; an estimate from Scottish surgeons. British Medical Journal **295**: 1382.

Callum MJ, Ruckley CV, Harper DR, Dale JJ (1985) Chronic ulceration of the leg: the extent of the problem and provision of care. British Medical Journal **290**: 1855–1856.

Cameron J (1995) The importance of contact dermatitis in the management of leg ulcers. Journal of Tissue Viability **5(2)**: 52–55.

Cameron J (1996) Venous and arterial leg ulcers. Primary Health Care **6(3)**: 23–30.

Cameron J, Powell S (1996) Contact kept to a minimum. Nursing Times Wound Care Supplement **92(39)**: 84–86.

Campbell J (1995) Making sense of clinical inflammation. Nursing Times **91(14)**: 32–33.

Carlson BM (1998) Stimulation of regeneration in mammals: pipe dream or realistic goal? Wound Repair and Regeneration **6(5)**: 425–433.

Carlson GL (1999) The influence of nutrition and sepsis upon wound healing. Journal of Wound Care **8**: 9.

Casteldine G (2001) New benchmarking toolkit reveals nursing's essence. British Journal of Nursing **10(6)**: 410.

Chapman CM (1983) The paradox of nursing. The Advanced Journal of Nursing **8**: 269–272.

Charles H (1991) Compression healing of ulcers. Journal of District Nursing **10(3)**: 4–8.

Charles H (1995) The impact of leg ulcers on patients' quality of life. Professional Nurse **10(9)**: 571–574.

Charles H (1999) Short stretch bandaging in the treatment of leg ulcers. Journal of Wound Care **8(6)**: 303–304.

Chen WYJ, Abatabgelo G (1999) Functions of hyaluronan in wound repair. Wound Repair and Regeneration **7(2)**: 79–89.

Cherry G (1990) Clinical comparison of a new compression bandage. Nursing Standard **4(39)**: 8–11.

Chisholm CD, Cordell WH, Rodger K (1992) Comparison of a new pressurised saline canister versus syringe irrigation for laceration cleansing in an emergency department. American Emergency Medicine **21**: 1364–1367.

Choucair M, Phillips T (1998) A review of wound healing and dressing material. Skin and Aging **6(6)(suppl)**: 37–43.

Christensen J, McMahon E, Stevenson A (1994) Enhancing nursing practice through the use of contemporary ideas, models and theories. In McMillan M, Townsend J (eds) Reflections on Contemporary Nursing Practice. Oxford: Butterworth-Heinemann.

Clark E, Hodsman N, Kenny G (1989) Improved postoperative recovery with patient controlled analgesia. Nursing Times 85(9): 54–55.

Clark M (1994) Problems associated with the measurement of interface (or contact) pressure. Journal of Tissue Viability 4(2): 37–41.

Clarke G (1997) The problem of pressure sores and how to treat them. British Journal of Therapy and Rehabilitation 4:11.

Cmiel P (1990) Postoperative management of the replant patient: monitoring, complications and education. Critical Care Nursing Quarterly 13(1): 47–54. Cited by Coull AF (1993) Using leeches for venous drainage after surgery. Journal of Wound Care 2(5): 2937.

Coleridge-Smith P, Thomas P, Scurr J, Dormandy J (1988) Causes of venous ulceration: a new hypothesis. British Journal of Medicine 296: 1726–1727.

Collett J (1994) Nutrition and wound healing. Educational Leaflet 2: 2.

Collier F, de Laet MH, Deconinck PG (1978) Anti–infection prophylaxis of infantile burns. Acta Chir. Belgium 77(5): 365–369.

Collier M (1993) Report for Addenbrookes Hospital, Cambridge, November 1993. Journal of Wound Care 8(2): 63–64.

Collier M (1994a) Anatomy of the skin and the natural healing process. Wound Care Society Educational Leaflet 2: 1.

Collier M (1994b) Assessing a wound. Nursing Standard Supplement 8(49): 3–8.

Collier M (1995) Pressure sore development and prevention. Wound Care Society Educational Leaflet 3: 1.

Collier M (1997) Know how, a guide to vacuum-assisted closure. Nursing Times Supplement January: 32–33.

Collier M (1999) Blanching and non–blanching hyperaemia. Journal of Wound Care 8(2): 63–64.

Collins F (1998a) Sitting pretty. Nursing Times 94(38): 66–73.

Collins F (1998b) Pressure Sores in the Elderly, What About the Armchair? Presented at the Tissue Viability Society Conference, Derby.

Collins F (1999) The contribution made by an armchair with integral pressure-reducing cushion in the prevention of pressure sore incidence in the elderly, acutely ill patient. Journal of Tissue Viability 9(4): 133–137.

Collins F (2000) Selecting the most appropriate armchair for patients. Journal of Wound Care 9(2): 73–76.

Collins F (2001a) Seating. Wound Care Society Educational Booklet 8: 1.

Collins F (2001b) Sitting: Pressure ulcer development. Nursing Standard 15(22): 54–58.

Collins F (2001c) How to assess a patient's seating needs: some basic principles. Journal of Wound Care 10(9): 383–6.

Collins F, Shipperley T (1999) Assessing the seated patient for the risk of pressure damage. Journal of Wound Care 18(3): 123–126.

Colombo AA, Perotti F, Boriolo P, Landi G, David PG, Del Forno M (1987) Chlorhexidine in the prophylaxis of surgical wound infections. Minerva Chir 42: 23–24.

Conly JM, Grieves K, Peters BA (1989) A prospective randomised study comparing transparent and dry gauze dressings for central venous catheters. Journal of Infection Diseases 159(2): 310–319.

Convatec (1993) Pressure Sore Blueprint. Convatec educational leaflet. Dublin: Convatec.

Cookson B, Farrelly H, Stapelyon P, Garvey R, Price M (1991) Transferable resistance to Triclosan in MRSA. Letter to the editor. The Lancet 337(8756): 1548–1549.

Cooper D (1993) Managing malignant ulcers effectively. Nursing Standard 8(2): 24–28.

Cooper R (1996a) The role of antimicrobial agents in wound care. Journal of Wound Care 5(8): 374–380

Cooper R (1996b) The prevalence of bacteria and implications for infection control. Journal of Wound Care 5(6): 291–295.

Cooper R, Lawrence J (1996) The isolation and identification of bacteria from wounds. Journal of Wound Care 5(7): 335–340.

Cooper R, Molan P (1999) The use of honey as an antiseptic in managing *Pseudomonus* infection. Journal of Wound Care 8(4): 161–164.

Cornwall J, Dore C, Lewis J (1986) Leg ulcers, epidemiology and aetiology. British Journal of Surgery 73: 693–696.

Coull AF (1993) Using leeches for venous drainage after surgery. Journal of Wound Care 2(5): 292–297.

Crow R (1988) The challenge of pressure sores. Nursing Times 84(38): 68–73.

Cruse PJ, Foord R (1980) The epidemiology of wound infection, a ten year prospective study of 62,939 wounds. Surgical Clinics of North America 60(1): 27–40.

Culley F (1997) Patient advocacy in relation to tissue viability services. Journal of Wound Care 6(1): 29–30.

Curtin L, Flaherty J (1982) Nursing Ethics: Theories and Pragmatics. London: Prentice-Hall.

Custronuovo JJ, Ghobrial I, Giusti AM, Rudoph S, Smeill JM (1998) Effects of chronic wound fluid on the structure and biological activity of Becaplermin (rhPDGF-BB) and Becaplermin gel. The American Journal of Surgery 176: 61s–67s.

Cutting K (1994) Factors influencing wound healing. Nursing Standard 8(50): 33–36.

Cutting K (1998) Wounds and infection. Wound Care Society Educational Leaflet 5: 2.

Cutting K (1999) The causes and prevention of maceration of the skin. Journal of Wound Care 8(4): 200–201.

Cuzzell J (1988) The new RYB colour code. American Journal of Nursing 88(10): 1342–1346.

Dale J (1984) Leg work. Nursing Mirror 159(20): 22–25.

Dale JJ, Gibson B (1997) Educating leg ulcer patients and their carers. In A Guide to Leg Ulcer Management. Hull: Smith & Nephew Healthcare.

Dale J, Cullum M, Ruckley CV, et al. (1983) Chronic ulcers of the leg: a study of prevalence in a Scottish community. Health Bulletin 41: 310–314.

Dalstra M (1997) Biomechanics of the Human Pelvic Bone. In Vleeming A, Mooney V, Dorman T, Snijders C, Stoeckart R (eds) Movement Stability and Low Backpain.

Daltrey D, Rhodes B, Chattwood J (1981) Investigation into the microbial flora of healing and non-healing decubitus ulcers. Archives of Internal Medicine 143: 2093.

Danielsen L, Cherry GW, Harding K, Rollman O (1997) Cadexomer iodine in ulcers colonised by Pseudomonus aeruginosa. Journal of Wound Care **6(4)**: 169–172.

David JA, Chapman RG, Chapman FJ, Locket B (1983) An Investigation of the Current Method used in Nursing for the Care of the Patient with Pressure Sores. Guildford: University of Surrey.

Davies K, Strickland J, Lawrence V, et al. (1991) The hidden morality of pressure sores. Journal of Tissue Viability **1(1)**: 18.

Davis E (1998) Education, microbiology and chronic wounds. Journal of Wound Care **7(6)**: 272–274.

Davis J (1992) Expanding horizons. Nursing Times **88(47)**: 37–39.

Davis M (1996) Wound-care training in medical education. Journal of Wound Care **5(6)**: 286–287.

Dealey C (1992) Pressure sores: The result of bad nursing? British Journal of Nursing **1(15)**: 748.

Dealey C (1994a) The Care of Wounds. London: Blackwell Science, p 128.

Dealey C (1994b) A problem solving approach to wound care. Journal of Community Nursing **November**: 26–30.

Dealey C (1997) How is exudate currently managed in specific wounds? In Cherry, C, Harding K (eds) Management of Wound Exudate. Proceedings of Joint meeting of EWMA and ETRS. London: Churchill Communications.

Dealey C, Earwaker T, Eden L (1991) Are Your Patients Sitting Comfortably? Journal of Tissue Viability **1**: 2.

Deane K (1993) CNS and NP: Should the roles be merged? Cancer Nurse **92(6)**: 24–30.

Defloor T (2000) The effect of position and mattress on interface pressure. Applied Nursing Research **13(1)**: 2–11.

Demling R, et al. (1996) Use of anti catabolic agents for burns. Current Opinions in Critical Care **2**: 482–491.

Demling R, De Santi L (1999) Involuntary weight loss and the non healing wound: the role of anabolic agents. Advanced Wound Care **12(1) (suppl)**: 1–14.

Dennis H (1998) Skin care in atopic eczema. Professional Nurse Study Supplement **13(4)**: S10–S13.

Denton GW (1991) Chlorhexidine. In Block SS (ed) Sterilization, Disenfection and Preservation 4th edn. Philadelphia: Lea & Febiger. pp 274–289.

Department of Health (DoH) (1993) Pressure Sores a Key Quality Indicator. London: HMSO.

Department of Health and Social Security (DHSS) (1972) Report of the Committee on Nursing. London: HMSO.

Desia H (1997) Ageing and wounds part 2. Journal of Wound Care **6(5)**: 237–239.

Devlin H (1994) The effect of hyaluronic acid scarring: a preliminary study. Journal of Wound Care **3(8)**: 375–377.

Dickerson JW (1993) Ascorbic acid, zinc and wound healing. Journal of Wound Care **2(6)**: 350–353.

Donlin NJ, Bryson PJ (1995) Hyperbaric oxygen therapy. Journal of Wound Care **4(4)**: 175–178.

Donnelly J (2001) Hospital-aquired heel ulcers: a common but neglected problem. Journal of Wound Care **10(4)**: 131–135.

Donovan S (1998) Wound infection and wound swabbing. Professional Nurse **13(11)**: 757–759.

Douglas M (1996) Necrotising fasciitis: a nursing perspective. Journal of Advanced Nursing **24**: 162–166.

Drucker M, Cardenas E, Arizti P, Valenzuela A, Gamboa A (1998) Experimental studies on the effect of Lidocaine on wound healing. World Journal of Surgery **22(4)**: 394–397.

Duby T, Hoffman D, Cameron J, et al. (1993) Randomised trial in the treatment of venous leg ulcers comparing short stretch bandage system and long stretch-paste bandage system. Wounds **5**: 276–279.

Duckworth G, Lothian J, Williams J (1988) Methicillin-resistant *Staphylococcus aureus*: Report of an outbreak in a London teaching hospital. Journal of Hospital Infection **11**: 1–15.

Dunford C (2000) Using honey as a dressing for infected skin lesions. Nursing Times **96(14)**: 7–9.

Dunn LJ, Wilson P (1990) Evaluating the permeability of hydrocolloid dressings to multi-resistant *Staphylococcus aureas*. Pharmacology Journal 248–250.

Duthie GS, Foster ME, Price-Thomas JM, Leaper DJ (1990) Bowel preparation or not for elective colorectal surgery. Journal of the Royal College of Surgeons Edinburgh **35(3)**: 169–171.

Dvorak HF, Detmar M, Claffey KP, Nagy JA, van de Water L, Senger DR (1995) Vascular permeability factor/vascular endothelial growth factor: an important mediator of angiogenisis in maliganancy and inflammation. International Archives of Allergy and Immunology **107(1–3)**: 233–235.

Dyson M, Young S, Pendle CL, Webster DF, Lang SM (1988) Journal of Investigative Dermatology **91(5)**: 435–439.

Dyson R (1978) Bed sores – the injuries hospital staff inflict on their patients. Nursing Mirror **146(24)**: 30–32.

Eagles M (1999) Compression bandaging. Elderly Care **11(2)**: 17–21.

Edmonds M (1999) Early use of antibiotics should not be ruled out. The Diabetic Foot **2(4)**: 122–125.

Edmonds M, Foster A (2000) Managing the Diabetic Foot. Oxford: Blackwell Science

Edwards M (1996) Pressure sore risk calculators: some methodological issues. Journal of Clinical Nursing **5(5)**: 307–312.

Effective Health Care (1999) Complications of diabetes: screening for retinopathy and management of foot ulcers. NHS Centre for Reviews and Dissemination, booklet 3:4. Plymouth: Latimer & Trent.

Ek AC, Gustavssen G, Lewis DH (1987) Skin blood flow in relation to external pressure and temperature in the supine position on a standard hospital mattress. Scandinavian Journal of Rehabilitation **19**: 121–126.

Elliott Pennels CJ (1997) Professional negligence. Professional Nurse **13(1)**: 50–51.

Emflorgo CA (1999) The assessment and treatment of wound pain. Journal of Wound Care **8(8)**: 384–385.

Emmott C (1992) How do we heal? Nursing Times **88(36)**: 78–84.

EPUAP (2001) Pressure ulcer classification. EPUAP Business Office. Wound Healing Unit. Department of Dermatology. Churchill Hospital. Oxford. www.epuap.org/gltreatment.html

Ertl P (1991) Incidence and aetiology of leg ulcers. Professional Nurse **December**: 190–196.

Ertl P (1992) Allow the ulcer to heal. Professional Nurse **7(6)**: 406–412.

Ertl P (1993) Planning a Route to Treatment. A framework for leg ulcer assessment. Professional Nurse **8(10)**: 675–679.

Esuvaranathan K, Kuan K, Kamarasinghe G (1992) A study of 245 infected surgical wounds in Singapore. Journal of Hospital Infection **21**: 231–240.

Exton Smith AN, Sherwin RW (1961) the prevention of pressure sores: significance of spontaneous bodily movements. Lancet **ii**: 1124–1126.

Falanga V (1998) Clinical trials experience with Apilgraf in chronic wounds. Presentation at Eighth Annual Meeting of the European Tissue Repair Society. Copenhagen.

Falanga V (2001) The dark side of evidence–based wound management. Journal of Wound Care **10(5)**: 145.

Falanga V, Eaglestein WH (1993) The trap hypothesis of venous ulceration. Lancet **341**: 1006–1008.

Faoagali J, George N, Ledistschke JF (1997) Does tea tree oil have a place in the topical treatment of burns? Burns **23**: 349–351.

Ferguson A (1993) Wound infection – the role of antiseptics. Accident and Emergency Nursing **1**: 79–86.

Fiers SA (1996) Breaking the cycle: the etiology of incontinence deramatitis and evaluating and using skin care products. Ostomy Wound Management **42(3)**: 32–40.

Fitzgerald V, Sims R (1987) A Positive Approach. Community Nurse **November**: 16–21.

Flanagan M (1991) Pressure sore prevention. Management and selection of equipment. Educational Leaflet 4. Huntingdon: Wound Care Society.

Flanagan M (1992a) The role of the specialist nurse in wound care. Journal of Wound Care **1(2)**: 45–46.

Flanagan M (1992b) Variable influencing nurses' selection of wound dressings. Journal of Wound Care **1(1)**: 33–43.

Flanagan M (1993) Pressure sore risk assessment scales. Journal of Wound Care **2(3)**: 162–167.

Flanagan M (1994) Assessment criteria. Nursing Times **90**: 35.

Flanagan M (1995) Pressure Sore Risk Assessment, Educational Leaflet, 3: 4. Huntingdon: Wound Care Society.

Flanagan M (1997) Wound Management. Edinburgh: Churchill Livingstone, p64.

Flannigan K (1997) Nutritional aspects of wound healing. Advances in Wound Care **10(3)**: 48–52.

Flemming KA, Cullum NA, Nelson EA (1999) A systematic review of laser therapy for leg ulcers. Journal of Wound Care **8(3)**: 111–114.

Fletcher A (1996) Equipment Selection, Educational Leaflet. Huntingdon: Wound Care Society.

Fletcher A, Callum N (1997) A systematic review of compression treatment for venous leg ulcers. British Medical Journal **315(7108)**: 576–580.

Fletcher J (2000) The role of collagen in wound healing. Professional Nurse **15(8)**: 27–530.

Fogg L, Gross D (2000) Threats to validity in randomized clinical trials. Research in Nursing and Health **23**: 79–87.

Foster ME (1994) Wound Healing – a surgical procedure. Journal of Wound Care **3(3)**: 135–138.

Fotherby M, Spanwick A, Gibbs S, Barclay C, Potter J, Castleden M (1991) Effects of various dressings on wound-healing in healthy volunteers. Journal of Tissue Viability **1(3)**: 68–70.

Fowler A, Dempsey A (1998) Split-thickness skin graft donor sites. Journal of Wound Care **7(8)**: 399–402.

Fowler BA, Norberg GF (1994) Silver. In Friberg L, Norberg GF, Vouc VB (eds) The Hand Book of Toxicology of Metals. New York: Bio Medical Press.

Fowler E, van Rijswijk L (1995) Using wound debridement to help achieve the goals of care. Ostomy Wound Management **41(7A Suppl)**: 23S–35S.

Fox SI (1996) Human physiology. Times Mirror Higher Education Group. C. Brown. USA.

Frazer D (1991) Collins Concise Dictionary of Quotations. Glasgow: Harper Collins, pp 111–120.

Frick WG, Seals RR (1994) Smoking and wound healing: a review. Tex Dentistry Journal **111(6)**: 21–23.

Frykberg R (1998) The diabetic foot ulcer: current concepts. Journal of Foot and Ankle Surgery **37(5)**: 440–445.

Galvan L (1996) Effects of heparin on wound healing. Journal of Wound Ostomy and Continence Nursing **23(4)**: 224–226.

Galvani J (1995) Surgical Wounds. Educational Leaflet 3.3. Huntingdon: Wound Care Society.

Galvani J (1997) Not yet cut and dried. Nursing Times Supplement **93(16)**: 88–90.

Ganong WF (1995) Review of Medical Physiology. London: Prentice Hall International.

Gardner A, Fox H (1983) The venous pump of the human foot – preliminary report. Bristol Medico Chirurgical Journal **1983**: 109–112.

Garibaldi RA, Skolnick D, Lerer T, Poirot A, Graham J, Krisuinas E, Lyons R (1988) The impact of preoperative skin disinfection on preventing intraoperative wound contamination. Infection Control Hospital Epidemiology **9(3)**:109–113.

Garrett B (1998) Re-epithelialisation. Journal of Wound Care **7(7)**: 358–359.

Gebhardt K, Bliss MR (1994) Preventing pressure sores in orthopaedic patients – is prolonged chair nursing detrimental? Journal of Tissue Viability **4(2)**: 51–54.

Getliffe K (1998) Developing a protocol for a randomised controlled trial: factors to consider. Nursing Researcher **6(1)**: 5–17.

Gibbings S (1993) Informed action. Nursing Times **89(46)**: 28–33.

Gibson J (1979) Modern Microbiology and Pathology for Nurses. London: Blackwell.

Gilchrist B (1990) The microbiology of leg ulcers treated by occlusion. In Fullerton E (ed.) Modern Wound Healing: The Pharmacist's Role. Littlewick Green: Burr Associates, pp 8–9.

Gilchrist B (1994) Treating bacterial wound infection. Nursing Times **90(50)**: 55–58.

Gilchrist B (1997) Should iodine be reconsidered in wound management? Journal of Wound Care **6(3)**: 148–150.

Gilchrist B, Reed C (1989) The bacteriology of chronic venous ulcers treated with occlusive hydrocolloid dressings. British Journal of Dermatology **121**: 337–344.

Gilliand EL, Dore CJ, Nathwanin N, Lewis J (1988) Bacterial colonisation and its effect on the success rate of skin grafting. Annals of the Royal College of Surgeons England **70**: 105–108.

Goldheim P (1993a) An appraisal of povidone-iodine and wound healing. Postgraduate Medical Journal (**Suppl 3**): S98–S105.

Goldheim P (1993b) In vitro efficacy of povidone-iodine solution and cream against methicillin-resistant *Staphylococcus aureus*. Post Graduate Medical Journal **69 (suppl)**: S62–S65.

Gottrup F (1999) Wound closure techniques. Journal of Wound Care **8(8)**: 397–400.

Gould D (1994) Understanding the nature of bacteria. Nursing Standard **8(28)**: 29–31.

Gould D (1997) Hand Care: Maintaining Standards. Hygenic Hand Decontamination. London: MacMillan.

Gould D, Campbell S, Newton H, et al. (1998) Setopress vs Elastocrepe in chronic venous ulceration. British Journal of Nursing **7(2)**: 66–73.

Graner JL (1997) SK Livingston and the maggot therapy of wounds. Mil Medicine **162(4)**: 296–300.

Green C (1993) Topical Streptokinase produces anti-bodies. The Pharmaceutical Journal **251**: 12.

Green SM, Winterberg H, Franks PJ, Moffatt CJ, Eberhardie C, McLaren S (1999) Nutritional intake in community patients with pressure ulcers. Journal of Wound Care **8(7)**: 325–330.

Greenwood JE, Parry AD, Williams RM, McCollum CN (1997a) Trigger-fired pinch-graft harvester for use in chronic venous ulcers. British Journal of Surgery **84**: 397–398.

Greenwood JE, Crawley BA, Clark SL, Chadwick PR, Ellison DA, McCollum CN (1997b) Monitoring wound healing by odour. Journal of Wound Care **6(5)**: 219–221.

Grey JE, Bale S, Harding K (1998) The use of cultured dermis in the treatment of diabetic foot ulcers. Journal of Wound Care **7(7)**: 324–325.

Griffiths-Jones A (1995) Methicillin-resistant *Staphylococcus aureas* in wound care. Journal of Wound Care **4(10)**: 481–483.

Grimshaw J (1995) Developing clinically valid practice guidelines. Journal of Evaluation in Clinical Practice **1(1)**: 37–48.

Groth KE (1942) Klinische Beobactungen des Dekubitus. In Bliss M (1993) Aetiology of pressure sores. Reviews in Clinical Gerontology **3**: 379–397.

Haines R, Blaire R, Osborn M (1997) The challenges of assessing outcomes in chronic pain. International Journal of Health Care and Quality Assurance **10(4)**: 149–152.

Hall Angeras M, Brandberg A, Falk A, Seeman T (1992) Comparison between sterile saline and tap water for the cleaning of acute traumatic soft tissue injury. European Journal of Surgery **158**: 347–350.

Hallbrook K, Lanner E (1972) Serum zinc and the healing of leg ulcers. Lancet **2**: 780–782.

Hallett A (1993) Fungating Wounds. Education Leaflet. Huntingdon: Wound Care Society.

Hallett A (1994) Barrier to invasion. Nursing Times **90(16)**: 90–92.

Ham R, Aldersea P, Porter D (1998) Wheelchair Users and Postural Seating, a Clinical Approach. Edinburgh: Churchill Livingstone.

Hambreaus A (1973) Transfer of *Staphylococcus aureas* via nurses' uniforms. Journal of Hygiene **71**: 799–814.

Hampton J (1996) The use of metranidazole in the treatment of malodorous wounds. Journal of Wound Care 5(9): 421–425.

Hampton S (1997a) Germ Warfare. Nursing Times 93(40): 74–79.

Hampton S (1997b) Sharp debridement. Journal of Wound Care 6(3): 151.

Hampton S (1997c) Treatment of macerated and excoriated peri-wound area with no-Sting Barrier Film. Presented in poster form at European Wound Management Conference, Harrogate.

Hampton S (1997d) Reliability in Reporting Pressure Sores. Professional Nurse 12(9): 626–630.

Hampton S (1997e) Venous leg ulcers: short–stretch bandage compression therapy. British Journal of Nursing 6(17): 990–998.

Hampton S (1997f) Best dressed wounds. Practice Nurse **February** 81–86.

Hampton S (1997g) Preventable pressure sores. Care of the Critically Ill 13(5): 193–197.

Hampton S (1998a) Film subjects win the day. Nursing Times 94(24): 80–82.

Hampton S (1998b) Can electric beds aid pressure sore prevention in hospital. British Journal of Nursing 7(17): 10–17.

Hampton S (1998c) Germ warfare. Nursing Times 93(40): 74–79.

Hampton S (1999) Efficacy and cost-effectiveness of the Thermo contour mattress. British Journal of Nursing 8(15): 990–996.

Hancock REW (1997) Research Interests. Vancouver: Hancock Laboratories.

Handfield-Jones SE, Grattan CEH, Simpson RA, Kennedy CTC (1988) Comparison of a hydrocolloid dressing and paraffin gauze in the treatment of venous leg ulcers. British Journal of Dermatology 118: 425.

Hansson C, Holm J, Lillieborg S, Syren A (1993) Repeated treatment with lidocaine/prilocaine cream (EMLA) as a topical anaesthetic for the cleansing of venous leg ulcers: a controlled study. Acta Derm Venereal (Stockh) 73: 231–233.

Harding K (1996) The use of antiseptics in wound care. Journal of Wound Care 5(1): 44–47.

Hart J (1999) Growth factors. In Miller M, Glover D (eds) Wound Management, Theory and Practice. London: Emap Healthcare.

Hashmi F (2000) Non-enzymatic glycation and the development of plantar callus. British Journal of Podiatry 3(4): 91–94.

Hastings D (1993) Basing care on research. Nursing Times 89(13): 70–76.

Haughton W (1996) The 30° tilt positioning technique. Journal of Tissue Viability 6(3): 87.

Haury B, Rodheaver G, Vensko J, Edgerton MT, Edlich RF (1978) Debridement: an essential component of traumatic wound care. American Journal of Surgery 135(2): 238–242.

Hayes M (1996) Understanding the aetiology of leg ulcers. Journal of Wound Care 5(9): 435–438.

Hayward J (1975) Information – A Prescription Against Pain. London: RCN Publications.

HEA (1994) Balance of Good Health. London: HEA/HMSO.

Healey F (1995) The reliability and utility of pressure sore grading scales. Journal of Tissue Viability 5(4): 111–114.

Hedin G, Hambraeus A (1993) Daily scrub with chlorhexidine reduces skin colonisation by antibiotic-resistant staphylococcus epidermis. Journal of Hospital Infection 24: 47–61.

Heggers JP (1998a) Defining infection in chronic wounds: methodology. Journal of Wound Care 7(9): 452–455.

Heggers JP (1998b) Defining infection in chronic wounds: does it matter? Journal of Wound Care **7(8)**: 389–392.

Herbert C, Kreutz D (1997) Seating issues in wound care. The Interdisciplinary Journal of Rehabilitation Management **109(3)**: 52–54.

Heys S, Gardner E (1999) Nutrients and the surgical patient: current and potential therapeutic applications to clinical practice. Journal of the Royal College of Surgeons Edinburgh **44(5)**: 283–293.

Hibbs P (1987) Pressure Area Care for the City & Hackney Health Authority. London: St Bartholomews Hospital.

Hibbs P (1999) A report completed by the NHS Executive on behalf of Eastbourne Hospitals NHS Trust. Eastbourne: Eastbourne Hospitals NHS Trust.

Hill J (1991) Assessing rheumatic disease. Nursing Times **87(4)**: 33–35.

Hill S (1995) The problems Tissue Viability Nurses have in advising their Health Authorities in the purchase of pressure relieving equipment. Journal of Tissue Viability **5(4)**: 127–129.

Himes D (1999) Protein calorie malnutrition and involuntary weight loss. The role of aggressive nutritional interventions in wound healing. Ostomy Wound Management **45(3)**: 46–55.

Hinchcliffe S (1995) Promoting learning: a helping relationship. In Schober J, Hinchcliffe S (eds) Toward Advanced Nursing Practice. London: Arnold.

Hinchcliffe S, Montague S (1988) Physiology for Nursing Practice. London: Balliere Tindall.

Hinchcliffe SM, Montague SE, Watson R (1996) Physiology for Nursing Practice. 2nd edn. London: Bailliere Tindall.

Hine P (1993) The mechanics of the medical negligence claim. Journal of Tissue Viability **3(2)**: 39–41.

Hoekstra MJ, Hermans M, Richters C, Dutrieux RP (2002) A histological comparison of acute inflammatory responses with a hydrofibre or tulle gauze dressing. Journal of Wound Care **11(3)**: 113–117.

Hoffman D (1996) Know how. A guide to wound debridement. Nursing Times Supplement **93(32)**: 22–23.

Hoffman R, Starkey S (1998) Plasmin generation by keratinocytes is reduced by wound fluid from venous leg ulcers due to the degradation of plasminogen. Presentation at Eighth Annual Meeting of the European Tissue Repair Society, Copenhagen.

Hoffman R, Eagle M (1999) The use of proteases as prognostic markers for the healing of venous leg ulcers. Journal of Wound Care **8(6)**: 273–276.

Hofman A, Geelkerten RH, Wille J, et al. (1994) Pressure sores and pressure-decreasing mattresses: controlled clinical trial. Lancet **343**: 568–571.

Hohn DC, Ponce B, Burton RW, Hunt TK (1977) Antimicrobial systems of the surgical wound. American Journal of Surgery **133**: 597–660.

Hollander D, Stein M, Bernd A, Windolf J, Pannike A (1999) Autologous keratinocytes cultured on benzylester hyaluronic acid membranes in the treatment of chronic full thickness ulcers. Journal of Wound Care **8(7)**: 351–355.

Hopf H (1999) The role of oxygen tension in wounds. Presentation at a Symposium on Thermoregulation in Wound Care. St Annes College. University of Oxford, Oxford.

Hopkins A (1998) A programme for pressure sore prevention and management. Journal of Wound Care **7(1)**: 37–40.

Hopkins S (1987) Prophylactic treatment for venous ulcers. Nursing Times **83(26)**: 45–46.

Hopkinson I (1992) Molecular components of the extracellular matrix. Journal of Wound Care **1(1)**: 52–54.

House N (1996) Patient compliance with leg ulcer treatment. Professional Nurse **12(1)**: 33–36.

Hoyman K, Gruber N (1992) A case study of interdepartmental cooperation. Decubitus **5(6)**: 12.

Hughes C (2001) Obstetric care. Is there a risk of pressure damage after epidural anaesthetic? Journal of Tissue Viability **11(2)**: 56–57.

Humphries D (1998) Disturbance and resilience: an overview of evidence based practice. Journal of Tissue Viability **8(2)**: 16–18.

Humphries D, Masterson A (1998) Practising at a higher level. Professional Nurse **14(1)**: 10–13.

Hunt J (1996) Guest editorial. Journal of Advanced Nursing **23(3)**: 423–425.

Hunt TK (1995) Disinfectants, antiseptics and antibiotics. In: Iodine and Wound Physiology: Proceedings of the Fifth Annual Meeting of the European Tissue Repair Society Meeting. Cambridge: Information Transfer.

Hunt TK, Pai MP (1975) The effect of varying ambient oxygen tensions on wound metabolism and collagen synthesis. Surgical Gynaecology and Obstetrics **135**: 561–567.

Hussian T (1953) An experimental study of some pressure effects on tissues with reference to the bed sore problem. Journal of Path Bacteria **66**: 347.

Hutcheson F (1999) Foot impulse technology in arteiovenous disease. Journal of Wound Care **8(9)**: 462–465.

Hutchinson JJ (1990) Infection in occluded wounds. In Fullerton E (ed.) European Hospital Pharmacy Workshop Series. Littlewick Green: Burr Associates, pp 10–11.

Hutchinson JJ (1992) Influences of occlusive dressings on wound microbiology. Interim results of a multi-centred clinical trial of an occlusive hydrocolloid dressing. In Harding KG, Leaper DJ, Turner TD (eds) Procedings of the First European Conference on Advances in Wound Management. London: Macmillan.

Hutchinson A, McIntosh A, Feder G, Home PD, Young R (2000) Clinical Guidelines for Type 2 Diabetes: prevention and management of foot problems. London: Royal College of General Practitioners.

Im MJ (1995a) Commentaar of 'pressure ulcers and wound management'. WCS–Nieuws **11**:18.

Im MJ (1995b) Evaluation of a new dressing on diabetic foot lesions. WCS–Nieuws **11**: 28.

Iocono JA, Krummel TM, Keefer KA, Allison GM, Ehrlich P (1998) Repeated additions of hyaluronan alters granulation deposition in sponge implants in mice. Wound Repair and Regeneration **6(5)**: 442–448.

Irizarry L, Merlin T, Rupp J, Griffith J (1996) Reduced susceptibility of β methicillin-resistant *Staphylococcus aureus* to cetylpyridinium chloride and chlorhexidine. Chemotherapy **42**: 248–252.

James H (1994) Exploring the role of the tissue viability specialist nurse. Nursing Standard **2(9)**: 60–63.

Jay E (1995a) How different constant low pressure support surfaces address pressure and shear forces. Journal of Tissue Viability **5**: 4.

Jay E (1995b) Pressure and shear: their effects on support choice. Journal of Ostomy/Wound Management **41(8)**: 36–45.

Jeffcoate W (1999) Use of antibiotics in uninfected ulcers may do more harm than good. The Diabetic Foot **2(4)**: 122–125.

Jeffs E (1993) The effect of acute inflammatory episodes (cellulitis) on the treatment of lymphoedema. Journal of Tissue Viability **3(2)**: 51–55.

Jeter KF, Lutz JB (1996) Skin care in the frail elderly dependent patient. Advances in Wound Care **9(1)**: 29–33.

Johnson A (1987) Treatment of infected wounds. Nursing Times **83(36)**: 60–62.

Johnson HM, Swan TH, Weigand GE (1930) In what positions do healthy people sleep? Journal of the American Medical Association **94**: 2058–2062.

Johnson R (1994) How to approach medical negligence in order to avoid it. Journal of Tissue Viability **4(1)**: 14–20.

Jones M, Thomas S (1997) Wound cleansing – a therapy revisited. Journal of Tissue Viability **7(4)**: 119–121.

Jones V, Milton T (2000) When and how to use hydrogels. Nursing Times Plus **96(suppl)(23)**: 3–4.

Jude E, Boulton A (1998) Foot problems in diabetes mellitus. British Journal of Podiatry **1(4)**: 117–120.

Kane K (1990) Prompt action on leg ulcers. Community Outlook **November**: 2–28.

Kaufman JP (1996) Nurse practitioners in general practice: an expanding role. Nursing Standard **11(8)**: 44–47.

Keachie J (1992) Compression Therapy. A Treatment in it's own Right. Educational Leaflet no. 9. Huntingdon: Wound Care Society.

Keeling D, Price P, Jones E, Harding K (1997) Social support for elderly patients with chronic wounds. Journal of Wound Care **6(8)**: 389–391.

Keh C, Soon Y, Wong LS (2000) Latex allergy: an emerging problem in theatres. International Journal Clinical Practice **54(9)**: 582–584.

Kelly J, Chivers G (1996) Built-in resistance. Nursing Times **92(2)**: 50-52.

Kelso H (1989) Alternative technique. Nursing Times **85(23)**: 70–72.

Kemp M (1994) Protecting the skin from moisture and associated irritants. Journal of Gerentological Nursing **September**: 8–13.

Ketovuori H (1987) Nurses' and patients' conceptions of wound pain and the administrations of analgesia. Journal of Pain and Symptom Management 2(4): 213–218.

Kiecolt-Glaser JK, Marucha PT, Malarkey WB, Mercado AM, Glaser R (1995) Slowing of wound healing by psychological stress. The Lancet **346(4)**: 1194–1196.

King B, Brereton L (1998) Using photoplethysmography as part of nursing assessment. Journal of Wound Care **7(10)**: 543–546.

Kings Fund Centre (1988) The Prevention and Management of Pressure Sores Within Health Authorities. Advisory Document. London: Kings Fund.

Kingsley A (1992) Assessment allows action on risk factors: infection and surgical wounds. Professional Nurse **July**: 644–648.

Klock G, Frank H, Houben R, et al. (1994) Production of purified alginates suitable for use in immunoisolated transplantation. Appl Microbil Biotechnol. **40:5** 638–643.

Knowles A (1996) Diabetic foot ulceration. Nursing Times **92(11)**: 65–67.

Kop P (2000) Understanding evidence based care. Professional Nurse **16(1)**: 853–857.

Kosiak M (1961) Etiology of decubitus ulcers. Archives of Physical Medicine and Rehabilitation **January**: 19–29.

Krasilovsky G (1993) Seating assessment and management in a nursing home population. Physical and Occupational Therapy in Geriatrics 11(2): 25–38.

Krasner D (1995) Minimizing factors that impair wound healing: a nursing approach. Ostomy Wound Management 41(1): 22–6, 28, 30.

Kreig T, Eming AS (1997) Is exudate a clinical problem? A dermatologist's perspective. In Cherry C, Harding K (eds) Management of Wound Exudate. Proceedings of Joint Meeting of EWMA and ETRS. London: Churchill Communications.

Kristofferson A (1998) Lidocaine–prilocaine cream (EMLA cream) as a topical anaesthetic for the cleansing of leg ulcers. The effect of length of application time. European Journal of Dermatology 8(4): 245–247.

Krizek TJ, Robson MC (1975) Evolution of quantitative bacteriology in wound management. American Journal of Surgery 130(5): 570–584.

Kruz A, Sessler DI, Lenhardt R (1996) Perioperative normothermia to reduce the incidence of surgical–wound infection and shorten hospitalization. The New England Journal of Medicine 334(19): 1209–1215.

Kucan JO, Robson MC, Heggers JP (1981) Comparison of silver sulphadiazine, povidone–iodine and physiological saline in the treatment of chronic pressure ulcers. Journal American Geriatric Society 29: 232–235.

Laing P (1998) The development and complications of diabetic foot ulcers. The Journal of American Surgery 176: 11s–19s.

Laing W, Williams R (1989) Diabetes. London: Office of Health Economics.

Landis CA, Whitney JD (1997) Effects of 72 hours sleep deprivation on wound healing in the rat. Research in Nursing Health 20(3): 259–267.

Landis EM (1930) Micro-injection studies of capillary blood pressure in human skin. Heart 15: 209–228.

Lansdown ABG (2002) Silver 1: its antibacterial properties and mechanism of action. Journal of Wound Care 11(4): 125–130.

Lansdown ABG, Sampson B, Laupattaraksem P, et al. (1997) Silver aids healing in the sterile skin wound: experimental studies in the laboratory rat. British Journal of Dermatology 137: 728–735.

Lawrence JC (1989) Treating minor burns. Nursing Times 85(26): 73.

Lawrence JC (1994) The use of alcoholic wipes for disinfection of injection sites. Journal of Wound Care 3(1): 11–14.

Lawrence JC (1996) The use of antiseptics in wound care. Journal of Wound Care 5(1): 44–47.

Lawrence JC (1997) Celullose dressings. Journal of Wound Care 6(1): 46–47.

Lawrence JC, Lilly HA, Kidson A (1992) An adherent semipermeable film dressing for burns. Journal of Wound Care 1(2): 10–11.

Layton AM, Ibbotson SH, Davies JA, Goodfield MJD (1994) Randomised trial of oral aspirin for chronic venous ulcers. The Lancet 344: 164–165.

Le KM, Madsen BL, Barth PW, Ksander GA, Angell JB, Vistnes LM (1984) An in-depth look at pressure sores using monolithic silicon pressure sensors. Plastic and Reconstructive Surgery 74(6): 745–753.

Leaper D (1987) Antiseptic solutions ples. Journal of Wound Care 1(4): 27–30.

Leaper D (1987) Antiseptic Solutions. Community Outlook 83(8): 30–34.

Leaper D (1988) Antiseptic toxicity in open wounds. Nursing Times 84(25): 77–79.

Leaper DJ (1992) Sutures and staples. Journal of Wound Care 1(4): 27–30.

Leaper DJ (1995) Risk factors for surgical infection. Hospital Infection **30(Suppl)**: 127–139.

Leaper DJ (1998) Defining infection. Journal of Wound Care **7(8)**: 373.

Leaper DJ, Simpson RA (1986) The effect of antiseptics and topical antimicrobials on wound healing. Journal of Antimicrobrial Chemotherapy **17(2)**: 135–137.

Leaper D, Cameron S, Lancaster J (1987) Wound care: antiseptic solutions. Community Outlook **11**: 30–34.

Leelaporn A, Pualsen I, Tennent J, Littlejohn T, Skurray R (1994) Multidrug resistance to antiseptics and disinfectants in Coagulase–negative Staphylococci. Journal of Medical Biology **40**: 214–230.

Lehninger A (1975) Biochemistry. 2nd edn. New York: Worth Publishers.

Letts (1991) Principles of Seating the Disabled. FL: CRC Press.

Levin M (1993) Pathogensis and management of diabetic foot lesions. In Levin M, O'Neal L, Bowker J (eds) The Diabetic Foot. Mosby: St Louis.

Lewis B (1996) Zinc and vitamin C in the aetiology of pressure sores. Journal of Wound Care **5(10)**: 483–484.

Leyden JJ, Karz S, Stewart R, Kligman AM (1977) Urinary ammonia producing micro-organisms in infants with and without diaper dermatitis. Archives of Dermatology **113**: 1678–1680.

Liedberg N, Reiss E, Artz CP (1955) The effect of bacteria on the take of split thickness skin grafts in rabbits. Annals of Surgery **142**: 192–196.

Lidowski A, Patterson P (1985) Cited by Young T (1997) Dressings selection: use of combinations of wound dressings. British Journal of Nursing **6(17)**: 10–18.

Lindholm C (2002) DVT the forgotten factor in leg ulcer prevention. Journal of Wound Care **11(1)**: 5.

Lindon O, Greenway RM, Piazza JM (1961) Etiology of decubitous ulcers: an experimental approach. Archives in Physical Medicine **46**: 378–385.

Littlejohn T, Paulsen I, Gillespie M, Tennent J, Midgley M, Jones I, Purewal A, Skurray (1992) Substrate and energetics of antiseptic and disinfectant resistance in Staphylococcus aureus. FEMS Microbiology Letters **95**: 259–266.

Lock P (1979) The effects of temperature on mitotic activities at the edge of experimental wounds. Proceedings of Symposium on Wound Healing. Chatham: Lock Laboratories Research.

Lockett B (1983) Post-operative wound care. Nursing **2(11)**: 309–310.

Lockyer-Stevens N (1994) A developing information base for purchasing decisions: A review of pressure-relieving beds for at-risk patients. Professional Nurse **9(4)**: 534–542.

Lorentzen H, Gottrup F (1998) Misclassification errors of ulcerative pyoderma gangraenosum. Presentation at Eighth Annual Meeting of the European Tissue Repair Society, Copenhagen.

Lowe GDO (1986) Blood rheology in arterial disease. Clinical Science **71**: 137–146.

Lowry M (1989) Are you sitting comfortably? Good seating requirements in a patient care setting. The Professional Nurse **December**: 162–164.

Lowthian PT (1970) Decubitus Ulcers: A Fresh Look at Some Perennial Nursing Problems. London: King Edwards Hospital Fund Centre.

Lucarotti ME, Lancaster JF, Jenkins AJ, Leaper DJ (1988) Laser-doppler velocimetry and photoplethysmography in the diagnosis of abnormal venous reflux. Phlebologie **41(4)**: 735–739

Lydon MJ, Huthchinson JJ, Cherry GW (1990) The scientific basis of wound healing. In Fullerton SE (ed.) European Hospital Pharmacy Workshop Series 1(1) 1–4. Littlewood Green: Prism International/Burr Associates.

MacClaine K (1998) Clarifying higher level roles in nursing practice. Professional Nurse 14(3): 159–163.

Macfarlane R, Jeffcoate W (1999) Classification of diabetic foot ulcers: the S(AD) SAD system. The Diabetic Foot 2(4): 122–125.

Madsen SM, Daneilson L, Rosdhal VT (1996) Bacterial colonisation and healing of venous leg ulcers. APMIS 104(12): 895–899.

MAFF (1995) Manual of Nutrition, 10th edn. London: The Stationery Office.

Majno G, Joris I (1996) Cells, Tissues and Disease: Principles of General Pathology. Oxford: Blackwell Science.

Mani R, White JE (1988) The use of oxygen sensors to study venous ulcers. Bioeng Skin 4: 229–242.

Marchant AC, Lidowski H, Dealey C (1990) How are you supporting your patients? Professional Nurse 6(3): 134–141.

Marieb EN (1998) Human Anatomy and Physiology, 4th edn. San Francisco, CA: Benjamin Cummings Science Publishing.

Marks-Maran D (1993) In Tschudin V (ed.) Ethics. Nurses and Patients. London: Scutari.

Marples R, Cooke E (1988) Current problems with methicillin-resistant *Staphylococcus aureus*. Journal of Hospital Infection 11: 381–392.

Marrs R (1990) An individual approach to ease frustration: support for people with eczema. Professional Nurse 5(10): 522–524.

Martin SJ (1996) Enzymatic debridement for necrotic wounds. Journal of Wound Care 5(7): 310–311.

Martin TA, Harding KG, Jiang WG (1998) Dermagraft regulates angiogenisis. Presentation at Eighth Annual Meeting of the European Tissue Repair Society. Copenhagen.

Martini FH (1998) Fundamentals of Anatomy and Physiology, 4th edn. New York: Prentice Hall.

Martini L, Borgognoni L, Andriessen A (1999) Comparison of two dressings in the management of partial–thickness donor sites. Journal of Wound Care 8(9): 457–460.

Mayall J, Desharnais G (1995) Positioning in a Wheelchair, 2nd edn. New Jersey: Slack.

Mayrovitz HN, Delgado M, Smith J (1997) Compression bandaging effects on lower extremity peripheral and sub-bandaged skin blood perfusion. Wounds 9(50): 146–152.

McCaffery M (1983) Nursing the Patient in Pain. London: Harper & Row.

McClarey M (2000) NICE: Your questions answered. Professional Nurse 15(98): 491.

McClemont E (1984) Pressure sores. Nursing 2(21): suppl1–3, 6.

McKay I, Leigh I (1991) Epidermal cytokines and their roles in cutaneous wound healing. British Journal of Dermatology 124(6): 513–518.

McLure A, Gordon J (1992) In–vitro evaluation of povidone–iodine and chlorhexidine against methicillin–resistant *Staphylococcus aureus*. Journal of Hospital Infection 21(4): 291–299.

McWhirter J, Pennington CR (1994) Incidence and recognition of malnutrition in hospital. British Medical Journal 308: 945–948.

Medical Devices Agency (1994) Static Mattress Overlays. Evaluation PS2 October. Norwich: HMSO.

Medical Devices Agency (1997a) The Effects of Posture, Body Mass Index and Wheelchair Adjustment on Interface Pressure. No 97/20. London: Department of Health.

Medical Devices Agency (1997b) Wheelchair Cushions Static and Dynamic, a Comparative Evaluation. Special Issue, No PS4. London: Department of Health.

Medical Devices Directorate (1993) Foam Mattresses. Evaluation PS1 August. Norwich: HMSO.

Meers SF, Law DW, Jeffrey PJ (1990) Factors affecting the incidence of post-operative wound infection. Journal of Hospital Infection 16: 223–230.

Mekkes JR (1998) Debridement of Leg Ulcers. Amsterdam: Academische Pers.

Melhuish JM, Wertheim D, Llewellyn M, Williams R, Harding KG (1998) Evaluation of compression under elastic tubular bandage utilized for compression therapy. Leg Ulcers: Physical Research. Wound Healing Research Unit. University of Wales. Cardiff.

Melzack R, Wall PD (1984) The Textbook of Pain. Edinburgh: Churchill Livingstone.

Merck (2000) The Merck Manual of Geriatrics, http://www.merck.com

MEREC (1998) Oral Nutritional Support Bulletin. National Prescribing Centre 9. 7 London.

Mertz P, Davis SC, Brewer LD, Franzen L (1994) Can antimicrobials be effective without impairing wound healing? The evaluation of a cadexomer iodine ointment. Wounds 6(6): 184–193.

Miles E, Calder P (1998) Modulation of immune function by dietary fatty acids. Proceedings of the Nutrition Society 57: 277–292

Miller M, Dyson M (1996) Principles of Wound Care. London: Macmillan.

Moffatt CJ (1992a) Compression bandaging – the state of the art. Journal of Wound Care 1(1): 45–50.

Moffatt C (1992b) A trial of a hydrocolloid dressing in the management of indolent ulceration. Journal of Wound Care 1(3): 20–22.

Moffatt C (1997) Know how. Four-layer bandaging. Nursing Times Supplement 93(16): centre pages.

Moffatt C, Franks P, Bosanquet N (1991) The Provision of Innovation in Venous Ulcer Management to the Elderly Population in the Community. (Report to the King Edwards Fund for London.) London: Kings Fund.

Moffatt C, Franks P, Oldroyd M, et al. (1992) Community clinics for leg ulcers and impact on healing. British Medical Journal 305: 1389–1392.

Moore D (1992) Hypochlorites: a review of the evidence. Journal of Wound Care 1(4): 44–53.

Morgan D (1992) Wound Cleansing Agents. Educational Leaflet No. 10(2). Huntingdon: Wound Care Society.

Morgan D (1993) Is there still a role for antiseptics? Journal of Tissue Viability 3(3): 80–84.

Morgan D (1996) Alginate dressings. Journal of Tissue Viability 7(1): 4–9.

Morgan D (1997a) Myiasis: the rise and fall of maggot therapy. Journal of Tissue Viability 5(2): 43–51.

Morgan D (1997b) Formulary of Wound Management Products, 7th edn. Haslemere: Euromed Communications Ltd.

Morison MJ (1992) Quality assurance and wound care in the community. Ostomy Wound Management **38(8)**: 38–44.

Morison M (1993) A Colour Guide to the Nursing Management of Wounds, 2nd edn. London: Mosby.

Morrison M (1989) Wound cleansing: which solution? Professional Nurse **4(5)**: 220–225.

Mortensen N, Garrard CS, Phil D (1996) Colorectal surgery comes in from the cold. The New England Journal of Medicine **334**: 1263–1264.

Mortimer PS, Regnard C (1986) Lymphostatic disorders. British Medical Journal **293**: 347–348.

Mulder GD (1995) Cost-effective managed care: gel versus wet-to-dry for debridement. Ostomy Wound Management **41(2)**: 68–74.

Murray KA (1997) Nutrition in wound healing a bio–psychosocial perspective. Clinical Nutrition: Oral Diet Therapies **32**: 4.

Naylor IL (1999) Ulcer care in the middle ages. Journal of Wound Care **8(4)**: 208–212.

Ndwadula EM, Brown L (1990) Mattresses as reservoirs of epidemic MRSA. Lancet **337(8739)**: 488.

Neal MS (1994) Treating patient's synergistic gangrene with hyperbaric oxygen. Journal of Wound Care **3(5)**: 218–222.

Nelson EA (1995) Improvements in bandaging technique following training. Journal of Wound Care **4(4)**: 181–184.

Nelson EA (1996) Compression bandaging in the treatment of venous leg ulcers. Journal of Wound Care **5(9)**: 415–418.

Nelson EA (1997) The selection and use of compression bandages. Journal of Wound Care **6(6)**: 297.

Newman V, Altwood M, Oakes R (1989) The use of metronidazole gel to control the smell of malodorous lesions. Palliative Medicine **3(4)**: 303–305.

NHS Centre for Reviews and Dissemination (1997) Compression therapy for venous leg ulcers. Effective Health Care **3**: 4.

Niitsuma J (2001) Aetiology of pressure ulcers using an animal model – an analysis of blood flow inhibition and recovery phenomena around compressed areas. Journal of Tissue Viability **11(1)**: 40.

Niwa Y (1987) The ratio of lipideperoxides to superoxide dismutase activity in the skin lesions of patients with severe skin diseases: an acute prognostic indicator. Life Sciences **40**: 921–927.

Noble-Adams R (1999) Radiation–induced reactions 1: an examination of the phenomenon. British Journal of Nursing **8(17)**: 1134–1140.

North West Thames Regional Advisory Committee (1989) Guidelines for pressure sores. Nursing Standard **4(10)**: 26–29.

Norton D, McLaren R, Exton-Smith A (1962) An Investigation of Geriatric Nursing Problems in Hospitals. London: National Corporation for the Care of Older People.

Norton D, McLaren R, Exton-Smith A (1975) An Investigation of Geriatric Nursing Problems in Hospital. London: Churchill Livingstone.

Nudds L (1987) Healing information: leg ulcers. Community Outlook **83**: 12–14.

Nursing Standard (1993) Survey shows hidden cuts. Royal College of Nursing Report. Nursing Standard **7(35)**: 23–24.

O'Connor H (1993) Bridging the gap? Nursing Times Supplement **8(32)**: 2–5.

Öien RF, Håkansson A, Ahnlide I, Bjellerup M, Hansen BU, Borquist L (2001) Pinch grafting in hospital and in primary care: a cost analysis. Journal of Wound Care **10**(5): 164–169.

Oliver L (1997) Wound cleansing. Nursing Standard **11**(20): 47–51.

Oryan A, Zaker SR (1998) The effects of topical application of honey on cutaneous wound healing in rabbits. Zentralbl Veterinarmed A **3**: 181–188

Otterlei M, Ostgaard K, Skjak-Braek G (1991) Induction of cytokine production from human monocytes stimulated with alginate. Journal of Immunotherapy **10**: 286–291.

Parekh SG, Trauner KB, Zarins B, Foster TE, Anderson RR (1999) Photodynamic modulation of wound healing. Lasers Surgical Medicine **24**(5): 375–381.

Parenteau NL, Hardin Young J, Isaacs C, Duff R, Sabolinski M (1998) Human skin equivalent: an active therapy for wounds. Presentation at Eighth Annual Meeting of the European Tissue Repair Society, Copenhagen.

Parker GE (1994) Hungry healers. Nursing Times **90**(24): 55–58.

Parker MJ (1979) Microbiology for Nurses. London: Balliere Tindall.

Partridge C (1998) Influential factors in surgical wound healing. Journal of Wound Care **7**(7): 350–353.

Peel K (1993a) Making sense of leeches. Nursing Times **89**(27): 33–35.

Peel K (1993b) Hypochlorite solutions. Journal of Wound Care **2**(1): 7.

Perdreau-Remmington F, Stefanik D, Peters G, Ruckdeschel G, Haas F, Wenzel R, Pulverer G (1995) Methicillin-resistant *Staphylococcus haemolyticus* on the hands of healthcare workers: a route of transmission or a source? Journal of Hospital Infection **31**: 195–203.

Perkins P (1992) Wound dehiscence: causes and care. Nursing Standard **6**(34): 12–14.

Perry C (1994) Care of central venous line exit sites. Journal of Wound Care **3**(6): 279–282.

Petch N (1993) Examining first aid received by burn and scald patients. Journal of Wound Care **2**(2): 102–105.

Phillips TJ, Al-Amoudi HO, Leverkus M, Park HY (1998) Effect of chronic wound fluid on fibroblasts. Journal of Wound Care **7**(10): 527–532.

Pontieri-Lewis V (2000) The role of nutrition in wound healing. Medsurg Nursing, http://www.ajj.com/jpi.

Potts RO, Guzek DB, Harris RR, McKie JEA (1985) Non-invasive, in vivo technique to quantitatively measure water concentration of the stratum corneum using attenuated total-reflectance infrared spectroscopy. Archives of Dermatological Research **277**(6): 489–495.

Poulton B (1991) Factors which influence patients compliance. Journal of Tissue Viability **1**(4): 108–110.

Presperin J (1992) Seating systems: the therapist and rehabilitation engineering team. Physical and Occupational Therapy in Geriatrics **10**(2): 11–45.

Preston KW (1988) Positioning for comfort and pressure relief; the 30 degree alternative. Care: Science and Practice **6**(4): 116–119.

Price P, Bale S, Newcombe R, Harding K (1999) Challenging the pressure sore problem. Journal of Wound Care **8**(4): 187–190.

Price P, Bale S, Crook H, Harding K (2000) The effect of a radiant heat dressing on pressure ulcers. Journal of Wound Care **9**(4): 201–205.

Prince HN, Noemaker WS, Nogard RC, Prince DL (1983) Drug resistant studies with topical antiseptics. Journal of Pharmaceutical Science **67**: 1629–1631.

Purvis P (1996) The prevalence of leg ulcers in mid-Essex. Equip **September**: 2.

Rabkin JM, Hunt TK (1988) Problem Wounds: The Role of Oxygen. New York: Elsevier.

Rainey J (1996) It's all in the sales pitch. Nursing Times Wound Supplement **92(39)**: 71–73.

Raman A, Weir U, Bloomfield S (1995) Antimicrobial effects of tea-tree oil and its major components on *Staphylococcus aureus*, *Staph. Epidermis* and *Propionibacterium acnes*. Letter to Applied Microbiology **21(4)**: 242–245.

Raman M, Sibbald RG (1998) Bacterial load as a predictor of primary Apligraf take for non-healing venous stasis ulcers. Presentation at Eighth Annual Meeting of the European Tissue Repair Society, Copenhagen.

Ramasasty S (1998) Chronic problem wounds. Wound healing: state of the art. Clinics in Plastic Surgery **25**: 3.

Ratcliffe P (1998) Under pressure to update research. Nursing Times Supplement **94(16)**: 59–61.

Rawls J (1973) A Theory of Justice. Oxford: Oxford University Press.

Rees C (1992) Practising research-based teaching. Nursing Times **88(2)**: 55–58.

Reiber GE, Lipsky BA, Gibbons GW (1998) The burden of diabetic foot ulcers. The American Journal of Surgery **17(2A)**: 5S–10S.

Reid J, Morison M (1994) Towards a consensus: Classification of pressure sores. Journal of Wound Care **3(3)**: 157–160.

Rheinwald JG, Green H (1975) Serial cultivation of strains of human epidermal keratinocytes: The formation of keratinizing colonies from single cells. **(6)**: 331–344.

Rice ASC (1994) Pain, inflammation and wound healing. Journal of Wound Care **3(5)**: 246–248.

Rieu S (1994) Error and trial. The extended role dilemma. British Journal of Nursing **3(4)**: 168–174.

Rithalia S (1996) Pressure sores: which foam mattress and why? Journal of Tissue Viability **6(4)**: 115–119.

Robinson B (1988) Aetiology and treatment of leg ulcers. MIMS Magazine **July (suppl)**: 2–3.

Robson MC (1979) Difficult wounds: pressure ulcerations and leg ulcers. Clinical Plastic Surgery **6**: 537–540.

Robson MC (1988) Wound Infection. A Failure of Wound Healing Caused by an Imbalance of Bacteria. Tampa, CA: University of South California.

Robson MC, Heggers JP (1969) Variables in host resistance pertaining to septicemia. I. Blood glucose level. Journal of American Geriatric Society **17(10)**: 991–996.

Roche S, Walker S (2000) Retrospective analysis of postoperative epidural analgeisia and pressure sores. Acute Pain **3(2)**: 77–83.

Rodheaver G (1989) Controversies in topical wound management. Wounds **1(1)**: 19–27.

Roe BH, Stoden PD, Taylor RS, Dormandy JA (1994) Reliability of ankle–brachial pressure index measurement by junior doctors. British Journal of Surgery **81**: 188–190.

Roitt C (1994) Essential Immunology. Oxford: Blackwell Science.

Rojas A, Phillips T (1999) Patients with chronic leg ulcers show diminished levels of vitamin A, E, carotenes and zinc. Dermatology Surgery **25(8)**: 601–604.

Roper N, Logan WW, Tierney A (1985) The Elements of Nursing. Edinburgh: Churchill Livingstone.

Rosenthal D, Murphy F, Gottschalk Baxter M, Nevin K (2001) Using a topical anaesthetic cream to reduce pain during sharp debridement of chronic leg ulcers. Journal of Wound Care **10(1)**: 503–505.

Rousseau P (1991) Comparison of the various physiochemical properties of various hydrocolloid dressings. Wounds **3(1)**: 43–48.

Rowson R (1993) In Tschudin V (ed.) Ethics. Nurses and Patients. London: Scutari Press.

Royal College of Nursing (1998) Understanding clinical governance. News Letter **Autumn**: 8–9.

Royal College of Nursing (2000) Clinical Practice Guidelines in the Management of Patients with Venous Leg Ulcers. York: University of York.

Royal College of Surgeons (1990) Commission on the Provision of Surgical Services: Report on the Working Party on Pain after Surgery. London: Royal College of Surgeons.

Ruckley CV (1998) Caring for patients with chronic leg ulcer. British Medical Journal **316(7129)**: 407–408.

Rund CR (1996) Non-conventional topical therapies for wound care. Ostomy Wound Management **42(5)**: 18–20.

Rutter PM, Carpenter B, Hill SS (2000) Varidase: the science behind the medicament. Journal of Wound Care **9(5)**: 223–226.

Ryan DW (1990) The fluidised bed 1: basic principles, bacteriology and wound care. Intensive Care World **7(2)**: 24–28.

Ryat MS, Quinton DN (1997) Tap water as a wound cleansing agent in accident and emergency. Journal Accident and Emergency Medicine **14**: 165–166.

Samuel J, Williams C (1996) *Pyoderma gangrenosum*: an inflammatory ulcer. Journal of Wound Care **5(7)**: 314–318.

Santy J (1995) Hospital mattresses and pressure sore prevention. Journal of Wound Care **4(7)**: 329–332.

Santy J (1998) Evaluation of pressure–redistributing replacement mattresses. Journal of Wound Care **7(1)**: 15–18.

Sato A, Zhidao X, Hughes MA, Cherry GW (1999) Basic research in warming and wound healing. A Symposium on Thermoregulation in Wound Care, St Annes College, University of Oxford.

Saxey S (1986) Nurses response to post-op pain. Nursing **3**: 377–381.

Schreibman IG (1990) The significance of haemolytic Streptococci in chronic leg ulcers. Annals of the Royal College of Surgeons of England **72**: 123–124.

Schubert V (1992) Hypotension as a risk factor for the development of pressure sores in elderly subjects. Journal of Tissue Viability **2(1)**: 5–8.

Schurr M, Turner J (1982) Nursing – Image or Reality? Sevenoaks: Hodder and Stoughton.

Scott E, Fintan GB, Leaper DJ (1999a) The use of intra-operative warming therapy with a dual purpose to reduce the incidence of post-operative pressure sores and wound infections. Presentation at a Symposium on Thermoregulation in Wound Care, St Annes College and Green College, Oxford.

Scott EM, Litt M, Earl C, Leaper D, Massey M, Mewburn J, Williams N (1999b) Understanding perioperative nursing. Nursing Standard **13(49)**: 49–54; quiz 55.

Scriven JM, Bell PRF, Taylor LE, et al. (1998) A prospective randomised trial of four-layer versus short stretch compression bandages for the treatment of venous leg ulcers. Annals of the Royal College of Surgeons of England **80**: 215–220.

Sebben JE (1983) Surgical antiseptics. Journal of the American Academy of Dermatology 9(5): 759–765.

Seedhouse D (1993) Ethics, the Heart of Health Care. Oxford: Alden Press.

Senior C (2000) Treatment of diabetic foot ulcers with hyperbaric oxygen. Journal of Wound Care 9(4): 193–197.

Settle JAD (1986) Burns – the First Five Days. Romford: Smith and Nephew.

Shahan MH, Chuang AH, Brennan WA, Dirkson TR, Van Dyke TE, McPherson JC (1993) The effect of chlorhexidine irrigation on tensile wound strength. Journal of Periodontology 64(8): 719–721.

Shakespeare P (1994) Scoring the risks. Journal of Tissue Viability 4(1): 21–22.

Sharp CS, Bessman AN, Wagner FW, Garland D (1978) Microbiology of deep tissues in diabetic gangrene. Diabetes Care 1(5): 289–292.

Sheikh W (1986) The activity of Hibiclens and Betadine in infected human wounds. Current Therapeutic Research 40: 1096.

Siana JE, Frankild S, Gottrup F (1992) The effect of smoking on tissue function. (And wound healing). Journal of Wound Care 1(2): 37–41.

Silverstein P (1992) Smoking and wound healing. American Journal of Medicine 93(1A): 22S–24S.

Simpson C (1997) Choose the right bandage. Pharmacy in Practice March: 133–138.

Simpson S (1992) Methicillin-resistant Staphyloccus aureus and its implications for nursing practice: a literature review. Nursing Practice 5(2): 2–7.

Sims M (1996) Protocols for the care of external fixator pin sites. Professional Nurse 11(4): 261–264.

Singer AJ, Hollander JE, Subramanian S, Malhotra AK, Villez PA (1994) Pressure dynamics of various irrigation techniques commonly used in emergency departments. Annals of Emergency Medicine 24(1): 36–40.

Sleigh JW, Linter SP (1985) Hazards of hydrogen peroxide. British Medical Journal 291: 1706.

Small JF (1994) The treatment of an indolent diabetic foot ulcer. Journal of Wound Care 3(1): 17–20.

Smith LN, Lait ME (1996) A study of postoperative wound management in nursing. British Journal of Nursing 5(19): 1162–1171.

Smith S, Griffin C (1998) The role of nutrition in wound healing. http://woundcare.org /newsvol2nl/nut3.htm

Souther SG, Carr SD, Vistnes LM (1974) Wheelchair cushions to reduce pressure under bony prominences. Archives of Physical Medical Rehabilitation 55: 460–464

Sparacino P (1992) Advanced practice: the clinical specialist. Nursing Practice 5(4): 2–4.

Stadelmann WK, Digenis AG, Tobin GR (1998) Impediments to wound healing. The American Journal of Surgery 176: 39s–44s.

Steed DL (1998) Foundations of good ulcer care. The Journal of American Surgery 176: 20s–25s.

Steele S, Harmon V (1983) Values Clarification in Nursing, 2nd edn. London: Prentice-Hall.

Stemmer R, Marescaux J, Furder C (1980) Compression treatment of the lower extremities particularly with compression stockings. The Dermatologist 31: 355–365.

Stephenson T, Thacker J, Rodheaver G, et al. (1976) Cleansing traumatic wounds by high pressure syringe irrigation. Journal of American College of Emergency Physicians 5(1): 17–21.

Stickler D, Chawla J (1987) The role of antiseptics in the management of patients with long term indwelling catheter. Journal of Hospital Infection 10: 219–228.

Stockport JC, Groarke L, Ellison DA, McCollum C (1997) Single–layer and multilayer bandaging in the treatment of venous leg ulcers. Journal of Wound Care 6(10): 485–488.

Stocum DL (1998) Regeberative biology and engineering strategies for tissue restoration. Wound Repair and Regeneration 6(4): 276–290.

Stoddard S, Sherman R, Mason B, Pelsang D (1995) Maggot debridement therapy. An alternative treatment for non–healing ulcers. Journal of American Podiatry Medical Association 85(4): 218–221.

Stotts N (1990) Nutrition and wound healing. AACN Clinical Issues 3: 585–594.

Stotts N (1996) Nutrition, perfusion and wound healing: An inseparable triad. Nutrition 12(10): 733–734.

Sugarman B, Hawes S, Mushner D, et al. (1983) Osteomyelitis beneath pressure sores. Archives of Internal Medicine 143: 683.

Surguna LS, Chandrakasan G, Ramamoorthy U, Thomas JK (1993) Influence of honey on biochemical and biophysical parameters of wounds in rats. Journal of Clinical Biochemistry and Nutrition 14: 91–99.

Svensio T, Pomahac B, Yao F, Eriksson E (1998) Acceleration of full thickness skin wound repair in normal saline. Presentation at Eighth Annual Meeting of the European Tissue Repair Society, Copenhagen.

Taylor JL (1990) Infection control at your fingertips: procedures for preventing and controlling MRSA. Professional Nurse 5(10): 547–551.

Taylor T (1974) Ascorbic acid supplementation in the treatment of pressure sores. Lancet 2: 544–546.

Tejero-Trujeque R (2001) Understanding the final stages of wound contraction. Journal of Wound Care 10(7): 259–264.

Telfer NR, Moy RL (1993) Drug and nutrient aspects of wound healing. Dermatology Clinic 11(4): 729–737.

Tengrove NJ, Stacey MC, McGechie DF, Mata S (1996) Qualitative bacteriology and leg ulcer healing. Journal of Wound Care 5(6): 277–280.

Terill PJ, Kedwards SM, Lawrence JC (1991) The use of Gor-tex bags for hand burns. Burns 17: 161–165.

Thomas AML (1999) The structure and composition of chronic wound eschar. Journal of Wound Care 8(6): 285–288.

Thomas S (1990) Wound dressings: legal implications. In Fullerton E (ed.) European Hospital Pharmacy Workshop Series. Littlewick Green: Burr Associates.

Thomas S (1992a) Alginates. Journal of Wound Care 1(1): 29–32.

Thomas S (1992b) Current Practices in the Management of Fungating Lesions and Radiation Damaged Skin. Bridgend: The Surgical Materials Testing Laboratory, p2.

Thomas S (1994) Low–adherent dressings. Journal of Wound Care 3(1): 27–30.

Thomas S (1997a) Assessment and management of wound exudate. Journal of Wound Care 6(7): 327–330.

Thomas S (1997b) Exudate – who needs it? In Cherry C, Harding K (eds) Management of Wound Exudate. Proceedings of Joint meeting of EWMA and ETRS. London: Churchill Communications.

Thomas S (1997c) Celullose dressings. Journal of Wound Care 6(1): 46–47.

Thomas S, Loveless P (1991) A comparative study of the properties of six hydrocolloid dressings. Pharmaceutical Journal **247**: 672–675.

Thomas S, Loveless P (1992) Observations on the fluid handling properties of alginate dressings. The Pharmaceutical Journal **248**: 850–851.

Thomas S, Jones M, Shutler S, Jones S (1996a) Using larvae in modern wound management. Journal of Wound Care **5(2)**: 60.

Thomas S, Jones M, Shutler S, Andrews A (1996b) All you need to know about … maggots. Nursing Times Wound Care Supplement **92(46)**: 63–76.

Thomas S, Harding KG, Moore K (1999) The structure and composition of chronic wound eschar. Journal of Wound Care **8(6)**: 285–287.

Thomlinson D (1987) To clean or not to clean? Nursing Times **83(9)**: 71–75.

Thompson P (1998) The microbiology of wounds. Journal of Wound Care **7(9)**: 477–478.

Thor International (1993) Laser Therapy Introductory Notes. Amersham: Thor Iternational.

Thornton F, Schaffer M, Barbul A (1997) Wound healing in sepsis and trauma. Shock **8(6)**: 391–401.

Thurman RB, Gerba CP (1989) The molecular mechanisms of copper and silver ion disinfection of bacteria and virsuses. CRC Critical Reviews in Environmental Control **8(4)**: 295–315.

Tingle J (1997) Pressure sores: counting the cost of nursing neglect. British Journal of Nursing **6(13)**: 757.

Topham J (1996) Sugar paste and povidone–iodine in the treatment of wounds. Journal of Wound Care **5(8)**: 364–365.

Topham J (2000) Sugar for wounds. Journal of Tissue Viability **10(3)**: 86–89.

Torrance C (1981) Pressure sores: pathogenesis, prophylaxis and treatment. 3. Medical management and surgical intervention. Nursing Times **77(12)**: suppl 1–4.

Torrance C (1983) Pressure Sores: Aetiology, Treatment and Prevention. London: Croome Helm.

Torrance C (1986) The physiology of wound healing. Nursing **5**: 162–166.

Torrance C (1990) Sleep and wound healing. Surgical Nurse **3(3)**: 16–20.

Torres A, Rossbach O, Vogt P, Steinau HU (1998) Immediate skin occlusion with silicone-sheets improves skin quality after skin transplant in burned patients. Presentation at Eighth Annual Meeting of the European Tissue Repair Society, Copenhagen.

Towler J (2001) Cleansing traumatic wounds with swabs, water or saline. Journal of Wound Care **10(6)**: 231–234.

Trevelyan J (1996) Wound cleansing: principles and practice. Nursing Times. **92 (16)**: 46–48

Trevelyan J (1997) Spirit of the beehive. Nursing Times Supplement **93(7)**: 72–74.

Tyler VE (1987) New honest herbal. USA. G Stickly Co. Cited by Trevelyan J (1997) Spirit of the beehive. Nursing Times Supplement **93(7)**: 72–74.

Tyrell W (1995) Shoes for people with diabetes. Journal of Wound Care **4(3)**: 123–126.

UKCC (1989) Exercising Accountability. London: UKCC.

UKCC (1992) The Scope of Professional Practice. London: UKCC.

UKCC (1996) Guidelines for Professional Practice. London: UKCC.

Unosson M, Ek A, et al. (1995) Influence of macronutrient status on recovery after hip fracture. Journal of Nutritional and Environmental Medicine **5**: 23–34.

US Department of Health and Human Services (1992) Pressure ulcers in adults: prediction and prevention. Decubitus **5(3)**: 26–30.

Van de Kerhof PCM (1996) Inflammation versus re-epithelialisation during wound healing. Wound Management **1**: 1–3.

Van den Broek PJ (1982) Interaction of povidone-iodine compounds, phagocytic cells and micro-organisms. Antimicrobial Agents and Chemotherapy **22(4)**: 593–597.

Van Luyn MJA, Van Wachem PB, Nieuwenhuis P, Jonkman MF (1992) Cytotoxicity testing of wound dressings using methycellulose cell culture. Biomaterials **13(5)**: 267–275.

Venables J (1994) Knowledge needed to educate patients about psoriasis. Nursing Times Supplement **90(23)**: 33–35.

Verluysen M (1986) How elderly patients with femoral neck fractures develop pressure sores within hospital. British Medical Journal **292**: 1311–1313.

Vickery C (1997) Exudate: what is it and what is its function in acute and chronic wounds. In Cherry C, Harding K (eds) Management of Wound Exudate. Proceedings of Joint Meeting of EWMA and ETRS. London: Churchill Communications.

Vistnes L, Pardoe R (1976) The effect of commonly used antiseptics on wound healing. Plastic Reconstructive Surgery **55**: 472–476.

Vosskuhler R (1999) Warm-up active wound therapy. Presented at a Symposium on Thermoregulation in Wound Care, St Anne's College and Green College, University of Oxford, February.

Vowden K (1998) Lipodermatosclerosis and atrophie blanche. Journal of Wound Care **7(9)**: 441–443.

Wallis S (1991) An agenda to promote self-care. Professional Nurse **September**: 715–716.

Walsh M, Ford P (1992) Rituals in nursing. We always do it this way. Nursing Times **85(41)**: 26–32.

Walshe C (1995) Living with a venous leg ulcer: a descriptive study of patients' experiences. Journal of Advanced Nursing **22**: 1092–1100.

Warner U (1986) Pressure sores: a policy for prevention. Nursing Times **April**: 59–61.

Waterlow J (1988) The Waterlow card for the prevention and management of pressure sores: towards a pocket policy. Care Science and Practice **6**: 1.

Waterlow J (1995) Pressure sores and their management. Care of the Critically Ill **11(3)**: 121–125.

Weiman TJ (1998) Clinical efficacy of Beaplermin gel. The American Journal of Surgery **176**: 74s–79s.

Wells L (1994) At the front line. Professional Nurse **May**: 525–530.

Wells RJ (1984) Controversial issues in wound care. Nursing (Suppl) **June**: 10–11.

West DC, Shaw DM, Lorenz P, Azdick NS, Longaker MT (1997) Fibrotic healing of adult and late gestation fetal wounds correlates with increased hyaluronidase activity and removal of hyaluronan. International Journal of Biochemistry and Cell Biology **29**: 201–210.

Westaby S (1981) Wound Care No 4. Nursing Times **16 December** Wound Care 13.

Wheston R (1996) Principles of doppler. Nursing Times Supplement **92(20)**: 66–70.

White J, Katz M, Cisek P, Kreithen J (1996) Venous outflow of the leg: anatomy and physiologic mechanism of the venous plexus. Presented at the Eighth Annual Meeting of the American Forum, San Diego, 22–24 February.

Whiteside MCR, Moorhead RJ (1999) Traumatic wounds: principles of management. In Miller M, Glover D (eds) Wound Management, Theory and Practice. London: Emap Healthcare.

Whitney J, Heitkemper M (1999) Modifying perfusion, nutrition and stress to promote wound healing in patients with acute wounds. Heart and Lung 28:2.

Wigfield A, Boon E (1996) Critical care pathway development: the way forward. British Journal of Nursing 5(12): 732–735.

Wilkes L, Bostock E, Lovitt L, Denis G (1996) Pressure sores in the older patient with fractured neck of femur: a challenge for the nurse in the acute care setting. Geriaction **Autumn**: 32–37.

Wilkinson E, Buttfield S, Cooper S, Young E (1997) Trial of two bandaging systems for chronic venous leg ulcers. Journal of Wound Care 6(7): 339–343.

Wilkinson M, Kirk J (1965) Leg ulcers complicating rheumatoid arthritis. Scotland Medical Journal 10:179–182.

Williams C (1993) Using water-filled gloves for pressure relief on heels. Journal of Wound Care 2(6): 345–348.

Williams C (1994) Kaltostat. British Journal of Nursing 3(18): 965–967.

Williams C (1995) Cavicare. British Journal of Nursing 4(9): 526–528.

Williams C (1996) Lyofoam. British Journal of Nursing 5(12): 757–759.

Williams H (1998) Common skin lesions. Professional Nurse Study Supplement 13(4): S8–S9.

Williams M (1992) One in the eye for care. Nursing Standard 6(43): 48–49.

Winter GD (1962) Formation of the scab and rate of epithelialisation of superficial wounds in the skin of a young domestic pig. Nature 193: 293–294.

Winter G (1978) Wound healing. Nursing Mirror Supplement **9 March**: 1–8.

Winter GD, Perins DJ (1970) Proceedings of the Fourth International Conference on Hyperbaric Medicine. Tokyo: Igaku Shoin.

Wipke-Tevis D, Stotts N (1998) Nutrition tissue oxygenation and healing of venous leg ulcers. Journal of Vascular Nursing 26(3): 48–56.

Wollina U (1997) Quality of life: an underestimated aspect of wound care. Journal of Wound Care (suppl) 6(3): 11.

Wood R (1976) Disintegration of cellulose dressings in open granulating wounds. British Journal of Medicine 1: 1444–1445.

Wound Care Journal (1995) Using potassium permanganate for wound cleansing 4(2): 64.

Wright M (1994) Hip blisters. Nursing Times 90(16): 86–88.

Wright S (1991) The nurse as a consultant. Nursing Standard 5(20): 31–34.

Wysocki AB (1996a) Wound fluids and the pathogensis of chronic wounds. Journal of WOCN 23(6): 232309–232310.

Wysocki AB (1996b) The effect of intermittent noise exposure on wound healing. Advances in Wound Care 9(1): 35–39.

Yalcin AN, Bakir Z, Bakici Z (1995) Postoperative wound infections. Journal of Hospital Infection 29: 305–309.

Young A (1991) Law and Professional Conduct in Nursing. Harrow: Scutari Press.

Young J (1992) Preventing pressure sores: does the mattress work? Journal of Tissue Viability 2(1): 17.

Young T (1995) Common problems in overgranulation. Practice Nursing 6(11): 14–15.

Young T (1997a) Use of a hydrocolloid in over-granulation. Journal of Wound Care 6(5): 216.

Young T (1997b) Dressing selection: use of combinations of wound dressings. British Journal of Nursing **6(17)**: 64–71.

Young T (2000) Factitious wounds. Presentation at Images of Wound Care: Restoring Damaged Tissue. Tissue Viability Society Conference, Nottingham.

Yura H, Walsh MB (1987) The Nursing Process: Assessing, Planning, Implementing and Evaluating, 3rd edn. New York: Appelton Century Croft.

Zacharkow D (1984) Wheelchair Posture and Pressure Sores. IL: Charles C Thomas.

Zamora JL, Price MF, Chaung P, Gentry LO (1985) Inhibition of povidone-iodine bacterial activity by common organic substances, an experimental study. Surgery **98**: 25–29.

Ziegler TR, Young LS, Mansom JM, Wilmore DN (1988) Metabolic effects of recombinant human growth hormone in patients receiving parenteral nutrition. Annals of Surgery **208**: 6–16.

Index

3